MEDICAL ETHICS:
EVOLUTION, RIGHTS AND THE PHYSICIAN

Episteme

A SERIES IN THE FOUNDATIONAL,
METHODOLOGICAL, PHILOSOPHICAL, PSYCHOLOGICAL, SOCIOLOGICAL, AND
POLITICAL ASPECTS OF THE SCIENCES, PURE AND APPLIED

VOLUME 17

Editor: Mario Bunge
Foundations and Philosophy of Science Unit, McGill University

Advisory Editorial Board:

The titles published in this series are listed at the end of this volume.

MEDICAL ETHICS:
EVOLUTION,
RIGHTS AND THE PHYSICIAN

by

HENRY A. SHENKIN

KLUWER ACADEMIC PUBLISHERS

DORDRECHT / BOSTON / LONDON

Library of Congress Cataloging-in-Publication Data

Shenkin, Henry A., 1915-
    Medical ethics : evolution, rights and the physician / Henry A.
Shenkin.
        p.   cm. -- (Episteme ; v. 17)
    ISBN 0-7923-1031-4 (HB : alk paper)
    1. Medical ethics.   I. Title.   II. Series: Episteme (Dordrecht,
Netherlands)
    [DNLM: 1. Ethics, Medical.   W 50 S546m]
    R724.S47   1990
    174'.2--dc20
    DNLM/DLC
    for Library of Congress   90-15594

ISBN 0-7923-1031-4

Published by Kluwer Academic Publishers,
P.O. Box 17, 3300 AA Dordrecht, The Netherlands.

Kluwer Academic Publishers incorporates
the publishing programmes of
D. Reidel, Martinus Nijhoff, Dr W. Junk and MTP Press.

Sold and distributed in the U.S.A. and Canada
by Kluwer Academic Publishers,
101 Philip Drive, Norwell, MA 02061, U.S.A.

In all other countries, sold and distributed
by Kluwer Academic Publishers Group,
P.O. Box 322, 3300 AH Dordrecht, The Netherlands.

Printed on acid-free paper

Printed in the Netherlands

TABLE OF CONTENTS

TABLE OF CONTENTS

TABLE OF CONTENTS

PREFACE

The subject of medical ethics is always current and offers an inviting theme, particularly for anyone who has spent his life in medical practice. But the subject of ethics is impossible to deal with unless one first asks its purposes.

Therefore, this book is divided into two parts, the first comprehends theoretical considerations and the second, pragmatic and empirical data on, and discussions of, current problems. Part One will be of greater interest to moral philosophers, philosophers and historians of science, and social scientists. Part Two should have greater appeal to physicians, medical students and medical planners. Nevertheless, it is hoped that the latter will look into Part One for the justification of the conclusions the author could reach on the material presented in Part Two. Likewise, it will become obvious why it is believed the solutions of many, if not most, ethical dilemmas are not always discernible at a given moment in time. Also, those who are more concerned with the theoretical material of Part One might find its application to current real-life problems interesting.

It should not be too much to hope that the entire book will appeal to many general readers. The bio-ethical problems presented are of frequent and growing personal concern, and are discussed almost daily in the news media.

PART ONE

AN EVOLUTIONARY VIEW OF ETHICS, RIGHTS AND THE DOCTOR-PATIENT RELATIONSHIP

INTRODUCTION

An evolutionary origin for ethics was proposed by Darwin and widely discussed in the latter part of the 19th and early 20th centuries. It was in eclipse and seldom discussed thereafter until revived by the sociobiologists over a decade ago. Their views have been vigorously questioned, and in particular, their assertion that culture, and therefore ethics, are totally under the control of the genes has been contested. Nonetheless, an evolutionary origin for ethics remains a viable conception[1], even if human culture is not dominated by genetic inheritance.

Medical ethicists, despite the plethora of their publications in recent years, never mention evolutionary ethics. The failure of bioethicists even to discuss an evolutionary origin for ethics might be ascribed to the fact that the vast majority of them had their training in philosophy and/or in the social sciences. These disciplines, under the influence of the behaviorist psychologists, were, and possibly are still, dominated by the belief that the impact of the environment on the individual is far more important than heredity. Those who had espoused the importance of evolution, through heredity, on the characteristics of individuals were identified with political reaction, and with being opposed to the liberal policies that have been the source of our democratic strength. Social Darwinism was, and to many still is, regarded as the most despicable label that can be applied to a social opinion. Over recent years the influence of heredity has slowly regained some ground, and it is fair to say the influence of the environment is not considered to be as overwhelming as presented by the behaviorists.

Bioethicists use only deontological (absolute duty) and/or utilitarian (consequentialist) systems (created before Darwin discovered evolution and evolutionary principles) in their approach to dilemmas. This is reflected in the controversy over which principle should dominate in the discussion of medical ethics - autonomy (duty to respect the patient's right to self-determination) or beneficence (physician's obligation to do the best for a patient). Evolutionary ethics, though broadly discussed for more than 100 years, is *never* mentioned. Perhaps a carry-over from the ostracism of Spencer and social Darwinism is still intimidating, and prevents a wider consideration of an evolutionary origin for ethics?

There really is little controversy within the coterie of medical ethicists on the relationship between patient autonomy and physician beneficence. The opinion is practically unanimous on the primacy of the principle of patient autonomy as the basis for all considerations in medical ethics. Doctor beneficence, while a desirable secondary principle, on the whole must be fought as being really paternalism. The medical ethicists have been so successful in their endeavors that they have convinced even the medical profession of the correctness of their position - patient autonomy is supreme, and physician beneficence rarely is justified as the basis for care. The incorrectness of this position, based on an evolutionary (or consequentialist) point of view, is a major consideration of Chapter Three.

Chapters One and Two offer a justification for an evolutionary origin for group characteristics such as ethics, customs and rights. This means that such characteristics evolve in a manner dictated by that which is best for society. This does *not* imply that it is necessarily a genetic process as stated by the sociobiologists; in fact the principal process involved is a cultural one which most observers agree is not genetic, at least in its greatest part. The important issue is that evolutionary ethics rests on the assumption that culture, despite not being genetically controlled, is subject in its development to evolutionary principles similar to those regulating biological change[2].

In this approach ethical principles and the rights of individuals when examined historically are discovered to have come about because they were in the best interests of the welfare of the group or society. Another way of understanding the evolutionary approach is that the establishment of an ethical principle or a right by a group or a community is an adaptation that is to the greatest advantage to society and not necessarily for any individual in particular. This is a difference from genetic evolution which, for the most part, operates through individuals to assure their survival and propagation.

One must be careful to differentiate between the connotation of the word "evolution" as used ever since Darwin propounded his theory, and the general meaning of the word "evolution": the process of developing, or working out in detail, what is implicitly or potentially contained in an idea or principle. Thus, we can say technology evolves: we even can talk about technological evolution as also occurring in fits and starts - rapidly propelled by the thrusts of war, and more evenly by peaceful competition between nations, as in space and commerce. But the difference between technological evolution and Darwinian evolution is that the former does not have to be to the advantage of the species. The ecologists know all about that, particularly those technological advances that threaten the environment. The atom bomb can destroy the species; but it might not be the bane of existence. Its threat has prevented war between the superpowers and its technological by-products well might be necessary to protect the environment and permit the species to thrive in the future.

Therefore technological evolution (advance) may be good or bad, or perhaps neutral (neither good nor bad). Society has to judge its good and bad uses, and judge in such a manner as to benefit society as a whole, and this is a Darwinian cultural evolutionary process. It is true that over the eons most species have become extinct and only a small fraction have survived but, when it was environmental changes that caused extinction of species in the past, it was never self-imposed.

An evolutionary ethics is a consequentialist one, and though allied to utilitarianism it differs from it in both origin and mode of operation. It originates in the inherited moral instincts and acquired cultural reactions of individuals; it is not the result of the thoughtful balancing of positive and negative factors for an action. It operates through what is good for the community as a whole and not through the accumulated happiness of individuals. Evolutionary ethics recognizes that biology permeates all aspects of life, the mind as well as the body and that the former is not the independent creation of an omnipotent, transcendental power. Viewing the classical deontological and utilitarian systems for ethics from an evolutionary perspective offers the probability that their differences are more apparent than real: both having arisen from what was perceived, from mankind's intuitions, to be for the good of society.

Spencer's and Sumner's advocacy of Darwinism as controlling in the behavior of man (social Darwinism) had been dismissed (and castigated) as only a justification for Western superiority, capitalism, and imperialism, and then as bad science to boot. Sociobiology, which recently has renewed the proposal for an evolutionary origin for culture (and ethics), seems destined for the same fate, say some biologists and most philosophers. Critics object principally to the sociobiologists' assumption that behavior is totally controlled by the genes. In addition, many philosophers are not convinced that the mind is of an evolutionary derivation, and therefore, they conclude, behavior certainly cannot be subject to evolutionary development.

An approach that culture *totally* results from an evolutionary process even if it is only partially under genetic control, would justify an evolutionary theory for ethics. Such an approach to culture assumes the brain, which is indisputely a biologically evolved organ, contains templates for behavior that provide partial control for the development of culture. Those parts of culture clearly acquired by individuals, even if shaped by the inherited templates, can be viewed as also products of a trial and error process controlled by what is for the benefit of the society in which the individuals exist[3].

The 1985 publication of Boyd and Richerson[2] expands and adds substance to the relatively recent renewed interest of anthropologists in an evolutionary theory for the origin of culture[4], and gives strong support for this position. Boyd and Richerson ally the evolutionary process governing culture more closely to the principles regulating biological evolution. Richards' recent history of Darwinism in relation to behavior[1], moreover, gives new believability to Spencer's views and reveals that he, and Darwin before him, constructed ideas of evolutionary ethics that "reanimate moral life". Richards further discloses how unjustified were the attacks of the behaviorists and social scientists on the ethics of Spencer. The eugenics movement, so talked about at that time, and up through WW II, undoubtedly helped to discredit evolutionary ethics.

The evolutionary approach of this book is optimistic: no matter what - that which is best for society will *eventually* triumph. Genetic evolutionists would call this compliance with their principle of "fitness optimization" or the "optimality assumption"[5]. The validity of this principle in biologic evolution is under serious debate, with, on occasion, unfortunate political overtones[6]. This debate does establish the necessity of defining what constitutes optimal fitness, and that such a definition should apply to evolutionary processes that are not genetic, if optimality is to be used as an end-point. Thus, it is to be assumed that when an ethical principle or a law becomes firmly established in a society and its general acceptance is taken as proof that it is in its best interest, it remains to be confirmed by whether the society is a successful one, and over a suitably long period of time.

The definition of what constitutes a successful society is certain to elicit a broad range of opinions. Physicians well might state that reduction in the death rate is the principal expression and index of human and social progress. Sociologists might offer the opinion that statistics on violence (homicide, etc.), as evidence of the quality of life, should be used for comparison among communities. Probably the degree to which a society participates in the recognized advances of the contemporary world, technologically and economically, would be a broader and therefore more acceptable criterion of a successful community. Such progress would be manifested by the totality of the well-being and creativity of its members, and these would include statistics such as death rates and the amounts of violence. The population size of a successful society should be sufficient and stable enough to assure the prosperity of its economy and its perceived power to defend itself, militarily as well as economically. Because of advances in communication, which make the world relatively smaller, criteria for the success of societies worldwide are more and more alike[7].

Attempts to define the term "well-being" has evoked much discussion and even an entire book[8]. When used as a criterion for an optimality endpoint of a cultural evolutionary process, it is not determined by that of an individual or even some individuals, but rather the well-being of the community as a totality. It is true that the well-being of the community often would be determined by the positive result of the addition of the degree of well-being in the totality of individuals; yet it is conceivable that such a summation of the effects of a cultural process could be negative and yet the process be beneficial for the group as a whole.

Universality among all, or most, successful societies is another way of granting the validity of an ethical principle or law. The law is included because, as is explained in Chapter Two, when an ethical principle is accepted widely enough in a community, it often is codified into law. Political scientists[9] recognize that the laws and rights which are the foundation of present industrialized nations serve their constituent individuals well. This is especially apparent when comparison is made with those of the states that preceded them. Political scientists describe these newer rights and laws historically and how good they are; but it is probable most of these political scientists understand less clearly how and, more importantly, why they came about.

Evolutionists have been concerned with predictability in their area of scientific endeavor. They recognize that the complexity in the initial and background conditions of most evolutionary processes, especially if social traits are involved, may be an overwhelming obstacle to evolution ever being a predictive science. They reach this conclusion from the appraisal of the influence that individual cultural traits have on genetic fitness and the reverse relationship - the degree of influence genetic inheritance has on individual cultural traits. Ethical principles and the customs of communities, such as in the area of individual rights, are group characteristics and matters of even greater complexity. To predict the eventual outcome of an evolutionary process in a group setting is analogous to trying to predict the weather (long term) or the economy - both latter phenomena now being recognized as belonging in the field of "chaotic dynamics of dissipative systems"[10]. Evolutionary processes are not predictable for similar reasons - a large number of variables being involved with minute differences between any of them at a given time, but capable of expanding exponentially to create an unpredictable state from an originally well-defined and ordered one.

Thus, if ethics are of evolutionary derivation, the analysis of dilemmas in this field may not yield either a short term solution or, even less likely, predict its eventual outcome. An evolutionary approach to ethics will make clear, however, that zealots (or fundamentalists) on any side of a question do not have the answers for certain either, and frequently exert a disruptive and/or delaying effect on achieving solutions. The source of the disruption is their certainty in their opinion and willingness to act, while moderates are relatively immobilized both because of their nature, and because often they realize that they cannot yet discern the correct solution of some dilemmas.

The fact that the solutions of ethical problems often cannot be predicted could account for the proclivity of many medical ethicists to believe their role in ethical dilemmas is to pose questions (often obvious ones) without the need to offer answers. This is, of course, a charitable interpretation of this inclination, since they offer no evidence that they are aware of the possibility for an evolutionary origin of ethics.

The discovery that many social scientists, including economists[11], political scientists[12], and anthropologists once again[13], and now scientists too[14], are currently trying to apply the principles of biologic evolution to explain situations and developments in their fields obviously not dependent on genetics, is most encouraging to one who is attempting to do the same for medical ethics. That social scientists utilize the evolutionary theory to better understand problems in their disciplines should please those biologists who have been exploring an evolutionary origin for ethics; it is surprising That bioethicists continue to ignore it. The latter should understand that physicians, when they think about ethical dilemmas tend to do so in consequentialist terms, a concept that is very close to the basic premise of evolutionary ethics. All of us might wonder: should ethical principles be imposed on physicians by ethicists who create them on an *a priori* basis, or should they arise from living in society and from life itself?

Structural anthropologists, together with other influential early and mid-twentieth century anthropologists such as Boas, Radcliffe-Browne and Malinowski, disclaimed an evolutionary approach for the understanding of social issues. The structuralists maintain that we cannot assume that modern societies represent the most advanced stage of progress nor that the West, despite a temporary scientific advantage, has any basis to claim intellectual superiority over the rest of the world[15]. Thus, they would dispute the criteria offered above for an optimality end-point of societal development. It is true that *Homo sapiens* has had the same brain capacity for the last 30,000 years and was able to think remarkable thoughts and make remarkable innovations long ago (the Neolithic Revolution was certainly as remarkable as the Industrial one). Structurally older and even primitive societies could have been as sophisticated as modern ones, and it can be understood they had different needs and therefore developed different emphases. Yet, it cannot be denied that the species has evolved: in population size, in all manners of techniques, and even in anthropological understanding. This is all Darwinian evolution, cultural if not biological. Ethical principles, too, can *evolve* in societies to help in adapting them to new situations.

A most important distinction between genetic and cultural evolution is the temporal difference required for a change to take place. Genetic evolutionary change in the higher animals, such as man, require tens of thousands of years and, this would be true for individual traits. Darwin did not have this problem since he died before the inheritance of acquired characteristics (Lamarckism) had been disproven. Cultural evolutionary change, to the contrary, can come about in a matter of years, even within a decade, but in most instances at least several decades are necessary for a change to be established.

A new book, "Evolution, the Grand Synthesis" by E.Laszlo[16], expands the reply to structural anthropologists. Laszlo avers that the Darwinian evolutionary paradigm can be applied to the development of all societal issues, as well as life itself. He postulates that technological revolutions push the "ineluctable advance of society along an evolutionary axis"; and "Through alternating epochs of stability, and now exponentially increasing technology-triggered bifurcations, societies in history evolve from the low energy and structurally relatively simple nomadic tribes of the Paleolithic to the dynamic, autonomous, and relatively complex technological nation-states of the contemporary age." His view of cultural evolution is similar to that of Boyd and Richerson[2]: "The dynamics of social evolution concern the progressive yet discontinuous development of society's collective information pool. The processes of history act on actual societies but they select cultural information pools, much as the processes of biological evolution act on actual organisms but select genetic information pools. This then is the deeper meaning of the term cultural evolution." My approach, too, is that cultural evolution is controlled, in the long run, by what best serves the evolutionary process of the species, but is expressed through that which operates directly for the benefit of the community (as ethics, rights and laws) rather than through only individual traits.

Laszlo must believe that social evolution is a predictive science. He implies that without the correct intervention of individuals in society, that which is good for society will never be achieved. The urgency expressed in this advice is unnecessary because, in my view, the correct solution will always be achieved - eventually. It can be agreed that the earlier those members of a society who happen to have the correct position are sufficiently numerous or politically potent, the more promptly the proper solution will be achieved. However, early on, it often is impossible to be certain of the correct solution, and advocating tolerance on all sides, until data are clear as to the proper solution, would be better advice, and reduce the stress in the community.

An evolutionary theory for ethics, as discussed above, utilizes the optimality assumption and therefore is a sanguine proposal. Some, taking exception to this perception of the human condition, would label it Panglossian, with its pejorative connotation of naivete. Yet the history of the species *Homo sapiens* can be charted as onward and upward, despite interruptions by many severe, and even prolonged, depressions on such a graph. While there are good reasons for pessimism from daily, monthly, yearly or even eral experiences, the overwhelming evidence from the broad sweep of history must be interpreted as optimistic. It does seem optimism dominates the attitude of anyone who is a firm believer in evolution[17]. In any event, such optimism is in line with the hopeful American philosophic approach of James and Dewey and opposed to the pessimism of Nietzsche and Foucault, even if their understanding of the evolutionary process is not the obvious source of their difference in attitudes.

CHAPTER ONE. ETHICAL THEORY

1. Introduction

Ethical codes have been promulgated for physicians since ancient times, but ethical problems in medical practice have never been of more concern or so widely discussed as at present. The applications of innovative technologies have brought forth new moral problems, and contemporary economic problems in the delivery of medical care have renewed discussion of old ethical considerations. Not only are medical ethics now the concern of patients and doctors but in many instances they have spilled over into the political arena and the law courts.

In response to this increasing number and importance of moral dilemmas in medical practice, hospitals have been advised to form ethics committees and appoint ethicists to their staffs. In 1985, 59% of 150 hospital surveyed in the United States had ethics committees, compared with 26% two years previously[1]. A survey of 200 other hospitals, also done in 1985, revealed that almost two-thirds had such committees[1]. The view from abroad[2], where the doctor-patient relationship remains stronger than in the United States and these committees have not yet appeared, is that the issues which have led to the formation of ethics committees in the United States are beginning to gain prominence in the United Kingdom and on the continent. These issues are an increasing concern for human rights, including the problem of informed consent before medical intervention, and the increased strength of the consumer movement with demand for better information on health care and various aspects of treatment. Whilst the physician in Europe is still often regarded as the arbitrator of medical decisions ("Whatever you think, doctor") this situation is probably changing along American lines. These factors, and relative lack of resources in the United Kingdom (they spend roughly a third as much per capita for medical care as does the United States) abetting the need for rationing, probably will cause the ethics committees phenomenon to spread in the United Kingdom. They believe they have the advantage of time to monitor the function of these committees in the United States for their advantages and disadvantages, before deciding whether to embark on their formation in the United Kingdom.

The term "ethics committee" under discussion should not be confused with ethics committees for research. The latter, initiated by physicians themselves, had become common in medical institutions in the United States and abroad over at least the last three decades and have served well in evaluating the objectives of intended research projects and protecting humans, and often, the animals to be used. Reports of the use of patients for non-therapeutic research without their consent[3] and the activity of anti-vivisectionists beginning in the mid-nineteenth century undoubtedly stimulated the early formation of ethics committees for research.

It might be asked: why should medical practice, alone among the professions, have attracted the full-time attention of so many ethicists? Why are medical ethics described as a "growth industry" in the U.S.[4]? An answer that immediately comes to mind is that the public is more concerned with their bodily health than with their financial or political well-being. A more plausible explanation is the change in the doctor-patient relationship, the affluence of the medical care system, and activities of the medical profession itself.

Up until the mid-twentieth century the relationship between doctor and patient was always one on one; public health problems were the province of epidemiologists and state officials. As long as this form of relationship persisted the attention of the public and ethicists was not attracted to medical practice. The introduction of "third-party payers" - medical insurance plans and the government (medicare and medicaid) - to pay medical fees altered the one on one relationship. Previously the cost of medical care was an individual responsibility and now it became a public concern. How hospitals operated, as well as how doctors practiced, became the business of the public. Another effect of the new system of payments was to increase the financial affluence of the medical care system. It now could afford a host of para-medical personnel (economists, sociologists, planners, administrators, as well as ethicists).

Another effect of this affluence was that hospitals (and/or medical schools) began to employ physicians, and corporations were formed to participate in the profits that were being made from medical care. These corporations also employ doctors; it is projected that as many as 90% of physicians in the U.S. will no longer be self-employed by 1993. This is diluting further the one on one doctor-patient relationship, employed doctors no longer being responsible only to their patients. Indeed, in many, if not most of these instances, the doctor's loyalty to patients only could be secondary.

Technological advances (and financial considerations) placed more and more of medical practice in hospitals. Responding to public questioning of their operation, hospitals turned to doctors, lawyers, clergymen, the laity and moralists to form committees to give answers to the dilemmas posed to them. It was soon obvious to philosophy students that medical schools and hospitals could afford ethicists, and they responded positively to offers to become full-time medical ethicists.

Another factor that has propelled ethics for medical practice ahead of ethics for other professions has been the activities of physicians themselves[5]. In 1904 the American Medical Association (AMA) created a Council on Medical Education which established "an ideal standard" for medical education. The Council inspected medical schools and urged the States not to license graduates from inferior schools. The AMA cooperated with the Carnegie Foundation's sponsorship of Abraham Flexner's landmark investigation of, and recommendations for, medical schools, a report issued in 1910. The AMA with the collaboration of the Association of American Medical Colleges saw to it that the recommendations were carried out. This was followed in 1916 by the American College of Surgeons taking the initiative and joining with the various hospital associations to upgrade hospitals by establishing "Minimum Standards for Hospitals". Survey teams were formed and inspections were done regularly. This endeavor was turned over in 1952 to a new organization, The Joint Commission for Accreditation of Hospitals (JCAH) composed of representatives of the AMA, the American Hospital Association, the Canadian Medical Association, the American College of Surgeons and the American College of Physicians. Various committees (credentials, tissue, records, etc.) were constantly being recommended by the JCAH as mechanisms for doctors to police themselves. The attention paid by physicians, through their organizations, to standards for themselves and hospitals did not escape general notice and, no doubt, played a role in attracting the public to bio-ethical discussions. The introduction of committees for policing doctors' activities was a gradual one and doctors grew accustomed to their presence with but minimal resistance.

A final reason for appointment of consultant ethicists to hospital staffs has been the severe increase in medical malpractice suits. It is not surprising that many physicians in the U.S., particularly those caring for infants or for adult patients who are dying, are increasingly uncertain where action based on their medical judgment should stop and legal concerns take over. "Largely in response to this a new profession has emerged - that of the clinical medical ethicist. By advising on the ethics of a situation it is hoped that open discussion will be encouraged and ethical solutions will be reached which, on the whole, will also, therefore, be legal."[6]

An implication of the formation of ethics committees and proliferation of medical ethicists is that there is an accepted theory of ethics the application of which, by individuals more learned in the field, would solve the practitioners' dilemmas. Physicians have found this not to be true[7] and even an ethicist questions the value of ethical consultations[8]. Another medical ethicist, professor of the subject in a leading university, confesses that medical ethics is a peculiar field, one that is not built on a factual basis[9]. He goes on to mention two "nasty secrets." One is that "there is no such thing as medical ethics as a discipline" in the sense that philosophy and theology are disciplines. Secret number two is that the field lacks concern for methodology. "Ethicists don't think in terms of what is right or wrong, we have arguments based on unproven premises. The only thing we can claim are these premises, followed by conclusions." "When I sat on the President's Commission on Bioethics our views would be reported by the media as either right or wrong, but to those of us on the committee, this was an inside joke. When I'm interviewed by the media, sometimes I can't help myself and I will give a point of view, knowing that my colleagues will say, 'Boy, has he deteriorated.'" Still other well-known medical ethicists admit "there is certainly no currently accepted credential for ethics consultants,"[10].

Consultation with ethicists and/or committees are of help in sharing the responsibilities for actions or inactions and in shielding physicians and the hospitals from legal assaults. The committees often by their discussion do elicit facts which had been overlooked or insufficiently considered and which when exposed, clarified the situation making possible resolution of a dilemma, which only had been an apparent one. Ethics committees are useful in setting guidelines in the rationing of new technologies with limited availability, as organs for transplantation. Aside from these advantages the doctor often finds little guidance from ethicists or ethics committees beyond what he has always known intuitively: to act with good conscience, to be of good character and behave with integrity.

The frequent advice of these committees and ethicists, who are generally unclear on the exigencies of the situations from the doctors' point of view, is that physicians hold extensive discussions with their colleagues, nurses and other paraprofessionals, and especially with their patients and/or patient's families before acting or not acting. An acknowledged medical ethicist states: "there is little evidence that training in the science of ethics improves one's ability to know what is moral."[11] More recently, the effectiveness of ethics committees (presumably in resolving dilemmas) has been questioned and a plea made for their empirical evaluation[12]. The usefulness of these committees often are negated by their questionable mode of functioning: their composition may be ill-considered; they may accept secondhand information uncritically; they may be subject to "groupthink" - too easily persuaded by forceful members, or a perceived need to come to a rapid recommendation despite inadequate information[12].

Contemporary texts on medical ethics most often avoid theoretical considerations or even argue against ethical theory in an effort to prove it cannot exist[13]. The authors of these texts go on to concern themselves with the application of normative principles to medical circumstances, either without a theoretical basis, or else, the occasional use of deontology and/or utilitarianism. Most often, their normative principles are derived from *prima facie* or *a priori* reasoning. The difficulties encountered by clinicians and practicing bioethicists in attempting to resolve real clinical problems by this method (application of normative principles without the basis of a clearly defined theory) cast doubt on this mode of procedure. It seems to lead to little more than the recapitulation of moral disagreements at a higher level of abstraction. It has been said that while scientific dilemmas are disputable there is always hope more information will become available to solve them, but moral disagreements often become basic irresolvable confrontations. A principal problem, then, appears to be the lack of consensus on a theoretical basis for ethics and failing this, a consequent diminution of authority for any of the proposed systems for morality.

Ethics is the systematic study of moral values. Morals concern the determination of right from wrong or what is good or bad in reference to actions. Implicit in this definition of ethics is that a theory underlies the organization of moral knowledge. The application of this theory should guide us in selecting those actions which are right or good and avoid those which are wrong or bad, even in new situations arising in the present or future. Williams[14] states: "An ethical theory is a theoretical account of what ethical thought and practice are...."[14, page 72]. Later he adds: "ethical theories are philosophical undertakings and commit themselves to the view that philosophy can determine, either positively or negatively, how we should think in ethics..."[14, page 74]. His critical examination of the entire question of ethical theory in his recent (1985) book confirms that presently there is no consensus for any theory offered by the best philosophical minds over the past 2500 years.

It appears there is a considerable division between many biologists and many philosophers in their approach to ethical theory. Even when philosophers accept naturalism, they are loathe to accept the evolutionary origin of ethics, lately reintroduced by sociobiologists. If these differences between biologists and philosophers could be reconciled then perhaps a universal agreement on a completely natural origin for ethics would be possible. Since physicians are specialized biologists by training, they tend to favor naturalism when they consider philosophical questions[15] and an agreement on a completely naturalistic theory for the origin of ethics ought to have great influence on the medical profession.

2. Philosophical Considerations

For many centuries widespread faith in religious principles and the omnipotence of a deity supplied authority for ethical conduct. Since the Enlightenment the discoveries of biology and physical sciences have undermined many religious doctrines. Contemporary philosophers for the most part have abandoned the metaphysical approach in their thinking, thus completing the destruction of the previous consensus that ethical concepts arise from divine command or by revelation. One line of reasoning is that if a supreme authoritative source existed (in terms of right and wrong) the inference should be drawn that ours is presently the best of all possible worlds[14]. "To accept any such notion, the numerous stupendous evils that have existed and those that are now presently evident must somehow be construed as not being evil. In view of this paradox, we cannot believe there is any such God without abandoning our good sense or good will. Of course, God may not have omnipotent power and then our intuitions for "good" are not derived from His power but from His goodness." But, as Williams[14, page 32] continues: "There is nothing wrong with the general shape of this account: it explains why one would have good reason to live the kind of life that respected others' interests. It is rather that we know that it could not be true -- could not be true, since if we understand anything about the world at all, we understand it is not run like that. Indeed many, including many Christians, would now say we know that it is not run at all." Even though the majority of informed persons still believe in a transcendental force giving origin to the universe, only a minority believe it to be omnipotent or revealing.

Moral philosophers in recent centuries have adopted a more natural approach in their quest for the origins of ethical thought. At first ethical sentiments were said to originate in mankind's nature and this placed there by the deity; Bishop Butler certainly had not abandoned religion. With the advance of political thought it became clear that the feudal order used God and the Church to sustain the position of the aristocracy. With the rise of the bourgeois class culminating in the French Revolution it was necessary to disaffirm theocracy to weaken the power of the aristocracy and emphasize freedom and equality.

It was also clear to many thinkers of the Enlightenment that the concept of God had been developed to explain the mysteries of the Universe and as their new science began to explain the workings of nature, religious concepts were weakened further. The advances in science ever since have continued the decline of reliance on religious faith by progressively greater portions of societies, into the modern era. It should be conceded that very, if not the most, important Enlightenment philosophers and scientists were deists. However, they either equated God with nature (Spinoza and Einstein) or viewed the deity as the creator of the Universe but who thereafter abstained entirely (Descartes) or almost entirely (Newton) from intervening in its direction. They all regarded the Universe to be directed immediately by the laws of nature, the deity being abstract or aloof.

A naturalistic view of ethics means a view according to which ethics is to be understood in worldly terms, without reference to God or any transcendental authority. It means the kind of ethical view from the general attitude that man is part of nature[14]. Ethical values were recognized to be innate in the individual, but how this nature was acquired could only be a matter of speculation. Influential English moral philosophers (G.E. Moore[16] and A.J. Ayer[17]) writing in the early part of this century continued to expand the naturalistic approach but nevertheless believed that there was no relation between empirical facts and the sense of value. Ethical values, just as aesthetic ones, were innate in the individual and could not be rationally disputed. Moore[16] forcefully stated the value sense of good, while easily recognizable as an intuition, nevertheless, was indefinable. He also believed even though "good" and "bad" were indefinable, we could investigate how these values are used. Philosophers could and should do this (pursue meta-ethics) but should not engage in telling one what they ought, or ought not, to do (normative ethics). If a person did not know of what good or bad consisted, they could not be told, since these values were simple, indefinable and irreducible. This point of view did limit and constrict ethical discussion and was an extension of the opinion of Hume that "the distinction of vice and virtue is not founded merely on the relations of objects, nor is perceived by reason"[18]. In other words, the way things ought to be, is derived from our intuitions and cannot be come upon by an examination of how things are.

Despite lack of agreement on a general theory for ethics, two systems have been recommended to physicians by the medical ethicists for help in solving their dilemmas: utilitarianism, particularly as developed by John Stuart Mill and a deontological system as most forcefully expounded by Kant. Deontology proclaims there are universal rules for behavior, *intuitively* understood by a rational man. By reflection, all rational persons know what is right or what is correct conduct. Kant believed there was one supreme moral law comprehending: one, all men should act only on those maxims capable of being willed as universal laws; and two, no person should be treated as a means, but always as an end, since all people have an intrinsic moral worth that needs to be respected.

More contemporary deontologists have expanded this monistic approach to a pluralistic one. They maintain that our common moral convictions are composed of a plurality of principles that cannot be reduced to one another or to some higher single principle. Ross[19] believes that many so-called *prima facie* moral obligations (obvious on the face of it, or at first sight) can be listed by reflection upon, and analysis of, our *intuitions*. In considering which of these *prima facie* principles took precedence over the others (in an effort to resolve dilemmas occurring when two or more such principles arise in the course of a single action) Ross believes one can only have an opinion from our *intuition*, never actual knowledge, on how they might be ranked. Rawls[20], on the other hand, believes it is possible to rank *prima facie* obligations in order of their priority and thus conflicts can be resolved. All agree that besides principles which apply to everyone, there are also particular duties that apply to those with special roles, as doctors. Physicians have a particular duty to their patients: to promote their health and respect their confidences.

Utilitarianism states morality is determined by what maximizes happiness or what minimizes misery. Another description is that it is a doctrine which states that the rightness or wrongness of an action is determined by the goodness or badness of its consequences[21]. While some have interpreted utilitarianism to mean assessing the consequences of an action to the individual perpetrating it (egoistic utilitarianism), the majority of utilitarians believe the morality of action is dependent upon a calculation of its impact on society in terms of its producing the greatest happiness for the greatest number (universalistic utilitarianism). It is self-evident in this system happiness is good and suffering is evil.

A most important division in utilitarianism has been created between what are described as "act" and "rule" utilitarianisms[21]. In the former, "actions" mean particular actions and the rightness or wrongness of an individual action is determined directly by the assessment of its consequences. When the word actions is interpreted to mean "sorts of actions" then it is rule utilitarianism that is invoked. Rule utilitarianism does consider the consequences of each particular action but also considers the consequences of adopting a general rule for actions. A rule for actions is adopted if the consequences of all such actions are better than those of the adoption of some alternative rule. In a sense rule utilitarianism can be considered deontologic, or Kantian, since one has a duty to act in a certain way based upon a theory (to produce the best consequences - the greatest happiness, or the best welfare, of society). Modern utilitarians have advanced their theory to state that the best way to maximize overall happiness is to maximize the satisfaction of individuals by favoring their autonomous preferences. This provides a basis for the rights of individuals and their autonomy and thus freedom. It has been pointed out that utilitarianism, particularly egoistic utilitarianism, seems to over-ride moral principles that are widely accepted: respect for honesty and openness, and promise keeping, and justice, and individual autonomy, etc. Utilitarians (more clearly, the more modern rule utilitarians) respond this is not so, because not to respect these principles is not conducive to the maximization of human happiness. Indeed, Mill had stated to respect the autonomy of the individual, insofar as compatible with autonomy for all, is a fundamental component of utilitarianism[22].

Each of these systems proposed for ethical conduct suggest that they should conform to mankind's "intuitions" or "common sense". "Just as physical scientists must start with our perceptions of physical objects, it has been stated that moral philosophers must start with our common sense ethical judgments, since they have no other data."[23] They must then bring their data into a system that will provide coherent solutions to problems.

From where do intuitions arise? If one accepts a natural approach to philosophical thought it is logical that an evolutionary process be considered. Mary Midgley[24], a philosopher, agrees that many aspects of our social relationships can be observed in animal behavior. "Had we known no other animate life-form than our own, we should have been utterly mysterious to ourselves as a species. And that would have made it immensely harder for us to understand ourselves as individuals too. Anything that puts us in context, that shows us as part of a continuum, an example of a type that varies on intelligible principles, is a great help"[24, page 18]. She further points out we differ from animals in that our instincts require completion by a culture. Instincts can be termed drives or programs and can be classified as open or closed ones. Closed instincts are behavior patterns fixed genetically in every detail and, particularly in lower species, will take place even if creatures are carefully reared in isolation from their own kind and from any helpful conditioning. Such genetic programming takes the place of intelligence. "Open instincts are programs with a gap. Parts of the behavior pattern are innately determined, but others are left to be filled in by experience"[24, page 53]. The gaps could, of course, be filled in by culture or modified by reflection, which require language and reason. The latter are human characteristics. Midgley believes there is true altruism in our nature and these come from our social instincts; instincts are not just egotistic as Hobbes believed. Ethics according to Midgley is a process to resolve conflicts within and between people. Ethics are a combination of feelings (deep, long lasting motivations, not just temporary moods) and rationality. Ethical principles cannot be understood by just introversion, but we must look around and see how others behave and also how other species behave. Throughout her writings she infers that all ethics are based on our nature to be human and we can only learn about ourselves by looking at other animals.

It is amazing then, that Midgley could have been so dismissive of evolutionary ethics[24, page 155], and in light of the enormous contributions made to this subject by biologists and philosophers who preceded her. Those contributions were recently resurrected in a scholarly book by an historian of science and philosophy[25]. He makes available to the non-cognoscenti, such as physicians (and as it turns out, to some ethicists and philosophers too), the enormous contributions made to ethics from an evolutionary point of view 100 years ago by Darwin, Wallace, Spencer, et al.

Darwin extended his concept of evolution to morals and community selection[26]. He believed that man in social groups evolved sets of instinctive responses to preserve the welfare of the community. Indeed these immediate, unthought responses were distinguished from utilitarian, calculated criteria of morality and they were designed not for the general happiness but "the general good of the community". Wallace in 1864[27] proposed that natural selection would operate to favor tribes with a high proportion of moral members, a proposal quite in line with Darwin's thoughts in the *Descent of Man*. These theses were developed subsequently, and enlarged upon by others, still long ago[28,29]. Thus, an evolutionary theory for ethics states that ethical principles are ultimately based upon what is best for the welfare of society. There are ambiguities in the positions of these early writers, and controversies over them, all of which is presented in detail by Richards[25].

Many modern philosophers accept an evolutionary (or natural) derivation for the human species but cannot accept that this applies to the mind[30,31,32]. The acceptance or denial of the evolutionary origin of the mind appears to be a fundamental difference between many biologists and most philosophers. Nagel[30], in discussing the conception of the mind and evolution, can understand why creatures with vision or reason will survive, but he believes that evolution cannot explain how vision or reasoning are possible. While his discussion touches on most of the fact offered by biologists in their approach to the development of the mind, he seizes on the so far incompleteness of their explanation to support his skepticism of it. Moreover, he states that in his opinion there *never* will be a satisfactory biological explanation of the mind. He admits he has no explanation of his own. He does not resort to the belief of divine creation, asserting he is a rationalist. Rationalism is a system of philosophical belief which states that human reason unaided is competent to attain objective truth. Rationalists believe moral ideas are innate and they support the claims of reason against those of revelation and theistic authority. He believes there needs to be "something fairly remarkable...an unheard of property of the natural order of things" that makes human knowledge intelligible.

Most scientists agree they are not yet close to simulating the mind, yet they do not dispute it is a natural, evolutionary development. Despite the mechanism of the workings of the mind not being clear to them at present, most believe that it will be simulated, even though that appears to be decades away. Yet it should be noted that a world famous neuroscientist, as late as 1989, still regarded the human mind (and the soul) as a supernatural creation "which is implanted into the fetus at some time between conception and birth"[(32A)].

It does seem Nagel's position, that the mind could not have evolved because it is too enormous a development to have occurred in that manner, can be countered by the enormity of other evolutionary developments he does accept. The evolution of even the lowest animals from unicellular precursors should be as mind-boggling as is the development of the mind in the evolution of the brain. Because we do not know the significance or meaning of the Universe does not mean we cannot understand, with our current scientific knowledge, the particular mechanisms of its development from the "big bang" to the infinite contraction or expansion that lies billions of years ahead, and our Earth and life upon it.

A more direct answer to Nagel's concern re the development of the mind along natural lines is that evolutionary changes need not always be equally gradual[(33)]. There are many examples of sudden rapid changes in biological evolution[(34)]. The gradual enlargement and increasing complexity of the brain in the numerous lower species, invertebrates to vertebrates and through the mammals to the primates and finally to man is apparent to all. It is not difficult to conceive the abrupt development of a mind to accompany this final additional enlargement and complexity.

In the evolution of the circuitry of the brain it is understandable that the complexity achieved in *Homo sapiens* could cause an unexpected quantum leap to the increased consciousness and ability to conceptualize, characteristics of this species. The change in human brain function accompanying the anatomic enlargement in *Homo sapiens* was so enormous that it acquired the qualities of representation and abstraction. The variety in its adaptations and possible responses gives it sufficient choice so that it can be termed freedom. The term "sudden rapid change" in the evolution of brain function to explain the development of the mind can be best be understood as a remarkable *qualitative* change appearing at, and accompanying, a certain level of *quantitative* enlargement.

Other philosophers who regard themselves as otherwise favoring naturalism also find it difficult to accept the evolutionary development of the mind and the view that it is only the result of a very complex, but nevertheless natural mechanism. Even Midgley[24] takes issue with E.O. Wilson[35], the sociobiologist, on his view that the mind is naturally evolved. She does so on his statement that the mind will become in time understood at the neuronal level, accusing him of extreme reductionism. He obviously does view the mind as a complexity of the whole, beyond the composition of an enormous number of neurons[35, page 77], no matter how he expressed it elsewhere[36]. Dr. Midgley, who otherwise intensely favors naturalism in her philosophic thinking, nonetheless seems to believe the mind has a mysterious origin, since she takes issue with Wilson by stating: "'Cognition' cannot be 'translated into circuitry'. Learning and creativeness cannot 'be defined as specific portions of the cognitive machinery'."[24, page 171]

Churchland in her recent book, "Neurophilosophy" gives an excellent presentation of this very subject: the unity of the science of the brain with the philosophic concept of the mind[37]. While there are large gaps to be explained in finally achieving her goal, it is clear there can be no *a priori* arguments against it. She does present in detail a believable means (from recent neuro-anatomical and neurophysiological findings and advances in "artificial intelligence") by which the brain in its evolutionary development could create the mind. It may be that the brain "is more complicated than it is smart" but philosophers must: "see that empirical discoveries in psychology, neuroscience, artificial intelligence research and so forth could mold and shape and perhaps transmit the language of the mental."[37] A biologist has more recently presented a plausible explanation of the mind as the most recent evolutionary development of the brain and relates the significance of this explanation to moral philosophy[38].

It is correct to say that the vast majority of scientists believe in neo-Darwinian evolution and in the evolutionary derivation of the brain and mind. To be fair however, it is only right to point out that there are those with impeccable scientific credentials, an astronomer and a mathematician, who question this statement[39,40] . The former does not believe that the human brain and mind has evolved on earth, at least not *de novo*. The latter does not believe it is possible for consciousness or the mind to be explained by neuroscientists or simulated by artificial intelligence efforts. He gives sophisticated mathematical reasoning for this opinion and disbelieves that an algorithmic process can be created to replicate the workings of the mind. Both agree that the earth has existed for an insufficient amount of time for these phenomena to have occurred through evolution.

Returning to Ethics, Churchland in her book[37, page 399] concludes: "At a minimum it is worth considering whether transformation in our moral conceptions to adhere more closely to the discovered facts of brain function might be no bad thing as well... It is at least conceivable that our moral and legal institutions will be seen by future generations to be as backward, superstitious, and primitive as we now see the Christian Church's doctrine of past centuries concerning the moral significance of disease and the moral propriety of anesthesia, immunization and contraception."

3. Biologic Considerations

The group of biologists, termed sociobiologists, had pointed out that social behavior can be demonstrated in many species and concluded that human social behavior is part of the evolutionary process. The sociobiologists, Ruse and Wilson[41], state unequivocally that the social behavior of all animals, including mankind and its culture, is firmly under the control of genes and has been shaped into forms that give reproductive advantage. Altruism (a cornerstone of ethical thinking) is interpreted by them as an individual animal favoring genes identical to his own even if present in other individuals.

They offer as an illustration ants who perform their duties in perfect harmony, without thought, but perform their actions as the result of the closed circuitry, or "hard-wiring", of their nervous systems. When something goes wrong in their environment, worker ants unhesitatingly sacrifice themselves in efforts to counter the environmental change. Incidentally, Darwin pondered about ants, and they served to explain to him the possibility for the evolution of ethics[25]. Ruse and Wilson reason, teleologically, that worker ants are cheap to produce and their sacrifice as the result of the rigidity of their hard-wired response matters little to the colony. They point out such a hard-wired response does not do for humans: because each human requires a great deal of parental investment and "it would be stupid in the literal sense if we were to go wrong at the slightest environmental quiver". On the other hand they reason further, if there was no underlying hard-wired circuitry (it is to be presumed they meant in the "old" brain - the limbic system and hypothalamus) and only a completely thoughtful, evaluative "new" brain (the neocortex working alone) every environmental stimulus would result in man weighing and assessing every possible reaction and we would be forever making up our minds. Ruse and Wilson say that man has evolved an innate disposition (genetically determined) for altruism; just as to fear heights and snakes and to avoid incest are innately in place because of their biological virtues.

The effort by sociobiologists to place human activity entirely under genetic control and extending this thesis to all human social and political development has done a disservice to what biologists do have to contribute to philosophic thought: that there is a genetic evolutionary basis for only some, or some parts of, social conduct and for only some ethical principles. The emphasis of sociobiologists that the social behavior of animals is determined by the genes and can and should be extrapolated to *all* human behavior, together with some of their political opinions being conservative, has precipitated severe rebuttal within the biologic community[42]. For instance, sociobiological dictum has been used to support superiority of intelligence of one race over another and as a basis for male dominance. IQ testing and studies done on twins have been purported to support the belief that intelligence is genetically determined and that there are differences in intelligence between races.

Their opposing biologic colleagues pointed out patent errors in extrapolating the results from IQ testing to genetic differences between the races and social classes. The errors were not only in interpretation of the inheritability of actual test results, but also lay in not taking proper account of the cultural differences between the groups being tested. The clearest evidence for the genetic determination of the IQ was the massive work of Cyril Burt. His work was principally based on the study of identical twins separated early in life and on the interpretation of tests administered, by the thousands, to pairs and relatives. Analysis of his data revealed numerical impossibilities and investigation of the bases of his contributions, including interrogation of his secretary and co- workers, led to the conclusion his work was totally fraudulent, a situation now admitted by even his originally staunchest admirers[42].

Studies of identical twins separated early in life done subsequently were shown also to have serious flaws and cannot be relied upon to demonstrate an heritable basis for IQ test scores. Studies of adopted children at first seemed to show that heredity has more correlation with IQ test results than does environment, but later, better designed studies did not confirm this inference. On the other hand, newer studies comparing the correlations of IQ tests between identical and non-identical twins did indicate a marked influence of heredity on the results. Even more recent studies of identical and fraternal twins give firm support to the inheritance of personality, interests and development[43,43A].

The social differences between males and females are another point of contention between sociobiologists and biologists who are opposed to them. Anthropologists have confirmed that there has been a universal division of labor in primitive societies that has persisted throughout history until the present time, with the usual result being that of male dominance. This has been interpreted by the sociobiologists as proof for an evolutionary basis for patriarchy, and that this cultural pattern is genetically determined. They further point out the anatomical and hormonal differences between males and females lead to differences in abilities and proclivities between men and women, demonstrated from early childhood through adulthood. The biologists opposed to the sociobiologists claim the data demonstrating that these male-female differences are genetically determined are often fallacious or merely inferential at best[42]. While some objections are well taken, it still does not dispose entirely of the arguments advanced to explain the biological origins of patriarchy. Nevertheless the manifest social injustices of sexism and the losses to our cultural development by permitting or condoning over-bearing male dominance is convincingly presented.

It might be added that cultural advance (civilization) introducing labor-saving devices in all walks of life minimizes the importance of difference in strength between men and women. Likewise, innovation has permitted women to have control over their reproductive process so they more fully can participate on equal terms with men in contemporary endeavors. These cultural changes neutralize some of the genetic differences between the sexes and do provide a plausible basis for the "feminist movement" that well might prove to be of greater consequence to its success than merely appealing for "justice".

The fundamental objection to sociobiology is its unequivocal acceptance of natural selection at the genetic level of the individual to explain all of human behavior. Indeed, natural selection does not seem to work in such a simplistic manner even for much of biologic variation[42]. That selection takes place is generally accepted, but the units of selection and how it operates are still matters of controversy[25]. That some cultural traits may be under genetic control, is no basis for extrapolating that all cultural traits are of genetic origin. Indeed, it seems far-fetched to assign such control for the greatest part of culture, and empirically unsound. It would seem reasonable to presume that the unit through which natural selection operates is the individual in some stages in the derivation of species, and groups of individuals (particularly when it involves cultural traits) at other stages of human development.

Wilson[35] rejects the ethical systems of philosophers because of their being based on man's intuitions. While this sociobiologist believes intuition is a product of the evolved brain, he goes on to reason that because different people have different evolutionary interests (personal interests) they will only "see" (intuit) what is in their own interests to "see". Therefore, he reasons, intuition can't be trusted to "see" or intuit the truth of what is good or bad. The total rejection of intuition as a basis for ethics by a sociobiologist is strange. If intuition is feeling what is right or wrong with an action or about a set of circumstances, it then must be a conscious reading of an emotional reaction. Stated otherwise, it is whether one (presuming one is a rational person) feels good or bad when reflecting on a situation. Hume[18] long ago wrote that a feeling of pleasure or pain in sympathy with others is the sentiment of morality and these feelings are universal and are the basis of morality. It is probable that such feelings arise from neural patterns forming templates in our brains favoring conduct for our own and our species' benefit. It then would seem reasonable to conclude that contemplated or actual behavior which yields emotional satisfaction is our intuition that it is good; and anxiety, if aroused by the contemplation of a behavior, is the basis of our intuition that it is bad. If true, this would be a biologic contribution to any philosophic theory for ethics.

In substantiation of the theory for an evolutionary origin of ethical intuitions are the evidences of the ontogeny of the human brain and neurophysiology. It is known that the phylogenetically old brain, the limbic system and hypothalamus, are the sites of emotional circuitry. This is, in all probability, relatively "hard-wired". Reflection and consciousness is possible only with the new brain, the neocortex, the evolutionary addition of which affords humans the ability to learn and to be flexible in reactions. There are connections between old and new brain, thought modifying emotions, and vice-versa, and more or less variable in influence in either direction from individual to individual, and in different circumstances. Thus, permitting emotions initiated in the "old brain" unrestrained by the "new brain" to dominate one's behavior might explain the activities of extremists (see under animal-rightists, Chapter Seven). Also, "innate dispositions", or the "epigenetic rules" of Ruse and Wilson[41], undoubtedly reflect specific circuitry genetically "wired" into the brain. As an example, it may be presumed that what is "good" for the group would be in terms of what was good for its survival and those groups would best survive where such "good" producing responses were fixed in the circuitry of the brains of its individuals. Thus, it is recognized universally that to sacrifice oneself for family or group is an act of the highest moral significance and such actions are observed in lower species possessing no possibility of reflection. Indeed, such acts are carried out despite obvious strong instincts for self preservation in most situations. In humans it is conceivable self-sacrifice occurs as an evolved emotion issuing from the "old" limbic system of the brain. In some circumstances even the thought of self-destruction might be pleasant.

On the other hand, in their obsession with their biologic account of morality and their insistence on its control by the genes, sociobiologists deny the independence of cultural development and its influences on man. They even state that in all cultural characteristics genetic control is decisive[35,44]. This makes their present formulation for ethics and morality difficult for philosophers to accept. For example, "by appearing not to be concerned with the well-being of the individual, but with its genetic fitness to leave offsprings, sociobiology's relation to ethics seems to be particularly far-fetched"[45]. Bernard Williams[14, page 44] states, "the important point is that evolutionary biology is not at all directly concerned with the well-being of the individual, but with fitness, which is the likelihood of that individual's leaving offspring. The most that sociobiology might do for ethics lies in a different direction, inasmuch as it might be able to suggest that certain institutions or patterns of behavior are not realistic options for human societies. That would be an important achievement, but first sociobiology will have to read the historical record of human culture much better than it does now".

Culture is an achievement of mankind made possible by the evolutionary process which developed their brain to use language, to have the ability to learn, and to be capable of reflection. Culture, where achievable in a species, needs to be taught to, and learned by, the individual. While bounded in some directions by the genes (through the influence of inherited circuitry), culture is truly transmitted generation to generation by instruction and by imitation. Perhaps communication at the level of language is a good example of genetic evolutionary traits interacting with individually acquired cultural ones. In the first place, the anatomical evolution of the vocal apparatus permits the production of a wide and rich variety of sounds by the human child. More interestingly, modern linguists have offered believable arguments for there being an innate capacity for language in the brain of each *Homo sapiens* child, demonstrated by its rapid and apparently untaught understanding of grammar and syntax, and serving as a template for the acquiring whichever is the language of its culture, the latter obviously done by imitation and teaching[46].

Culture is a mechanism to permit very rapid adaptation to changing circumstances and gives humans plasticity in their reactions, helping to account for their biologic success. Culture in its transmission changes too rapidly to be under genetic control. Nevertheless, and most interestingly, it may in its transmission be governed by forces essentially similar to those of the genetic evolutionary process. This is the subject of a recent book by Boyd and Richerson[47] that adds considerable substance to the evolutionary theory for the development of culture[48]. They support the plausible theory that cultural development is governed by rules paralleling those of the Darwinian theory for biologic evolution. They point out how natural selection is an important force in changing the frequency of different cultural variants and that random errors in the transmission of cultural traits are analogous to mutations in genetic evolution. Of course cultural variations can occur in, or even within, one generation and this difference in the temporal rate of cultural changes as compared with genetic evolutionary changes is because it comprehends the inheritance of acquired characteristics, which genetic evolutionary change does not. Since items of information in cultural transmission can be regarded as equivalent to the genes in biology, the current constantly increasing speed of informational transfer is creating a "smaller world" and the opportunity for ever increasing rapidity of cultural change.

In the view of Boyd and Richerson, "natural selection" in cultural transmission often even can reduce ordinary genetic fitness. Individuals may be forced to decide between increasing their genetic and their cultural fitness. For instance, modern middle-class young adults seem to delay marriage and reduce their number of children so as to direct resources to the achievement of their own and their children's professional success. In agricultural societies, parents often manipulate their children in order to live a comfortable old age. When age confers high status in a culture, elders could be sacrificing their genetic interest in their children and grandchildren for the chance to be active in oblique transmission (the acquiring of cultural traits from non-parental adults or conversely, the transmitting of cultural traits to other than one's genetic offsprings). "In evolving a reliance on cultural transmission, the human species may well have 'traded' high rates of random error caused by individual learning in variable environments for a lower rate of systematic error (with respect to genetic fitness) due to the partial autonomy of cultural evolution."

That cultural evolution includes the inheritance of acquired characteristics might make it even more typical of the original Darwinian theory than biological evolution. The original Darwinian theory presumed linear improvement in the adaptability of a species through the mechanism of the "survival of the fittest" individuals; but evidence has been offered recently suggesting that biological evolution occurs more by chance, with a pruning of species from the "bush of life" and in a "punctuated equilibrium" manner[48A].

Having reviewed many opinions and the empirical evidence pro and con, Boyd and Richerson conclude that a dual inheritance theory for biological and cultural evolution can clarify issues in explaining human behavior. Boyd and Richerson, being scientists, are concerned with the predictability of the theory they support as evidence for its correctness[49]. They recognize to insist upon the proofs required in empirical sciences, such as physics, may be impossible to fulfill for the social sciences, but "to give up on empirical tests and prediction would be to abandon science and retreat to speculative philosophy." There aims may be unduly stringent: firstly, the number and complexity of the variables may relegate the predictability of the theory to the newly recognized field of "chaos", as with economics and the weather[50]; secondly, the theory can be useful retrospectively in historical analysis when, by elimination, no other possibility as an explanation could be creditable.

Thus, if it could be agreed that culture develops according to the evolutionary principle of what is best for the welfare of the group, we would have important support for a natural origin of ethics. Such a theory for ethics would state that ethical principles ultimately are arrived at according to what is best for society at a given time.

Molecular biologists[51,52] have recognized the independence of culture from full genetic control, but decry this independence. In their view, whatever autonomy is possessed by culture is the cause of self-delusion, psychic pain and social instability and violates mankind's true biologic nature; therefore culture independent of biology is to be regretted since it is not beneficial for species adaptation. This view is opposed to the theory of the evolutionary origin of culture discussed above. It may be the molecular biologists have arrived at their conclusion from too short an observation of the historical process. Or even if their conclusion on the evil effect of some of the surviving cultural traits that are independent of genetic control is correct as far as individuals are concerned, the total effect on species adaptation might not be crucial. On the other hand, the explosive reproductive success of man over the last two hundred years has to be the result of the industrial and technological revolution achieved by a culture which could not have been under total genetic control. The dual evolutionary theory for culture and biology as outlined above gives a more rational explanation of our species' success and should give confidence that mankind will survive any of the emotional and/or moral dilemmas that arise. This cannot, it must be feared, give reason to believe that the possibility of succumbing to some complication of technological advances (nuclear war or decimation of the environment) will be avoided.

That ethical principles are bound up with cultural practices not under genetic control seems undeniable, and just as undeniable is that the non-genetic, but nevertheless evolutionary, development of culture is likely to be the predominant factor in the ethical code of any society. But it must be reiterated that non-genetic culture is not the only source of morality. In order for culture to develop, people must work together in a giving and sharing manner. To be able to do so implies that an altruistic template existed in mankind's brain prior to the onset of culture. Also, altruism has been shown by the sociobiologists (and Darwin long before them[25]) to be hard-wired in lower species and it can be expected to be relatively so in man (only relatively in humans because the large neocortex undoubtedly can inhibit or modify any such circuits in lower brain areas). Therefore, it is proper to accept a genetic factor in morality. As another example: In the discussion above on the acquisition of language it was pointed out how the brain circuits were genetically in place to form a template in each human child for developing the particular language of its culture. Indeed, we are told that all languages, no matter how primitive the people or their culture, are equi-potential, and how complex it becomes depends upon the cultural development of its users[53].

Universals in cultural behavior, that is patterns of behavior or categories of behaviors found to be present in every culture no matter how far dispersed, have been thought by anthropologists to be indicative of their inherited origin. This has been mentioned for over sixty years. Wissler[54] believed that "the pattern for culture is just as deeply buried in the germ plasm of man as the bee pattern in the bee". Thirty years later, Kluckhohn[55] stated: "The attention of anthropologists throughout the world appears to have been directed overwhelmingly to the distinctiveness of each culture and to the differences in human custom as opposed to the similarities. The latter, where recognized, were explained historically rather than in terms of the common nature of man and certain invariant properties in the human situation". Other anthropologists have pointed out many cultural universals such as family organization, marriage, incest avoidance, religion (resulting from attempts to come to grips with the finitude of life and the death of the individual, as well as yearnings to transcend the natural), a natural division of labor, language (equally developed in all societies in their potential for expression), aesthetic expression, etc. Even an understanding of individual property rights appears to be universal in all cultures.

Raanon Gillon[56], in combating the belief of some that philosophical medical ethics is not possible since there is no agreement on ethical principles, directs attention to widespread agreement on many behaviors of ethical significance. His inference is that to inflict pain or harm on other people, or to kill people, or deprive people of their liberty, or to coerce people to do things against their will, unless there is good reason for any of these actions, is held to be wrong universally. He also states the list could be extended. A moral code has been said to be present in all cultures: Hallowell[57], an anthropologist, states that: "All cultures are infused with appraisals that involve cognitive, appreciative and moral values".

Kohlberg's[58] empirical observations also supported the thesis that there is a univerality in moral judgments and individual development in moral reasoning. He is disdainful of the assumption by the behaviorists (and other cultural relativists) that there is relativity in moral reasoning and principles. Indeed, if Kohlberg had had the opportunity to consider, and could have agreed with, an evolutionary origin for ethics he would have found his philosophical assumptions made easier in the formulation (and verification) of his theory for the moral development of children[59].

Students of jurisprudence in their efforts to ascertain the origin of laws turned to the studies of anthropologists and archaeologists and developed a line of inquiry called comparative jurisprudence. A.H. Post[60] examined how societies throughout the world - Hovas, Zulus, Maoris, Tunguses, Hindus, Teutons, Jews, Egyptians - handled problems in various legal situations. The startling result, to him, was how people, even those entirely cut off from one another and at different planes of development, resorted to similar expedients in similar situations.

Philosophers use the terms universal values and ethical relativism. The former implies there are ethical principles that hold for all people and at all times despite the fact of variations in cultural development. Ethical relativism asserts that no universal moral principles are valid for all persons in all circumstances or at all times; that moral rightness and wrongness are relative to the particular cultural or historical niche in which they happen to be operating.

However, most moral philosophers do not appear to be ethical relativists. Though likely to be unaware of the recent view that culture evolves, moral philosophers nevertheless tend to be skeptical of moral relativism[58].

The problems encountered by people, either as individuals or as a community, are likely in many, if not most, instances to be similar around the world. The similarity of so many of the responses, in terms of customs, ethical principles and laws, in so many societies (many unknown to each other) is an indication that these responses were dictated by the common necessity to continue to exist. The universality of so many ethical principles (and of customs and laws) therefore speak for their evolutionary origin.

It is up to the social scientists: anthropologists, archaeologists, sociologists, psychologists and historians to further verify (or refute) the proposition that ethical principles which are universal are of benefit to mankind. Further, that others which vary, either from group to group or with time in a single society, are adaptations to special or unique circumstances which, if not of obvious benefit in their variations to diverse societies, are at least indifferent in their consequence to the welfare of any society.

4. Discussion

Why have molecular biologists and sociobiologists been so critical of philosophers? The most obvious reason is the great success scientists have had in elucidating the many mysteries of the Universe and the failure of philosophers to make any real advances in their own epistemological enterprise since the period of Enlightenment. This does not mean in these past few centuries that great philosophical minds have not been put to the problem, but rather without new tools and only the use of their reflection, philosophers could not contribute any meaningful new knowledge of the world. The concentration on the dissection of the writings of others or on the meaning and use of language add to the frustration of scientists, since much of either enterprise could be termed quibbling. J.D. Watson has recently written[61]: "we must not automatically assume that because philosophers' arguments are increasingly subtle, they represent serious advances beyond the commonplace ideas about deduction and induction first formulated...by Francis Bacon. I am uncomfortable with much of this unneeded complexity." An astrophysicist comments[62]: "...the people whose business it is to ask why, the philosophers, have not been able to keep up with the advance of scientific theories. ...science became too technical and mathematical for the philosophers, or anyone except a few specialists. Philosophers reduced the scope of their inquiries so much that Wittgenstein, the most famous philosopher of this century, said 'The sole remaining task for philosophy is the analysis of language.'"

As scientific contributions have become increasingly fruitful, it also has become clear that many issues (such as the nature of matter or even the mind) can only be explained by science. Over the past fifty years even some philosophers have expressed the conviction that their discipline cannot answer the perennial questions and enigmas that have confronted them[63,64]. Perhaps this position of some philosophers has emboldened molecular biologists and sociobiologists to proclaim that only advances in their disciplines will provide an acceptable ethical theory and a moral code for behavior.

The direct forays of the molecular biologists and sociobiologist against philosophy (indeed, to the point of rejecting philosophers totally) has aroused hostility. The negative feeling of philosophers towards scientists is certain to be inforced by the serious conflict among biologists themselves on the value of sociobiologic observations. This conflict among biologists has already been alluded to: the insistence by sociobiologists that the gene alone controls human nature and culture, plus unwarranted political extrapolations. Biologists opposed to sociobiologists are not just content to do so on scientific grounds, but add to the fury of the conflict by giving vent to their own political polemics[42].

If the assaults could be overlooked and the biologic controversies resolved, contemporary moral philosophers probably would utilize the positive contribution of evolutionary biologists on the development of individuals and societies to strengthen their obvious feelings for a naturalistic approach to a theory for ethics.

If an evolutionary origin for ethics be accepted, what then would be the answer to the perennial question which must be asked when considering any possible theory for ethics: why should anyone lead an ethical life or live within a system of morality?

Aristotle's position was that the good life for an individual, since we are social beings, rests on one's relation to others. For fulfillment of this social role, individuals are required to have the familiar moral virtues. This has been the general position of most moral philosophers ever since. Religious philosophers believe that God created mankind and dictated that their moral behavior is to be the path to salvation. Philosophers, since the Enlightenment, have conceded that morality is part of man's nature and more recently many have denied the latter to be of divine origin.

Most contemporary thinkers believe in the evolutionary origin of man, and to varying extents, of his nature and of his ethics. Williams[14] in his recent book, "Ethics and the Limits of Philosophy" concludes: "While ethical thought will never entirely appear as what it is, and can never fully manifest the fact that it rests in human dispositions....".

Why one should lead an ethical life is inexorably concerned with the answer to what is the purpose of life and even further, the purpose of the Universe. Philosophers and scientists have considered these questions without reaching conclusions that can satisfy everyone. Ultimately for those who propose answers, they have to appeal to our faith. Theologians appeal for religious faith; others to the faith that it is the use of the mind (in the acquisition of knowledge; continuing reflection; acquiring aesthetic experience) that is the ultimate purpose for mankind[16,65].

Scientists have pondered these questions without arriving at answers. Steven Weinberg[66], the astrophysicist, writes: "The more the Universe seems comprehensible, the more it also seems pointless. But if there is no solace in the fruits of our research, there is at least some consolation in the research itself. Men and women are not content to comfort themselves with tales of Gods and giants, or to confine their thoughts to the daily affairs of life; they also build telescopes, and satellites and accelerators, and sit at their desks for endless hours working out the meaning of the data they gather. The effort to understand the Universe is one of the very few things that lifts human life a little above the level of farce, and gives it some of the grace of tragedy." Thus he finds no purpose in the Universe nor in the meaning of life and the only relief for human existence is to study and acquire knowledge.

In any event, faith in a theory cannot guarantee its correctness. Faith in a transcendental deity continues to originate in the incomprehensibility of natural phenomena, arrived at a level depending upon the educational background of the individual. To one, the extraordinary capability of the human hand is incomprehensible; to a more informed person, such as the philosophers alluded to in the earlier pages of this chapter, it is the development of the mind that is incomprehensible[30,31]; to still others, even if the entire Universe is understandable, it is what preceded the big bang or what will follow its ultimate fate (billions of years from now) that is incomprehensible. There certainly is not sufficient evidence at present that can recommend to a rational person faith in any particular theory for the purpose of life or of the Universe. As impressive as is the reciprocal relationships and mutual fitness between organisms and the environment, all that this can do for a biophysicist is to suggest purpose, without even being able to hint a why[67]. Since there is no satisfying answer to these questions (as to the purpose of life and the Universe), reason to lead an ethical life has to be sought elsewhere.

A reasonable conclusion from present evidence is that mankind is a species of mammal that has evolved a brain with sufficient memory and selection in recall to permit conceptualization. This conceptualization is further modified (or colored) by an inherited emotional circuitry. This, then, is the basis for the phenomenon labeled the mind, an unexpected "side-effect" of the massive circuitry for memory, recall and emotion; truly a quantum leap from other species. Another result of the development of this massive brain is that we are able to communicate with one another more precisely through language. Memory and language permit the development of culture, with evidence that this too evolves according to laws resembling those of genetic evolution. We all inherit a mind, but it varies from person to person in its qualitative capability, perhaps by genetic chance on how it is put together, or how it is used (cultural chance). The result is we are all individuals. That all this will be fully substantiated empirically is the expression of my faith, and that of others[37,38].

Appreciation of the vast potential of the human mind makes it understandable that most people would believe there must be a more complicated purpose for life than the simple, biologic evolutionary one of preservation and propagation of the species. This is particularly true for those minds sufficiently elite to contemplate this question. Those who believe the purpose of life is in the experiences of the mind, either with knowledge or aesthetically or religiously, are looking only into their own minds and concluding that life's purpose must be that which yields their talented minds satisfaction. The disparity in their conclusions, that they are only conjectural, and finally that the vast majority of people, who admittedly have minds (even if untalented ones), cannot participate in any of these so-called "higher purposes" of life - negate elitist opinions on life's purpose. It may be said the elitists suffer from "false consciousness", a term applied in the past, by Marxists, to lesser people.

It does seem, then, the only certain conclusion that can be drawn is that the object of life is life itself: for its maintenance and survival, and to assure its propagation. The creation of the mind by the evolutionary process has provided *Homo sapiens* with a clear advantage for this purpose. Early in the evolution of *Homo* they began to live in groups (just as many other mammals), and this is an evolutionary advantage, an advantage that the development of the mind enhances. Thus, for the human species the purpose of life is to further the well-being of the entire group (which by now probably means the nation), if not necessarily for an individual. The adherence of all individuals to an ethical code, nevertheless, contributes to the well-being of the group and therein lies the evolutionary purpose for (and origin of) ethics.

The same evolutionary process has provided a diversity of minds - some scientifically talented, others especially capable artistically - all contributing to the welfare of their communities. Yet even if there is no other purpose for life than life itself, nature has given each individual of our species, talented or not, sentience and the ability to raise it to an exquisite level by reflection. The fact that mankind's sentience is "exquisite" makes utilitarianism, the maximization of happiness and the minimization of misery for the greatest numbers, in many if not most instances, particularly attractive for the well-being of society and consonant with the evolutionary purpose.

The evidence[36] is good that inherited circuitry in the *Homo sapiens* brain offers a basis for altruism and reciprocity, but culture undoubtedly provides the major impact on ethics. It also seems reasonable to assume culture develops according to laws similar to those of biologic evolution. If these premises could be accepted by philosophers, then there could be a reasonable consensus on the conclusion that the purpose of ethics is for the well-being of society and thus for its survival.

Williams[14, pages 47,48] has observed that it is clear to him that it is natural for mankind to live in societies and that: "The formation of ethical disposition is a natural process in human beings." He goes on to explain how these innate dispositions need to be educated and require "upbringing", this being the function of society's culture (an independent expression of the dual evolutionary theory?). Also Williams says: "It is natural to human beings to live by convention...We wish, consequently, to bring up children to share some of these ethical, as of other cultural, conceptions, and we see the process as good not just for us but for our children, both because it is part of our conception of their well-being...". Ethics, then, are not the result of God's will, nor of *a priori* moral imperatives, but based on the shared qualities of evolved human nature. This approach, in many ways, is the antithesis of "social Darwinism", but it is "evolutionary ethics" nevertheless.

It is even suggested that "ethical conduct" is good for business. The dean of the Wharton School of the University of Pennsylvania recently reports[68] that a study done in his school on the connection between ethics in the workplace and productivity concluded that negative ethical attitudes "can permeate the entire organization and result in increased labor costs, loss of good will, major losses due to theft and purposefully counterproductive behavior, and direct market share losses". Indeed, in an inquiry into the economics of medical practice[69] one conclusion reached was that the ethical practice of medicine has a positive economic value to society. Ethics, in any event, are to "grease" social functions and are of value in achieving the well-being of society.

It is true that evolutionary ethics is a consequentialist theory and thereby close to utilitarianism. However it differs from it in both origin and mode of operation. Evolutionary ethics originates from the inherited moral instincts and acquired cultural reactions of individuals; it is not the result of the thoughtful balancing of positive and negative factors for an action. It operates through what is good for the community as a whole and not necessarily through the accumulated happiness of individuals - indeed, it is probable that evolutionary ethics could dictate a course of action that would be to the detriment of some individuals.

From an evolutionary ethical standpoint it is understandable why philosophers have debated how society's welfare can best be achieved: whether by deontological rules, social contracts, utilitarian calculations, etc. The minds of all philosophers are the products of the same evolutionary biology and react to the same rule of cultural development. Therefore the ultimate objective of their varied ethical systems, arrived at by reflection in these similarly derived minds, must have been the same: the well-being of society. However, it could be expected that, in pursuing these varied systems, often conflicting details would be derived; such conflicts would arise from the lack of insight by deontologists, and utilitarians too, into the origin and purpose of their intuitions. That, indeed, is what has been attempted to be made clear in this chapter. As a pertinent example, it will be seen below (Chapter Three) that in a leading medical ethical controversy, the relationship between patient-autonomy and doctor-beneficence, ethicists can derive a formula in favor of the former on an *a priori* basis and without feeling a need for any empirical verification.

If it could be agreed intuitions arise through the evolutionary process (biologic and cultural) then it might be possible to unify the ethical systems previously propounded. Utilitarianism can be supported if the well-being of the group can be identified with the accumulated happiness of its individuals. Also, deontology can be construed to be correct, insofar as rules for behavior that make for the well-being of society are the ones that cause men to have emotional response of good feeling or satisfaction and are the basis of intuitive rightness. The connection between utilitarianism and deontology had been pointed out by J.S. Mill[22] who stated: "The principle of utility, or as Bentham latterly called it, the greatest happiness principle, has had a large share in forming the moral doctrines even of those who most scornfully reject its authority...I might go even further, and say that to all *a priori* moralists...utilitarian arguments are indispensable". Mill also stated that in deciding between higher and lower qualities of pleasure one must refer to "innate human values".

In practice, medical ethicists when deliberating on dilemmas will often, and easily, permute their reasoning so as to bring their conclusions into accord, whether they be deontologists or utilitarians. For example, R. D. Redmon[70] considered the questions of whether children may be used as subjects in medical research which is not intended to benefit the individual child subjects. He did so from a deontological perspective based on Kant's categorical imperative: act so as to treat humanity, whether in your own person, or in that of another, always as an end and never as a means only. Some authors have argued from this injunction that research should not be undertaken on humans incapable of giving consent, such as children, unless the research is intended to benefit each human involved. Redmon suggests if one can reasonably expect a child in later life to identify with the objects of the research, feeling that involvement in the research was a worthwhile activity, then non-therapeutic research on that child is permissible. It is likely that the child's parents would identify with the research in a similar manner to the child in the future, so their consent may be taken as evidence of such identification. His conclusion about non-therapeutic research on children is therefore similar to the conclusion of a working group of the Institute of Medical Ethics on this subject using essentially an utilitarian argument[70].

Even a contemporary medical ethicist, who favors a social contract theory for ethics *a la* Rawls, in answer to the question "why should people agree to such a basic moral framework?": stated that it is a natural law to do so, like the laws of gravity and that "it is simply the way of the Universe..."[71]. This bioethicist apparently never heard of evolutionary ethics, at least he never mentions it, but his above quoted sentiment, nevertheless, best does conform with a purpose for life discerned to be that basic evolutionary principle: the maintenance and propagation of life itself through the well-being of the group.

An objection was made to deontology and utilitarianism, at the beginning of this chapter, because often they did not solve medical moral dilemmas. The inference might be taken that evolutionary ethics would accomplish such tasks. Unfortunately, it all too often cannot because, as was explained in the introduction, there are usually too many biologic and cultural variables to be able to predict, at any given moment, which will be crucial to attaining the target of optimality. Evolutionary ethics, however, does have a rational explanation for its lack of predictability, and at the same time spells out why extremists have a disruptive effect and aggravate tensions and delay solutions. Isaiah Berlin in a recent address, "On the Pursuit of the Ideal", reached a similar conclusion on fundamentalism of any origin, from a much different approach[72]: "The search for perfection does seem to me a recipe for bloodshed, no better even if it is demanded by the sincerest of idealists, the purest of heart.... To force people into the neat uniforms demanded by dogmatically believed-in schemes is almost always the road to inhumanity."

The dual evolutionary theory for the origin of ethics is a statement: what in our culture *eventually* survives, is what, for the welfare of the group, ought to survive. Such a statement can be attacked as Panglossian and therefore unreal. It is understandable that all the tragedies and injustices that have, and still, beset our world invalidate the statement: that what is, is what ought to be. It is the changing of "what is" to "what eventually is" that answers such criticism. An optimistic reading of history that describes the course of human affairs as erratic but nevertheless generally for the better over the very long run would confirm the is-ought statement as revised above. Unfortunately, for the reasons discussed in the introduction, optimal solutions for ethical dilemmas all too often are unpredictable. Nevertheless, it does seem anyone who firmly believes in evolution is an optimist. Lewis Thomas[73] stated it well: "If we like, we can sit tight, trusting nature for the best of possible worlds to come."

The thesis that ethics originates in nature and is passed on by heredity and culture is essentially the same as promulgated by the sociobiologists[41]. However, it differs, insofar as culture is relatively autonomous and independent of genetic evolution, and that the group and not the individual is the unit for the evolution of cultural characteristics, including ethics. Biologic evolution is concerned with the survival and propagation of species, cultural evolution has as its target the well-being of mankind's societies. The fact that culture development is postulated to follow laws similar to those of biologic evolution and to operate at the level of the group for the most part, may make the differences from the sociobiologic theory for ethics not always too obvious, but possibly more plausible to the community of moral philosophers.

5. Conclusions

A review of the history of moral philosophy, particularly in the last three hundred years, and the introduction of the concept of a dual evolutionary origin for biology and culture lead to the perception that ethics could, and probably does, have an evolutionary origin and purpose. Application of evolutionary ethics even permits a reconciliation of deontology and utilitarianism, particularly in the latter's generally most acceptable "rule" form. This is so because the reasoning of the proponents of both theories arose from their intuitions. Their intuitions can be viewed as derived from their inherited instincts and their cultural experiences, and so the goal of these high-minded philosophers had to be the well-being of society. It is difficult to conjecture why medical ethicists, when writing about ethical theories, completely ignore the possibility of an evolutionary purpose for ethics. Indeed, two bio-ethicists writing in 1990 stated: "Without the contribution of Kant's moral works, Mill's work, or Rawls' A Theory of Justice, modern ethics and medical ethics would simply not exist."[74]

The acceptance of the possibility, if not probability, of an evolutionary purpose for ethics demands that the doctor-patient relationship and the discussion of individual rights in the context of bioethical dilemmas be re-examined.

CHAPTER TWO. DUAL EVOLUTION:
ETHICS, THE LAW, RIGHTS

1. Ethics and the Law

Mankind lives in groups, a characteristic shared not only with other primates and some other mammals, but also birds in flocks, locusts in swarms, bees in hives and ants in hills. It is commonly agreed that this evolutionary development favors the welfare of the group and survival of the species. Human societies emerged from family groups: closely related individuals held together by their innate good feelings for other family members, a quality called altruism. This good feeling consists of a willingness to submerge, even sacrifice, one's interests on behalf of others. As groups of families expanded to form tribes, then ethnic groups, the altruism for the immediate family was extended, eventually to provide the basis for the concept of patriotism in nations. A major contribution of the sociobiologists has been to show that altruism is an inherited characteristic. In humans, in all probability, it is a circuit in the ontogenetic "old brain" that forms a template shaping the fabric of altruism as it exists in each individual - strong in some and more or less frayed in others - depending on a host of other factors. Such factors are the relative strengths of other inherited circuits for innate characteristics, and the influence of the environment on the strengths and interplay of these circuits.

In family groups and tribes, custom provided the moral code and was sufficient for cohesion and survival. With the development of larger political entities, laws needed to be promulgated for the same purpose as formerly served only by customs and ethical rules: to enable society to continue to exist - certainly an evolutionary objective. Consequently there is a close relationship between ethics and morality and the law, and a goodly portion of the latter is derived from the former. Laws can be legislated by the state, so-called statutory law, or delineated by judicial action and called case law.

Morality is concerned with the actions of individuals that are enforced by inner directives and re-enforced by individuals' knowledge of what will be approved or disapproved by others. In a sense, ethics operates in what can be called the private sphere. The law prescribes rules for action enforced by the collective power of a political entity, such as the state, and thus lies in the public domain.

Moral directives when given the re-enforcement of state power, are called natural laws. Experts in jurisprudence state that the natural law arises from "reason" discerning the basic inclination of human behavior[1]. If it can be agreed that the prime objective of behavior is the evolutionary one of survival and propagation of individuals (at the human level, achieved through that which is best for the welfare of their group) then the natural law can be said to have an evolutionary origin. The natural law must have universal approbation and cannot be the morality of only a segment of the population. Thus divorce is not recognized by the Catholic religion but it can be made unlawful only in countries where the overwhelming proportion of individuals are practicing Catholics (presently only Paraguay, San Marino, Ireland, Malta, The Philippines and Andorra). Even in predominantly Catholic countries as Italy, Spain and Argentina, divorce is legal.

Problems arise when a segment of the population with strong moral feelings, such as against abortion, try to impose these feelings on the entire population by attempting to convert their personal moral sentiments into laws. In other words, threat to societal organization arises when moral issues become transferred to the public sphere either prematurely or, perhaps, invalidly. The transfer from private to public spheres would be invalid if the transfer should never be attempted, as for instance in the case of a practice or belief whose morality was so confined to a particular region or group that it had no chance of becoming universal, even within the specific political entity involved.

The portion of the law not of natural derivation is enacted for administrative purposes, that is for the orderly conduct of society, i.e., a law stating on which side of the road one should drive a motorcar. Administrative law is generally created by legislation or by directive from an authorized portion of the state apparatus.

Judicial decisions which become law generally result from conflict in situations too complicated, or not of sufficient agreement within the polity, for legislative action. Perhaps the matter before the courts involves ethical principles that are universal in the community but not yet a matter of legislative action. In such instances, the solution of the conflict is easily reached by judges and juries. However if the conflict involves ethical issues not yet a matter of consensus, or perhaps never will be, a satisfying solution cannot be reached. In frustration, the partisans to such dilemmas repeatedly appeal to the courts and decisions are rendered on technical grounds, and convincing precedents for the issues in question are not established. Thus the issue of euthanasia when arising either in the aged or infirm or in malformed new-borns has been referred on repeated occasions to the courts. Also, if legislated law or directives of government agencies are unclear in certain situations or contradictory to legal or moral principles, the courts can be appealed to for interpretation or remedy.

It would seem legal judgments involve the kind of moral decisions that everyone is entitled to make. There is nothing to prevent judges from using only their own views in making their decisions, but at least matters can be argued in the open by lawyers prior to a decision. In the case of a jury trial it is presumed the jury will interpret the facts of a situation and the merits of the contending sides according to popular morals or customs.

Customs are often the basis of judicial decisions and indeed the British Common Law is largely of such derivation. "Customs are the prevalent beliefs and attitudes in a social group as to the rightness or wrongness of certain types of conduct... The expectation of each member of the group that the others will conduct themselves in accordance with previous practice...customs are conventions and give rise to claims having the same ethical basis that promises have"[2].

The law is cognizant of Kant's concern with the motivation or the intention of the individual as a criterion in assessing the rightness or wrongness of an act. It also distinguishes between "malice" and "good faith", "unknowingly" and "knowingly", etc., on the part of a perpetrator of an act. However the consequences of an act, evaluated in the best utilitarian manner, is thought to be of greater relevance to the specific content of the law[3].

In the last 100 years courts have tended more and more to insist that the content of legal rules be determined by their consequences, that is: How do they work? This is contrary to the previous tendency to rule simply on what appeared to be most obviously right or wrong with a particular type of conduct[3]. Dworkin,in his recent book[4], confirms the utilitarian bias of contemporary jurisprudence. His book, devoted principally to what he believes the law is and what it should be, recommends that judges should make their decisions according to principles that bind the community together. That is, the law should serve the welfare of society.

It would seem the experts in jurisprudence recognize the same basis for the origin of the law that was advocated for ethics in Chapter One: the evolutionary principle of what is good for society, and hence for individuals.

2. The Concept of Rights

A right is defined by the Oxford Dictionary as: "the standard of permitted and forbidden action within a certain sphere; law; a rule or canon; that which is consonant with equity or the light of nature; that which is morally just or due." Rights not only can be described by existing legal arrangements but also by demand, on moral grounds, that such arrangements should exist. Thus legal rights are conferred by political authority and enforced by the strength of government. They may be agitated for or against, but as legal questions they should not pose dilemmas in medical practice insofar as physicians have no alternative but to obey. Institutional rights are akin to legal rights promulgated by organizations, governmental or otherwise, and generally useful to its beneficiaries. Their acceptance is usually voluntary and they are rarely enforceable. Like legal rights, institutional rights can be created and abolished by the appropriate persons or groups of persons.

Moral rights are derived from the intrinsic entitlement of an individual as perceived by the entire community and are not subject to alteration by force. It is generally perceived to be right that an individual not be killed, enslaved, or dispossessed. Mill in his account of justice in *Utilitarianism* infers moral rights are those that are vital to human survival and well-being as opposed to, as an example, a right to beneficence, which is helpful to individuals but merely a matter of social expediency[5].

Individual rights to life and freedom, including the right not to be subjected to torture and the right to free expression, are often labeled human rights. The term "human right" is used to evoke greater emotional support than the terms individual right or civil right, etc., this despite the obvious speciesism involved that has been objected to by some. The term first appeared in the Preamble to the Declaration of the Rights of Man and of the Citizen promulgated by the French Revolution. Human rights as a term is thought to indicate universality insofar as they are possessed by every human being and are of such great importance[6]. Some now believe (as in the Western democracies) human rights primarily refer to the civil and political sphere; others (in Marxian-Leninist societies) believe they apply to the economic and social sphere; lastly in the Third (undeveloped) World some believe it is the collective right of groups on which human dignity depends and to which the term should apply[6].

There are positive rights: the right to benefits, such as medical care; and negative rights: the right of an individual not to be interfered with, as are the rights to life, liberty and property. A right might be negative and positive: the right to medical care can mean no interference by others between patient and doctor, or positively it means the right to be treated if ill. Rights in its various forms, because of their inherent relationship to morality, will arise in any discussion of medical ethics. Discussions of autonomy, beneficence, abortion and birth control, detection of communicable disease, surrogate parenthood, euthanasia, etc. all begin with, or shortly thereafter involve, a discussion of rights.

The concept of rights is of relatively recent origin. Actually it is a product of the Enlightenment and its development has paralleled the progressive liberalization of government, particularly in Britain and the United States, ever since the English Civil Wars. Moreover, "The Anglo-American liberal tradition has evolved, since the seventeenth century, in such a way as to view certain substantive characterizations of the terms in the relation, certain ways of talking about rights, as central and basic to moral and political philosophy."[7]

Shapiro in his recent book, *The Evolution of Rights in Liberal Theory*,[7] uses the word evolution in the sense of development or elaboration but, in certain contexts, he also infers its Darwinian connotation as well. He does believe the writers whose works he analyzes (Hobbes, Locke, Rawls, Nozick) generally report and elaborate on ideologies arising in society and do not create them. A Darwinian evolutionary approach to the origin of ethics, as discussed in Chapter One, would agree that such an interpretation of history is generally correct. However, it also might be deduced that Shapiro believes the writings of philosophers do contribute to the creation of individual rights that are legalized in the formation of subsequent political organizations. For instance, drafters of The Declaration of Independence and the Constitution of the United States and its Bill of Rights were undoubtedly influenced by John Locke's perception that personal freedom requires the private ownership of property as well as the rights to life and liberty, to work and enterprise, and to religious toleration.

Nevertheless, the crucial issue for the eventual survival of these governmental policies depend on whether the rights granted by law, work: providing for the increased well-being and advancement of society. Shapiro specifically mentions Darwinian evolution as a basis for his analysis: "A third reason for an historical approach derives from the fact of evolution. From an intellectual point of view (though not necessarily from an ideological one) the modern arguments can be thought of as lethal mutations of the earlier ones."[8] He is arguing that contemporary writers have fragmented an older tradition by appropriating parts of it and leaving behind crucial premises - and that does not work.

Nonetheless, it does appear that some contemporary political scientists are of the opinion that philosophers and/or political scientists by their reasoning create rights[9], or even invent forms of government[10].

What is the origin of the concept of rights? Considerations of this question from earlier times have concluded that rights are derived from the natural law which was thought to be either divinely inspired or intuitively known. While it is agreed that the concept of rights interplay with moral principles, the origin of the latter is far from settled, as previously indicated. Thus much of the discussion in Chapter One on ethical theory does apply to the discussion of the origin of rights.

Utilitarianism is proposed by some[11,12] as the basis for rights. Shapiro[7] points out[7, page 273] that rights-based theories of modern liberal ideology have always coexisted with powerful utilitarian commitments and "a history of utilitarianism could be written that would bring out its reciprocal dependence on the evolving language of individual rights... The nature of the term "right" is such that reference to the substance and purposes of rights is inevitably entailed by its use."

Those who dispute a utilitarian basis for rights particularly object to leaving such important concepts to trade-offs that would be at the mercy of utilitarian arithmetic. They assume that rights are basic principles of political organization that can be ascertained intuitively[13] or that participants in society theoretically agree to a mutually beneficial contract, which delineates their rights[14].

The close relationship between the concepts of individual rights and ethical principles would indicate that the origin of one should be related to the origin of the other. In Chapter One a line of reasoning was introduced that led to the conclusion that ethical principles originated on the evolutionary basis of what was propitious for the continuation and propagation of the species through survival of those principles which favored the welfare of society. In the same manner of reasoning the dual inheritance theory for biology and culture[15] can provide a plausible explanation for individual rights arising on a completely natural basis with the objective of favoring the welfare of society.

The definition and extent of individual rights are determined by the political organization of a society. History tells us that political changes, particularly over the last few centuries, have been more and more in favor of increasing the rights of the individual and this most obviously can be correlated with the success of the Western liberal democracies. Insofar as political changes can be counted as cultural ones and if culture is subject to evolutionary development then human history would seem to state that increasing rights for the individual are for the well- being of society. It is to be reiterated that cultural evolution, because it comprehends "inheritance" of acquired characteristics, can change far more rapidly than biologic evolution - and change within even one life-time.

The advance of civilization (particularly Western civilization) over the past millennium, and increasingly so over the past 300 years, appears to have accompanied the development of political forms of government favoring increasing rights to more and more individuals in society. If this relationship be accepted as true, and if cultural traits are governed by the evolutionary principle of survival of the fittest (or of those most beneficial for society) then the fear that the masses do not have sufficient genetic potential for democratic societies to "work" must be ill-founded.

This is an amazing conclusion! Heretofore it seemed plausible to favor the propagation of the elite (at least the intellectual one) on the basis that this small percentage of the population were the ones that created the success of societies and advanced civilization. Even if it is true that the elite are responsible for advances, it must be that the broadening of opportunity for development of the masses is what increases the number and quality of elite minds produced. In other words, *favoring the genetic pool of the entire population by increasing opportunity for all individuals is more effective in producing a greater number of elite minds than favoring just the elite portion of the population.* An increased number of elite minds is necessary for the continuing advance of civilization, particularly when it becomes dependent on high technology. This thesis is firm support for liberal political tenet of "equal opportunity". The elite of a community might yield a higher percentage of elite minds, but the masses (given "equal opportunity") will produce a greater number of elite minds, even if the percentage of their offsprings so endowed is smaller. The reasoning that "affirmative action" supports, or eventually leads to, "equal opportunity" is more remote, and therefore more debatable.

Australia provides an outstanding confirmation of these suggested relationships: "For much of the 200 years since it was first settled...the place was a sump into which Britain poured its undesirables.... Australia was settled by an 'excrementitious mass', projected as far out of sight as possible in an effort to rid Britain of its criminal class. Never before or since has so much filth been swept under such a distant carpet."[16] Despite this inauspicious beginning, Australia in a relatively short time has turned out well, a full partner in the great advances of Western civilization. "In terms of prosperity, democracy, contentment and tolerance, Australians today have few rivals."

Another mechanism that could be operative, if the dual evolutionary theory for biology and culture is correct, is that freedom for individuals in society gives more opportunity for asymmetric transmission of cultural traits of the elite[15]. That means it is more likely and profitable for individuals to imitate elite, non-parental, individuals than their genetic parents.

Kort[17] has presented the hypothesis that civil rights and liberties are the product of the evolution of behavior. In his view culture, and hence human behavior, is controlled by Darwinian evolution and Mendelian genetics. He states this is "in contrast to established conventional thinking in the humanities and social sciences - they (rights and liberties) *are not* the result of cultural development mistakenly conceived as being independent of biological foundations." This extreme approach, favoring a genetic basis as the sole determinant for culture, is one of the principle sources of contention between the sociobiologists and their biologic and philosophical critics. In Chapter One of this book the opinion also is expressed that this concept of total genetic control of culture is far-fetched. Moreover, since it is agreed that rights have an evolutionary origin, it is feared that Kort's approach will discredit it. Kort does recognize that placing culture totally under the control of the genes causes difficulty in explaining changes in human behavior over the past 30 thousand years, a period during which there has not been any significant human genetic or morphologic change. An approach that recognizes that cultural changes do conform to the familiar evolutionary purpose even if they are devoid of genetic control, ought to make the theory for an evolutionary origin of rights more widely acceptable.

On the basis that society and civilization are advanced by elite minds, many molecular biologists and sociobiologists have advocated eugenic programs which favor the minority of the elite in society, and thus their social views are generally conservative. However, if the overall greatest number of elite minds result from the political organization which increases the rights of the mass of society, then this so-called liberal point of view must be more correct. A further political conclusion that may be drawn from a theory for an evolutionary origin of rights is that if cultural evolution is allowed to proceed - that is, not terminated by the side-effects of technological advances which are occurring *parri-passu* - the political forms of government most beneficial for individual opportunity will be the ones to survive.

Such an approach provides a theoretical basis for those seeking equality of opportunity for women in society. Success of the feminist movement in this endeavor automatically would double the human pool for the recognition and use of capable and elite minds. It provides an "evolutionary" justification (despite the use of this term appearing to be paradoxical in this context) for women to gain control over their reproductive process through contraception and abortion. Control of their reproductive process enables women to maintain their other contributions to society, and be on a more equal footing with men in this regard. Also, the evolving of labor saving devices reduces the importance of the greater physical strength of men, as well as freeing women from many of the traditional toils of child-rearing and home-making.

J.S. Mill in his epochal treatise on the rights of women written in 1861 was unaware of the current broadened evolutionary concepts presented above, but nevertheless utilized them[18]. "Is there such a great superfluity of men fit for high duties, that society can afford to reject the services of any competent person? Are we so certain of always finding a man made to our hands for any duty or function of social importance which falls vacant, that we can lose nothing by putting a ban upon one half of mankind, and refusing beforehand to make their faculties available, however distinguished they might be?" Again[19]: "the addition to the amount of individual talent available for the conduct of human affairs, which certainly are not at present so abundantly provided in that respect that they can afford to dispense with one-half of what nature proffers;" Mill also expressed the awareness that equal opportunity for all segments of society widened the range of choice of individuals and had "the stimulating effect of greater competition on the exertions of the competitors" to the benefit of all.

A recent article by Piel[20] on the origin of the U.S. Constitution and its role in the success of this country offers additional evidence for an evolutionary origin of individual rights. It does so by supporting the direct relationship between the breadth of opportunity for all individuals and the number of elite minds a society will produce. Interesting questions are restated by Piel: "Why did the scientific-industrial revolution get underway only so recently, and in Western Europe? Why did it not start 2000 years ago in the high civilizations of the Mediterranean basin and Asia?" A.N.

Whitehead[21] previously answered that in primarily agricultural civilizations: "The normal structure of society was that of a comparatively affluent minority subsisting on the labors of a teeming population checked by starvation and other discomforts." He cited India and China as "instances of civilized societies which for a long period of their later history maintained themselves with arrested technology...". Cantor [22] stated: "Though Rome produced great statesmen, politicians, and lawyers, like other ancient world states it failed to undergo an industrial revolution....The availability of slave labor discouraged the invention of new machinery or industrial techniques. Thus it might be said the primary fault of the Roman economic system was that it was based on slave labor." Though the Greeks knew the principles of the steam engine, it was never put to industrial use, for the same reason.

These remarks do not indicate for certain it was a lack of elite minds that was the reason for not having an industrial revolution in previous civilizations. However Piel does observe that the political development of greater freedom for the many, starting in Europe in relatively modern times and reaching its greatest expression in the U.S. through its Constitution and Bill of Rights, provided the basis for scientific advance and the industrial revolution.

Conservative political philosophers have asserted that duties and obligations of individuals have priority over their "rights". They base this on their interpretation that the principles of authority, hierarchy, allegiance, law and tradition are historically self-justifying features of society[23]. Heretofore liberal political philosophers have appealed for support for individual rights and equality to the moral (*a priori*) obviousness of the correctness of their position[24]. The reasoning offered above for an evolutionary origin of individual rights offers a more satisfying explanation for the liberal position, by providing an underpinning for the demand for equal opportunity. It is interesting that Hobbes[25] assumed rights arose from nature - anything which is necessary to an individual's self-preservation. This, in a manner, foreshadowed a natural theory for rights based on their beneficial influence on the welfare of society with the preservation and propagation of the species.

A theory that rights depend upon what is good for the human species is obviously a consequentialist concept allied to utilitarianism. Mill did make the connection between individual freedom and the welfare and progress of society as a whole. He states in *On Liberty*[26]: "Where, not the person's own character, but the traditions or customs of other people are the rule of conduct, there is wanting one of the principal ingredients of human happiness, and quite the chief ingredient of individual and social progress." He goes on to compare Europe with China (in 1859) and points out that the organized form of the educational and political systems of China make their people alike while these systems in European nations had permitted the development of a diversity of individuals. This made "the European family of nations an improving, instead of a stationary portion of mankind" as in China[27].

From the above, one may truly wonder if J. S. Mill had known that the theory of biologic evolution was incontrovertible, whether he would not have suggested cultural traits also survive on the basis of their benefit to mankind, and that individual rights depend upon their benefit to society. Indeed. he possibly would have been more sanguine on the prospects for the European nations which he felt in 1859 were "advancing towards the Chinese ideal of making all people alike"[28]. He would have taken comfort, had he known it, from the evolutionary dictum: those traits survive which are most fit - applies to culture as well as biology.

Governments, too, are determined (eventually) by what is best for society. The legitimacy of government depends no longer on the ancestry of the monarch or on the approval of heaven or on the general will, but "simply on the attainment of an acceptable rate of economic wealth."[29] Present day industrial and affluent societies are not based on great wealth as such, but on the perpetual and sustained growth of wealth. Wrigley goes on to observe: "What had seemed inconceivable to (Adam) Smith and intolerable to Marx developed into an acceptable commonplace. National product could rise without apparent limit, and be so divided as to assure most men of rising real incomes."

Wrigley recognizes a distinction between the modernization and industrialization of European society and that the former preceded the latter. However he has difficulty in defining modernization and, as he uses the term, it does little more than label the changes that occurred in European society between the 16th and 19th centuries. The biggest social change that occurred in this period was the development of individual rights broadening the opportunity of more and more of the population for development and this, probably, was the "modernization" that provided the basis for technological advances that resulted in industrialization.

Modern developments in the economic programs of China and the Soviet Union ("glasnost" and "peristroika") seem to confirm Wrigley's observations. Might not such economic changes in these socialist states (made necessary to compete, now that war between the superpowers has been made suicidal for the leaders as well as deadly for the entire population) be labeled evolutionary ones?

Another inference that might be drawn from the theory presented is that cultural evolution progresses as a result of a marketplace of ideas, and is dependent on the transfer of information. Democracy permits wide opportunity for information transfer and thus provides a true marketplace for cultural evolution; dictatorships try to suppress information (increasingly difficult in the present world), and therefore in the long run cannot compete. Thus the Soviets have to have "glasnost" before they can have "perestroika". Information is to cultural evolution what mutations are to genetics! Moreover, with the recent increases in the ease and speed of informational transfer, it can be expected that cultural change throughout the world will rapidly increase. In instances of political and economic changes they will be evolutionary ones, since they will be for the benefit and welfare of a society as perceived by its members when comparing their standard of living to that of other societies.

While cultural evolution progresses more rapidly than biologic evolution, it still is not always so fast or so obvious that one can perceive which cultural traits are best for humanity and should be supported (to help the evolutionary process along). As an example, the Western democracies presently support as basic in the realm of human rights those that apply to an individual's civil and political condition, while the Marxist-Leninist states look upon economic and social rights as fundamental[6]. Presently it cannot be predicted which attitude to the individual will prove to be more correct (or perhaps some combination of the two). According to the dual evolutionary theory presented above, it will be that system's attitude towards rights which is most beneficial to society that will thrive and survive. This, of course, providing society does not destroy itself, through the side-effects of technology, before the outcome is determinable.

Similarly, in other conflicts between rights - such as between the right to individual privacy and the right of communities to protect themselves by testing for drug usage or AIDS - the correct solution of the utilitarian equation involved most often has to await the accumulation of sufficient data. Prior to this, the evolutionary theory for rights cannot pick out for certain a proper course of action, no matter how vociferous are the opponents on the subject. If all this could be agreed to, it would be clear that the ancient recommendation of Aristotle for moderation is now more than ever in need of being observed by opposing factions. Aristotelian moderation in appraising the pros and cons of issues, together with a position that supports equal opportunity for all, might just be the best definition for the political concept of "liberalism", especially as opposed to "fundamentalism". The phylogenetic division of the human brain, as discussed in Chapter One, offers a biological explanation of the Aristotelian mean: it is the suitable constraint (or inhibition) of the emotional circuitry of the old brain by the evaluative new brain, the neocortex.

The predominant theme of Western political philosophy since the mid-seventeenth century (principally Anglo-American) has been a progressive liberalism with an emphasis on individual rights[7]. The principles of equality and personal liberty were affirmed in the formation of the United States and are described in initial American documents as "inalienable rights". Subsequently, inalienable rights have been defined as those that a person has no right to give up or trade away, nor that can be ruled against by law. The change in theoretical political discussions, in this period, from emphasis on duties and obligations of the individual to that of individual prerogatives and rights has carried over to bioethics. Modern discussions in medical ethics concentrate on the rights of patients, superseding physicians' beneficence, as a principal theme. Presently, the autonomy of the patient is the over-riding consideration in efforts to solve medical ethical dilemmas, replacing the Hippocratic tradition of physicians' duties (see Chapter Three).

Support for individual rights cannot be challenged morally or politically unless they conflict. The source of many current medical ethical dilemmas are conflicts in differing perceptions of rights and these conflicts often spill over to the political arena (abortion, etc.). If the evolutionary origin of rights is correct, one can be confident, over time, these conflicts in the perception of rights will be resolved in favor of those interpretations which are most favorable to the welfare of society.

3. Conclusions

In this chapter the position is established that individual rights too, as well as ethical principles, have an evolutionary origin based on what is in the best interests of the community. Current medical ethical dilemmas, in a large measure, are dominated by varying interpretations of the rights of patients, of the individual, and that of the entire community.

The correct solution of these dilemmas due to varying perception of rights most frequently must be delayed until adequate data is available and, most importantly, society must have time to evaluate the effect of the various possible solutions on its well-being (including its competitive position vis-a-vis other societies or nations). Some people, devoted to one or another position (extremists), cannot await the outcome and feel the need to impose their personal preference, even by force. The outcome of some of the conflicts may well have no crucial impact on the welfare of society and these will continue to be contested indefinitely or be settled by force, as by law (as is the question of divorce in overwhelmingly Catholic nations).

CHAPTER 3. BASES FOR MEDICAL ETHICS

1. Origin of Medical Ethics and the Doctor-Patient Relationship

The ability to reflect not only permitted humans to develop culture but also allowed them to contemplate their frailty, including illness and death. In all primitive societies these issues were joined with that of the mystery of the Universe and so the functions of the shamans included "medical practice" along with their religious role. Even in more advanced societies priestly practice most frequently included medical care. At some point these functions became separated and in many ancient civilizations it was felt desirable to verbalize a special ethic for medical practice. This long preceded enunciated moral codes for other specialists in society or the development of the concept of individual rights.

The Code Of Hammurabi (circa 2250 B.C.) touched on the ethics of physicians and the Hippocratic Oath was a product of the classical period of ancient Greece. The inscription on the Asklepion of the Acropolis states: "(The physician) should be like a God; savior equally of slaves, of paupers, of rich men, of princes; to all a brother, because we are all brothers." The ancient Hindu Oath reads: "You shall assist Brahmins, venerable persons, poor people, women, widows and orphans and anyone you meet on your rounds as if they were your relatives." The Chinese Code of Sun Ssumiao (200 B.C. - 200 A.D.) affirms: "Aristocrat or commoner, poor or rich, aged or young, beautiful or ugly, friend or enemy, native or foreigner, educated or uneducated, all are to be treated equally."[1]

The Hippocratic Oath, which most medical graduates are asked to repeat even today, contains three elements: first, a code of duties to patients; second, a covenant on obligations to teachers; and thirdly, the swearing of agreement to the first two parts by an oath to the Gods, specifically the Gods of healing. The duties of physicians toward their patients are that they must always act for their benefit according to their best judgment and ability, and more generally to keep patients from harm and injustice. Physicians must not assist patients in attempts at suicide or abortion, nor breach their confidence, nor perform acts of injustice or mischief toward patients or their household (including sexual misconduct). The covenant sets physicians' obligations to their teachers, their teachers' children and their own children. They are required to accept full responsibility for their teachers' personal and financial welfare and to transmit without fee their art and knowledge to their teachers' progeny and their own, and others who take the oath. The doctor-patient relationship according to the Hippocratic formula rests almost exclusively on the principle of physicians' beneficence to their patients.

The moral rules of the Hippocratic Oath have undergone considerable development and modification by the successive declarations of the World Medical Association from 1948 through 1983. These are elaborations on the essentials of the Oath, often in light of modern problems: on research; abortion (1983 revision of the Declaration of Geneva changed the clause: "maintain utmost respect for human life from the time of conception" to "utmost respect for human life from its beginning"); patients' rights (including "to die in dignity" and that "clinical interest lies not in the state of preservation of isolated cells but in the fate of the person"); torture; psychiatric ethics; transplantation.

Why the physician should have such verbalized moral commitments so early, is not entirely clear. Primitive communities did consider medical practice a sacred function, as indicated by its association with religious rites and priestly duties. When medical practice became separated from the priestly function the commitment of priests did not need to be verbalized or codified because the sacredness of their activity was always clear. Perhaps, however, it was felt necessary to remind physicians that their relationship to society also was a sacred one, since it was believed that their power too, was derived from the deities. Priests in their sacred position related to the entire community, physicians to the individual. This, then, well might be the origin of the very special doctor-patient relationship which has been the basis for most of the parameters of medical ethics ever since. Alterations in this relationship in recent years, and most notably in the U.S., inevitably has had a serious effect on the ethics of doctors.

Health was looked upon by all societies as an expression of harmony with the Universe: an aspect of an individual's well- being, effectiveness and luck. That which caused disease might also cause ill luck in hunting, or failure of the crops, or any other misfortune or natural calamity. The priest was looked to for the necessary rites to prevent or ameliorate all of these problems including disease. Later health of body and mind were separated out to become the responsibility of physicians, with little or no diminution in the sacredness of their function nor their relationship to the Gods. Restoration to health in primitive societies may require "bribing" the appropriate Gods with sacrifice or performance of specific acts. Anthropologists point out that a physician's right to treat often must be validated, perhaps by supernatural sanction or perhaps by payment. "Often the treatment itself is thought to be ineffective unless the patient makes some payment. This conception is quite prevalent, and may be important in ensuring the patient's faith in the treatment given by a physician."[2]

The emotional comfort concerned physicians can offer their patients remains an important part of their function and is not to be underestimated. Traditionally, individuals and families turned to their family physician for support at times of stress. Indeed, physicians participated with the clergy in this priestly activity and a discarding of this role in recent decades is part of the explanation for the contemporary decrease in respect for the profession. The clergy, untainted by the pursuit of financial reward, still continue in high regard and are viewed with respect, at least morally.

Another facet of the usefulness of physicians being held in high regard is that this is necessary in order for them to serve a proper role in recommending a proper lifestyle to their patients. It has been well expressed by Derek Bok, President of Harvard University, in his recommendations for changes in medical school pedagogy[3]: "Physicians have a special competence to discover risks that patients unwittingly run in their daily lives. They also have a special status and authority that can help them persuade individuals to alter their habits." Another university president, Steven Muller of Johns Hopkins[4], discussing the commercialization of medical schools and their hospitals states: "I detect and share a sense of loss among some members of medical school faculties. There is a sense that a physician is somehow meant to be more than a skilled medical craftsman; that medicine is, or should be, a learned profession, as opposed to a scientific, vastly demanding, and socially prestigious trade or craft; that the physician as a healer needs some unidentified dimension of social poise and human depth that goes beyond medical science." Another point of view in this regard is that with the diminished impact of religion in our civilization, practicing physicians have the opportunity to a "far greater priestly role than any of their predecessors"[5].

Despite scientific advances with the reduction of mortality rates, most of the time and efforts of physicians are devoted to improving the quality of life of their patients. In opting for change in our present mode of delivering medical care, it should not be in a direction that will diminish the regard of the public for doctors, but in the direction that will preserve it, so that patients may have the full benefit of their physicians' services and the community gain from the role doctors can play in rationing (see this chapter and Chapter Eleven).

Until the modern era physicians had but limited ability to affect the course of disease. Their use to society lay principally in giving moral support to their patients when threatened with illness (and to patients' families). No doubt a physician's greatest effectiveness was dealing with psychosomatic illness, which still is the basis of a goodly proportion of the complaints of present-day-patients. Therefore, up until the current era, the effectiveness of physicians rested almost completely upon their relationship to the individual. The doctor-patient relationship was cultivated by the strength of personality on the part of the physician and the faith placed in this relationship by the patient. Of course this gave great power to physicians and it was expected that patients would be protected by the ethics (beneficence) of the profession. Societies' early realization of this power of physicians in relation to their patients might be another reason for requiring, even in ancient time, that ethical codes for physicians be inscribed. Evidence of strict adherence to the ethical code by physicians no doubt advances their effectiveness by increasing their trustworthiness.

It is obvious that the doctor-patient relationships have deteriorated severely in the past several decades, especially in the

United States. This deterioration has occurred despite the accompanying scientific advances that have made it possible for doctors to be therapeutically effective, practically for the first time. The great advances of the 19th and early 20th centuries in medical science, to the contrary, were expressed most clearly in the fields of public health and preventive medicine. The paradox of deterioration in the doctor-patient relationship during the period of rising scientific effectiveness of physicians is explainable as an unforeseen side-effect of several economic and political changes: changes that only were meant to broaden benefits to the masses of people in our society. It has also been claimed that practicing scientific medicine has dehumanized doctors: the great demands of having to keep abreast of scientific knowledge has made doctors behave like applied scientists. "The need to be factual divorces them from all considerations of value"[6].

The agony produced by the world-wide economic depression of the 1930's followed by World War II, a war more clearly fought for democratic principles than preceding wars, led to the liberalizing era (in political terms) from 1945 to 1970. In this period the rights of the individual were perceived to include equal access to health care. In order to achieve this, funding had to be provided. In the U.S. this was done by broadening voluntary insurance plans, principally Blue Cross and Blue Shield, and government funding of health care for the aged (Medicare) and the indigent (Medicaid). The worthwhile objective of these measures was diluted by the manner in which the providers of health care were paid: hospitals became essentially cost-plus operations and physicians were allowed to set their own fees. Overall health care became the single greatest industry in the U.S. and by 1988 consumed more than 11% of the gross national product.

Medical practice became the most remunerative of professions and many physicians were seduced by the system that made their large incomes possible. The making of money was generally not the main issue for doctors previously, but it has become the unbridled passion for some, reflecting poorly on the entire profession. Contributing to some physicians' abuse of the system was the divorcing of direct responsibility of the patient for payment for services rendered. When the patient personally pays the doctor most physicians are restrained from over-charging or from offering unnecessary services.

The obvious affluence of physicians has changed the attitude of the public towards them. The respect with which the profession had been viewed changed to resentment and condemnation. The fact that the system made it much more remunerative to be a specialist than a general practitioner furthers this effect. As a result there are more than twice as many specialists in the U.S. than general practitioners, a ratio that is the reverse of what exists in other countries, as for instance in Great Britain. Consequently, too few physicians are personal doctors, and available around the clock for consultation or home visits. This circumstance has been especially erosive of the doctor-patient relationship and of the public's respect for the profession. However, it should be pointed out that a more legitimate reason contributes to the reluctance of physicians to make home visits, namely the great technological advances in medical care that have occurred in recent decades. In previous eras no more could be done for patients seen in hospital emergency rooms or physicians' offices than could be accomplished at home; this is no longer true.

The new system of funding for medical care also has a deleterious influence on the doctor-patient relationship from the patient's circumstance. The substitution of indirect payment (via "third parties") for direct payment by the patient is thought by many to reduce the value of a physician's treatment. An anthropologist had observed that in many cultures direct payment for services was believed to be a necessary ingredient for a doctor's effectiveness[2]. Moreover the belief of patients that medical care is of no cost to them leads to their abuse of the system, by the frequency and extent of their demands. Even though the increased services requested are remunerative, the respect of physicians for such patients is inevitably diminished. On the other hand, resistance to unjust demands of patients frequently encourages conflict.

Yet another deleterious effect of a fee-for-service funding by insurance plans is the ability of third party payers to intrude into medical practice. For instance Medicare, in a cost containment effort, disallowed payment for visits to a woman terminally ill with cancer of the lung because the doctor was not contributing to her treatment[7]. That the doctor's visits were contributing to her comfort and peace of mind was of no interest to the anonymous Medicare employee.

In the distant past, patients depended on doctors to intervene with the Gods on their behalf. Despite the present emphasis on having informed consent before proceeding, doctors to be effective still need a patient's faith. Presently the scientific basis of medicine is so massive and intricate that no matter how much effort is made to inform, patients most frequently must rely on their doctors' judgment. This is not dissimilar to other professionals with such intricate and extensive knowledge that the laity must depend upon their faith in the professional's expertise and adherence to an ethical code, for assurance that they will receive proper professional service. A profession has previously been defined[8]: "Any profession is characterized by a monopoly in its chosen area of practical service on the basis of a defined and standardized body of intellectual knowledge and expertise; considerable individual autonomy; altruism; esprit de corps." Altruism, which most moral philosophers look upon as the key ingredient of ethics, is thought to be innate in humans. Sociobiologists, in particular, believe this is so because it is a trait useful to social animals and thus is favored by the evolutionary process. Physician beneficence (v.i.), a principal requirement in their ethical code, is an expression of altruism and therefore can be looked upon as having a firm basis in human nature.

Some economists have erred recently in assuming that the doctor-patient relationship can be described in purely business terms. They do this to give substance to their objective of reducing the cost of medical care by introducing more competition among doctors and other providers. This recommendation of medical economists has found much favor in some government circles and among insurance executives. (And, in 1989, in Great Britain when the Government issued its "White Paper" on reform for the National Health Service - see this chapter below.) The publicity generated for this approach and actual changes introduced in the U.S. based on creation of more competition among doctors are other factors eroding the patient-physician relationship.

The effort of government to control costs by replacing the cost-plus system of reimbursing hospitals with pre-payment according to patients' diagnoses (the DRG: diagnosis related group, system), while probably accomplishing its objective, nevertheless, has caused a further deterioration of the doctor- patient relationship. The DRG system reimburses hospitals with the same amount, no matter how long or short the hospitalization. Consequently, hospital administrations in order to make a profit, or limit losses, place inordinate pressure on their physicians to shorten their patients' stay in hospitals. Patients frequently are discharged from hospitals long before they, or their families, believe they can be cared for at home and the frequency of early readmissions has markedly increased.

The corporate takeover of the delivery of physicians' services, reducing doctors to hired hands - medical proletarians, albeit highly paid - working for large medical enterprises, including hospitals and health maintenance organizations (HMO's), is becoming rampant in the U.S.[9] It is estimated that up to 90% of physicians will be employed by some corporate enterprise (for- or not-for-profit) by 1992. Thus the erosion of professional autonomy feared by physicians 35 years ago to be the result of government action (advancing socialism), actually now is occurring from corporate expansion (extending capitalism)! These physicians will work, most often, the usual business hours and this is an attraction for doctors to this type of employment; but there is much reduced continuity of care of one physician for one patient, as exists when physicians practice independently.

Staff physicians that now are employed full-time employees of academic medical centers, regarded by many as paradigms for medical care, all too readily delegate a large part of, if not the entire, responsibility for the care of their patients to their immature staffs of residents, fellows and interns, purportedly for the purpose of "enhancing the training program". The following of this example by doctors is another item that has a deleterious effect on the bonding between patients and physicians.

The obsession of the news media with medical practice increases the fears of the public and their demand for medical services. While increased information to the public on medical matters has a beneficial effect in many ways, it often does pose a strain on the patient-doctor relationship. Partial information, misinformation, misunderstood information or inapplicable information will reduce the authority of the physician and often cause the seeking of attention from multiple physicians (especially if insurance will pay for it).

While in many instances multiple opinions are justified (500,000 physicians in the U.S. cannot all be equally qualified or all be always correct) the overall benefit of encouraging this activity has to be weighed against the inevitable erosion of the patient-doctor relationship that results. The widespread publicity encouraging it (second opinion campaigns) causes patients to become distrustful of their doctors, far more often than a diagnosis or treatment initially offered is proven to be incorrect. Of course, the practice of physicians and surgeons maximizing their incomes by unnecessary treatments, which the system encourages, is the real object of the campaigns to require multiple medical opinions. Since second-opinion programs have not proven to be cost-effective in correcting this abuse, it would seem that it would be better to change the system[9].

Another effect of the increased attention of the media to medical matters is to raise the expectations of the public as to what medical care can do for them - thus placing a greater strain on their relations to physicians. This factor, aggravated by the aging of the population (increasing the symptoms of chronic and degenerative diseases), together with the commercialization of medical care are cited as important causes of the declining satisfaction of the public with their health care[10].

Whether erosion of doctor-patient relationships led to the increase in malpractice actions against physicians in the U.S., or vice-versa, is unimportant since clearly the situation now is that of a vicious circle. The result is that physicians find it difficult or impossible to accept responsibility for decisions in their care of patients, despite it being well known that patients in general want doctors to make decisions[11]. The widespread assault on the medical profession via malpractice actions is now placing physicians in an adversarial relationship with patients and weakening the sense of responsibility doctors have had for patients.

This "sense of responsibility" insofar as it invokes paternalism and is part of the concept of beneficence, has been further weakened in recent times by civil libertarians and medical ethicists in favor of the concept of patients' autonomy (v.i.). While probably total suppression of beneficence is not intended, nevertheless the traditional utilitarian model of the beneficent physician is being replaced by the deontological model of the autonomous patient. One medical ethicist[6] believes that the great advances in sciences and the liberalizing changes in social relationship make necessary the change in the proper model for the moral relationship between the professional and lay communities. He favors the contractual model with recognition of the patient's autonomy as a principal basis for the contract and thereby the obligation of the professional to keep promises, tell the truth and have respect for freedom and justice.

The efforts of medical ethicists to replace beneficence by patients' autonomy as the principal basis of the doctor-patient relationship is understandable to most physicians. However most physicians believe ethicists over-emphasize the rationality of the vast majority of patients, especially when ill. The ethicists demand for "informed consent" at all stages of the patient's care appears too difficult a standard to satisfy in the daily conduct of their practices[12,13,14].

The more the emphasis is placed on patients' autonomy and the greater the attack on physicians' beneficence as unwanted paternalism, the more inevitable is it that physicians' responsibility to the doctor-patient relationship should weaken. Indeed, reliance on patient autonomy as the keystone of medical ethics means that the doctor is excused from exercising moral judgment in treatment, since the patient has the final word anyway. It is not clear these trends to dissolution of the special doctor-patient relationship and reduced ethical responsibility of physicians are worthwhile for society, especially when consideration is given to the positive economic value of professional ethics and this added to the balance sheet (discussed below).

Other social scientists specializing in health care deprecate the value of the Hippocratic model of the doctor-patient relationship. Starr[15], in his book on the social transformation of American medicine, views negatively the dependence that patients have on their doctors and the high regard of the public for physicians, which reached its apogee in the United States during the first part of the twentieth century. He rightly points out that these were the elements through which the medical profession established its autonomy and physicians achieved societal privilege and power. His discussion of these aspects of the doctor-patient relationship is detailed: its historical development, sociologic origin and deleterious consequences. However, he does not mention, or is unaware of, any positive value that is derivative of patient dependence on, or their high regard for, physicians. The resented "power" and "monopoly status" of doctors are not recognized as the necessary attributes of any profession[16]. Specifically to eliminate a profession's monopoly and abridge its power in its area of expertise also will reduce or eliminate other characteristics always expected of a body of specialists by society[8]. In that event, the most certain attribute to be lost will be its professional ethics.

A recent empirical inquiry into the apparent discrepancy between medical decisions for individual patients and for groups confirmed the fact that physicians give more weight to the personal concerns of patients when considering them as individuals and more weight to general criteria of effectiveness when considering them as a group[16A]. "From the individual as compared with the aggregate perspective, physicians are more likely to order an additional test, expend time directly assessing a patient, avoid raising some troubling issues, and recommend a therapy with a high probability of success but the chance of an adverse outcome." As a consequence of this obvious beneficent behavior of doctors: "the discrepancy between the aggregate and individual perspectives may create tension between health policy makers and medical practitioners even when the pertinent facts are accepted by both."

It is common knowledge that most U.S. physicians, and certainly their organizations, resisted all schemes for private or public insurance that they perceived would come between them and their patients. Physicians believed that insurance plans, and government ones in particular, by controlling their fees would be a lever to eventual erosion of their autonomy. Autonomy has always been conceived to be a necessary ingredient for maintenance of a professional ethic, as pointed out above. It was also argued that "third parties" becoming the payers of physician's fees would come between doctors and patients and erode this relationship. In order to appease the medical profession and blunt their opposition, the drafters of insurance plans, including Medicare, agreed to pay physicians by a scale dependent on their "usual and customary charges" and the norms already in existence for their services in the various regions of the country.

The spread of these insurance plans provided physicians with guaranteed full fees for services to patients, many of whom had been previously unable to afford them, particularly the elderly who were the sickest and, and at that time, the least affluent portion of the population. In the preceding era the less affluent portions of society

depended upon the ethics of the medical profession to provide them
with what medical care they received for reduced fees or in many
instances at no cost at all, albeit if this was through a hospital clinic.
The relief for the poor from dependence on charity for their medical
care, undoubtedly has been most important in improving this care
(for those eligible to have access to it), and as importantly, has
provided for maintenance of their dignity.

The evolving system of the delivery of medical care has already
gone a long way to erode the doctor-patient relationship. The
continued growth of corporations as providers of medical care is
likely. In this atmosphere, the non-profit hospitals are taking on the
character of the for-profit organizations: taking over or merging with
each other (horizontal expansion); expanding vertically (assuming
provider functions other than acute hospital service); and increasingly
are employing physicians[17]. The non-profit hospitals are taking
seriously the desire of many medical economists for more competition
between them, and their administrators are paying close attention to
"marketing". The atmosphere formerly created by their eleemosynary
purpose is now almost completely gone. Insofar as charity partakes
of altruism and altruism is the basic principle of ethics, that loss now
particularly is regrettable. As will be discussed below under autonomy
and beneficence, physicians' ethics are under siege from presumably
well-meaning, para-medical professionals (ethicists, sociologists,
economists, etc.) destroying the basis for physician altruism.

With further breakdown of the special relationship between
doctors and patients and private practice more and more replaced by
corporate delivery of medical care, the corporate ethos (maximize
profits) will certainly further displace medical ethics[18,19,20]. In the
climate of cost containment the result will be tiering of medical care
to an extent beyond any present conception. The wealthy and fully
insured patients will continue to have as much care as, and probably
more than, they need. The increasing number of uninsured (already,
in 1988, said to have exceeded 37 million Americans) plus the
under-insured, will have the quality of their care further impaired by
less and less medical ethics to protect them. Today, the deteriorating
quality of care (because of increasing financial constraints) for even
the insured individual is in the forefront of discussion.

Physicians in the U.S., despite their large incomes which are the
envy of doctors around the world, are an unhappy lot. This is the

result of all the factors mentioned above threatening their professional autonomy. In a manner, their affluence has defeated them: they now would like both, their large incomes and their autonomy. Professional autonomy and the societal respect it implies, of which everyone was aware in years past, often had been what attracted people to medical practice in the first place. Also, their large incomes has bred dissatisfaction among colleagues - surgeons earning far more than most non-surgeons, and some surgeons earning more than others. Moreover, they are assailed by para-medical personnel (economists, administrators, etc.) on items that have partial validity, sufficient to be intimidating and disuniting - as medical ethicists who rail on the subject of patient autonomy. These internal tensions prevent U.S. doctors from concentrating on what is their common complaint, their loss of professional autonomy. Add to all this the severe discommoding effect of malpractice suits and it is easy to appreciate the unhappiness of the American doctor. The point is that unhappy, perhaps unfulfilled, doctors more and more deprived of their professional autonomy cannot be looked to for maintenance of professional ethics.

An opposite situation in England might be confirmation for the arguments above. English physicians, despite lesser incomes in a system dominated by a National Health Service, are on the whole contented and appear to be more satisfied with their circumstance. They are more united in maintaining professional autonomy, and certainly the doctor-patient relationship is stronger, with their professional ethics better preserved. (However, see this chapter below, for efforts by the British Government to alter the workings of the NHS that could alter the doctor-patient relationship in the U.K.)

The heretofore open-ended reimbursement for providers in the insurance based system of the United States perpetuated a tendency to an over-supply of medical care for those insured. It is a system behaving as though medical resources and the ability to pay for them were infinite. It was realized by the early 1980's this was not so, and some form of rationing had to be inevitable[21,22]. Reinhardt pointed out that when national resources are recognized not to be unlimited, their allocation inevitably produces conflicts[23]. Any plan for allocation is a form of rationing and even a return to a complete marketplace economy in the delivery of medical care (as advocated by some medical economists) represents a form of rationing - depending upon the ability of the individual to pay for it.

In considering the problem of rationing it was recently concluded[24] that the U.S. must look to Great Britain for a probable solution. This was based on the fact that although there are differences between us, the "shared language and the common elements in our political and medical cultures" indicate we will react similarly to what is observed now in Britain when these necessary limits on the availability of medical care are set. The study centered on the use of several special technologies. The object was not to determine what was their proper use, but rather how their rationing were accomplished in the United Kingdom. It was found that physicians were aware of what was available, limited their indications for treatment accordingly, and for the most part accepted the limitations as to what their country could afford. The authors stated that the public was accepting of their doctors' decisions, "because of the respect that most patients have for physicians" and their "affection for the National Health Service". Unfortunately, the optimism of these authors, that what is being done abroad by physicians with regard to rationing can be done here, is unwarranted at the present time. It does point up the thesis that a high regard for physicians and the ethics of physicians, protecting the quality of their care for patients in their role of rationers, is of economic value to society. Unless our system is so altered as to restore medical ethics and the special doctor-patient relationship, the marketplace will impose rationing on the basis of financial considerations, rather than considerations of equity and quality of care for all citizens.

Some time ago the Economist, a British publication and a determined advocate of free enterprise and a marketplace economy, stated when discussing the nationalized health system: "Some kinds of public spending - most defense budgets for example - seem to involve great waste; others - like health - seems to achieve better value for money than their private counterparts." Isn't it probable the vital element in this difference between the value to the British government in their expenditures on defense and health is the difference between British physicians and munitions-makers? British physicians are motivated by a highly professional ethic protecting the quality of their "product" no matter what price they get for it and the munitions-makers are motivated only by the corporate ethos, which is profits regardless of quality.

In summary, the changes in the financing of the medical care system in recent decades has severely eroded the doctor-patient relationship. The ethics of the medical profession has deteriorated, and the effectiveness of doctors in many areas of medical practice dependent on the well-being of the doctor- patient relationship has suffered. Despite agreeing that the doctor-patient relationship has been severely eroded by the "transformation of American health care", authors nevertheless *call* upon physicians to exert their beneficence for "people who are ill and receiving care, those who are economically and socially disadvantaged and have limited access to care ...."[25]. The presumption is, one might surmise, that all that need be done is to make the *call*.

The question of what is the proper form of the doctor-patient relationship is constantly under discussion, at least in the United States, the United Kingdom and Western Europe. The matter may not always be specifically stated as such, but most of the principle topics of concern to medical ethicists fundamentally deal with parameters of this relationship. It is not of much concern elsewhere: the impression of those who have visited the socialist states of eastern Europe is that medical power and paternalism rule to a much greater extent than in the West. "Doctors made up their own minds and patients just had to accept the decision"[26].

A leading U.S. medical ethicist, in discussing models for the doctor-patient relationship, concluded that physicians' obligations are derived from the nature of medicine. Thus the physician's aim and the purpose of medicine should be the same: humanity and a love of mankind[27]. Another ethicist endorsed a contractual model for defining the doctor-patient relationship to be used for the analysis of medical ethics[28]. This model acknowledges the difference in decision making capacity between the well and knowledgeable doctor and the sick and relatively ignorant patient. However, both are free moral agents with the responsibility for medical decisions allocated to the doctor, and personal or moral value decisions affecting the life of the patient, to the patient.

Some would base the rights (or autonomy) of the patient above the doctor's opinion, declining to rely on the doctor's beneficence.

But this stress on the equal worth and dignity of every individual, powerful though it is, tends to immobilize the doctor. To treat everyone with equal consideration as prescribed by the Hippocratic Oath means a physician's help is tailored to the needs of his patients rather than to their demands or interests. A right, by definition is an *option*. To choose to exercise it is sometimes to defeat the very interest it is designed to protect. Doctors and patients treating each other with mutual respect (doctors too, are ends, not means) will get a better result than each standing on their rights. Basing medical ethics on patients' rights causes the doctor-patient relationship to be a static, even adversarial, affair, while the Hippocratic tradition by emphasizing beneficence and mutual respect creates a dynamic relationship. The former concentrates on preventing misbehavior of a small minority of doctors with deleterious effects for the vast majority of patients. Emphasis on the latter approach is aimed at increasing that majority of patients who could benefit from physicians' beneficence and a firm doctor-patient relationship.

Excessive malpractice actions provide another example of the undesirable consequences of over-emphasizing rights. Such litigations are based inevitably on the rights of patients and lead physicians to concentrate on practicing defensive medicine (some call it slot-machine practice). Surgeons avoid high-risk cases: a survey by the American College of Surgeons revealed that 40% did so, and 28% reported they were not performing certain procedures at all; obstetricians retire early (54% by age 55) and 45.4% avoid high-risk obstetrical cases[29]. Ethics dictated by jurisprudential considerations cannot be as good as an ethic based on doctors' humaneness and feelings of responsibility to their patients. There is no evidence that the pervasive climate of medical malpractice litigations in the U.S. has improved the quality of medical care. Indeed, for reasons noted above, the quality of medical care has been affected adversely, and certainly this includes its costs.

An important fact, brought out in the discussion above, is that professional ethics have an economic value to society. In other words, professional ethics protect society from being exploited by those with specialized skills and knowledge. The economic value of medical ethics is enhanced by the necessity for the containment of the costs of medical care and the need to ration it. No nation, not even the U.S., can afford the amount of medical care that can be demanded whenever the patient is not directly responsible for its cost. In the U.S. rationing is done by the marketplace technique of denying access to those who cannot pay for it: 37 million people in 1989 had no insurance, and many others were under-insured. In the U.K. there is universal access to medical care but the doctor, knowing what is available, limits its use; the government provides funding for the NHS, turning it over to doctors to expend it. The latter method of rationing is agreed to be more just and more humane, and it depends upon the professional ethics of the physicians.

If it be true that medical ethics depend upon the quality of the doctor-patient relationship and the professional autonomy of its practitioners, then governments should be careful that their plans for the delivery of medical care comprehend the preservation and even the bolstering of these items. So far, in the U.S., medical economists and medical ethicists have exerted their influence on politicians in the opposite direction.

Even though Great Britain expends less on health care than any other industrialized nation, about one half (as GNP) of that expended in the U.S., in early 1989 the British Government issued a White Paper on extensive plans to revise the NHS and the delivery of medical care in the U.K.[30]. Following the advice of an American medical economist, it favored increasing competition in the delivery of medical care as the means for cost containment and reducing queues (and in answer to the accusation that it was underfunding the NHS)[31]. This advice was being accepted even though this route in The U.S. already had proven deleterious to the quality of care, was reducing the caliber of the doctor-patient relationship and was not limiting its cost. The White Paper was in line with the Thatcher approach of promoting competition in business and privatization of public enterprises, and marked a continuation of recent efforts to replace administration of the British health delivery system, by management of the system.

To repeat, it was hoped by the British government that they could increase the efficiency of their health care system through the introduction of an "internal market" which would introduce competition among the medical providers. It was hoped this would overcome the deeply resented queuing. Also, the intention was to increase consumer choice; this despite it having been shown that patients are loathe to exercise choice[32]. The British Government, in view of their dependence on doctors to ration medical care (and thus contain its costs), should be careful that their new plans for medical care do not weaken the doctor-patient relationship. This is because a strong doctor-patient relationship is the *sine qua non* for doctors to be able to function in their capacity as rationers. Even a brief view of the doctor-patient relationship in the U.S., in a milieu of increased provider competition and consumer choice, should convince them to accept this advice.

A final point favoring physician-beneficence is that beneficence, insofar as it reflects altruism, is ingrained in human nature by the evolutionary process. There undoubtedly is a template for it in our brains that make it an automatic response, as when a person in an emergency, unhesitatingly, risks his or her life to save another. The quality of being aware of the personal autonomy of others is unlikely to have such a natural basis - it must be taught to individuals, and reiterated again and again, for people to apply such a principle. Therefore, it ought to be more dependable to base an ethical code, and the doctor-patient relationship, on beneficence rather than so impair it in favor of patient autonomy, as is presently the situation in the U.S.

An evolutionary approach to medical ethics is pragmatic and requires no hypothesis as to whether one principle rather than another should dominate the doctor-patient relationship. In this context, the special characteristics of the doctor-patient relationship arose because of their perceived need by society, over a long period of time. The needs of the situation should determine the proper mix of beneficence with autonomy and not the *a priori* pronouncement of ethicists.

The principle of patient autonomy gains its power from it being associated with rights for the individual, the moving force in the advances of Western democratic society. It is not necessarily correct that it be the dominant principle in every situation, especially if it is to be justified by the fallacy in reasoning by extrapolation or analogy (slippery-slope reasoning). That patients' autonomy had been neglected in many situations in the past cannot be denied. But, if at present it is being so emphasized as to diminish beneficence and thus yield a net poorer result in medical care, then we can be certain, over time, adjustments will be made.

There are situations around the world where the delivery of medical care is less costly and more equitable, and where the autonomy-beneficence balance is the reverse of what it is in the U.S., that can serve as paradigms for a change in the U.S. On the other hand, the solution of many medical ethical dilemmas may not be so crucial to the overall welfare of society for a change of direction in a specific situation to occur. Or else a final solution to a specific moral dilemma could take a very long time for evolutionary principles to exert their influence, depending upon their overall importance to the welfare of the community. Indeed it is one of the tenets of this book that the solutions of bioethical dilemmas cannot always be discerned at any given moment.

2. Rights and the Practice of Medicine

Rights, when discussed by medical ethicists in the context of the doctor-patient relationship almost always are applied to the patient. Perhaps this is in recognition of the relatively weaker position of the general public vis-a-vis professionals when an encounter takes place in the realm of the specialized knowledge of the latter. The rights concerned in the doctor-patient relationship are those of autonomy and informed consent, beneficence, non-maleficence, justice, confidentiality (or privacy), and the rights to medical care or to refuse treatment.

2.1 Autonomy and Beneficence

These are discussed together because consideration of the one almost always evokes the other. They appear frequently to conflict as already noted, a conflict which in itself poses a moral dilemma for medical practitioners.

Autonomy is defined[33]: "as the capacity to think, decide and act on the basis of such thought and decision freely and independently and without...let or hindrance." Autonomy thus comes under freedom, but it incorporates that specific attribute of mankind, rationality. This involves the concept of personhood: ascribed only to humans because of their ability to reason.

Insofar as the principle of autonomy prescribes the duty to respect persons, it is viewed as a deontological one, in accordance with the ethical theory of Kant. Some modern philosophers[34,35] believe the concept of a person as an autonomous agent must play a central role in any ethical theory. This concept in medical practice places an obligation on physicians to respect the values of patients and not let their own values influence decisions in treatment[36]. All of medical ethics may be viewed to exist to protect patients from ill treatment or exploitation. Imposing the duty on physicians to observe the autonomy of patients therefore can be viewed not only as an ideal philosophical principle, but also, pragmatically, as a mechanism for protection of patients from exploitation.

Observance of the autonomy of patients requires observance of the corollary principle of informed consent. Not only must the (simple) consent of a patient be obtained for a proposed mode of care, but complete information must be provided the patient so that the consent can be "informed". The information provided the patient should consist of the complications and expected results of the proposed treatment or procedure, as well as available alternative modes of care, or the possible results of no treatment. "Only if patients have complete information can they make intelligent decisions and their autonomy be properly recognized."

Beneficence is a principle that a physician is under obligation to do what is in the patient's best interest. Insofar as a duty is placed upon the physician to observe the patient's right to proper treatment, beneficence can be considered a part of the deontological view of ethics. However, since it involves a calculation of what is the patient's best interest, it is more generally considered to be derived from a consequentialist, or utilitarian, approach to ethical theory.

The ethics of medical practice traditionally have been based on beneficence as expressed in the Hippocratic Oath (q.v.). In recent decades this has come under attack by medical ethicists as really paternalism and a denial of the personhood of the patient. In their view the keystone in formulating the code of medical ethics has to be patient autonomy. This is based on the fact that no matter which theory for ethics is adopted, deontology or utilitarianism, respect for persons and their autonomy must be the basic premise. Deontology states that humans are rational individuals with wills of their own and as such are ends in themselves. This imposes the duty on physicians to respect the freedom of patients to make their own personal decisions just as physicians would wish their own freedom not to be compromised. ⁷⁄

Utilitarians also see a moral obligation to respect individual autonomy since it, as a political principle, increases opportunities for all and thus maximizes human welfare. Mill long ago stated that individual freedom, from which personal autonomy is derived, is a prerequisite for not only individual development and good, but also for societal good[37]. On the other hand Mill does condone paternalism in some circumstances[38]. He writes that unsophisticated persons often need to be governed as though they were children, but only after first having made "every effort to raise them up from this circumstance." He even endorses benign despotism if the population is in a barbarous state, since it would be in the best interests for all.

Autonomy as the overwhelming fundamental principle of medical ethics is so attractive because it is supported by the reasoning of Kant and Mill and conforms with the liberal political theory of the Western democracies[8]. However, this is *a priori* reasoning and need not be necessarily correct. Even if individual autonomy be a cardinal political principle it need not apply to every area of human endeavor, particularly the more specialized technical ones[39]. Medical ethicists ought to observe the verification principle of Ayer[40], and use empirical methods to substantiate their opinion that patient autonomy should be the pervasive over-riding tenet of medical ethics. For instance, it should be relatively easy for ethicists, now located full-time in medical institutions (in the U.S.), to place themselves in the clinics and offices of practicing physicians and collect data determining to what degree autonomy is possessed by patients and how much is it in their "vital interest". Perhaps the apparent aversion of medical ethicists to empirical observations is contributed to by most having obtained their preparatory training in philosophy. Many scientists have noted that contemporary philosophers avoid the collection of empirical data, preferring to use the reasoning ability of their, admittedly, powerful intellects.

The aversion of medical ethicists to empirical observations is clearly indicated in their failure to evaluate the effectiveness of their own ethics committees, even though they have functioned now for a number of years[41]. By 1988 only one such report of ethical problems had appeared[42]. This study was done in the general medicine teaching office practice operated by the division of general medicine of a university medical center. The question posed above, as to the degree of autonomy possessed by patients, was not specifically addressed. However, even the material they presented in their limited study indicated that fully a third of patients were devoid of the greatest part of their personal autonomy before they entered the doctor's office.

Fewer people would disagree that patients with psychiatric disturbances might well have their autonomy impaired, but even here there are professionals, the anti-psychiatrists, who dispute this (see Chapter Six). A study of 50 newly-hospitalized psychiatric patients to determine their competency to consent to voluntary admission found all had "severe impairment of competency"[43].

That autonomy often can be impaired by lack of sufficient rationality of individuals in specific situations has been repeatedly stated[12,13,14]. Hobbes went so far as to write that most men do not use their reason because reason is subordinate to the demands of the appetite and aversions[44]. He felt that reason was little used by most individuals in their "common life". Lindley[39] recently observed that autonomy was generally a matter of degree and was relative to our particular beliefs, desires and actions.

The necessity of rationality as a prerequisite for autonomy was given special significance in the discussion of the concept of "false consciousness"[45]. "False consciousness" is the failure of an individual to recognize the real motive forces by which he or she is impelled. Many, including the radical socialists, have stated that false consciousness was a characteristic of the masses of society. But, the principle of false consciousness also should dictate that healthy ethicists be aware, when looking into their own psyche for justification of their opinion that patient autonomy be the overwhelming principle of medical ethics, that they do not represent but a fraction of the individuals in any physician's practice. Perhaps the philosopher Berlin's reflection[46]: "I wish my life and decisions to depend on myself, not on external forces of any kind. I wish to be the instrument of my own, not of other men's, acts of will" applies very well to him and persons of his intellectual level but not to the masses of individuals, particularly when ill. Elitists could be confusing the issue of patient autonomy in the same way that distorts their contemplation of the purpose of life (see Chapter One), that is they identify their musings with the desires of the vast majority of people. How many healthy Berlins, or for that matter what percentage of people at the level of a healthy medical ethicist, are in the practice of most physicians?

Medical ethicists in their demand that respect for patients' autonomy be the over-riding principle in physicians' behavior write as though all patients have backgrounds equivalent to theirs[47]. Each patient's encounter with a doctor is taken to be the same as ethicists' own visits to physicians, and the resentment aroused in ethicists by such encounters is easily discerned in their writing. They believe the erosion of the doctor-patient relationship results from this resentment toward the overbearing, paternalistic attitude of doctors, and they believe that all patients possess this same resentment. Doctors fail to inform patients precisely of their condition or prevent them from participating in all decisions concerning their own treatment. No data is presented that ordinary patients have the same resentment to doctors as expressed by ethicists, and none of the other factors that affect the doctor-patient relationship are mentioned.

Perhaps a biological manner of regarding autonomy is to point out that it ought to reside in the activity in the circuitry of mankind's phylogenetically new brain, the cerebral neocortex. A characteristic conferred on humans by their cerebral cortices is their ability to contemplate and, to a greater or lesser degree, inhibit the emotional circuitry residing in their phylogenetically old (lower) brain. The less the activity of the cerebral cortex, for whatever reason, the less the autonomy of the individual.

The pervasive advance of liberalism in modern Western society with its emphasis on individual freedom unquestionably contributes to autonomy replacing beneficence as the fundamental basis of medical ethics. Western culture values highly the autonomy of persons because of its emphasis on freedom from authoritarian rule and the dislike of totalitarian practices.

Beneficence is translated to paternalism and this has become patently unacceptable to medical ethicists and indeed now when used by them it is most often in a pejorative sense. Paternalism is said to result from a lack of knowledge by the patient or a lack of communication skills on the part of the doctor[48]. Resentment of the perceived power of the medical profession in society[15] undoubtedly also contributes to the success in convincing the articulate of society that the medical profession needs to change the orientation of its ethics. Those who demand that the power of the marketplace be introduced into the delivery of medical care by increasing consumer choice should be aware that *patients* are loathe to exercise choice[32].

One physician perceived resuscitation of severely demented aged patients as harmful, and not do to so as an act of beneficence. However, to use this analysis permits not-to-resuscitate in such a situation to be criticized as paternalism, and therefore he suggested that to withhold resuscitation of such patients better should be described as compassion[49]. It seems that presently physicians cannot discuss paternalism with ethicists or educated laymen without a *mea culpa* on their lips. Indeed physicians can be trapped no matter what principle they use: an ethicist[50] within the same paragraph stated first and unequivocally: "the ultimate choice of treatment is the patient's" and then: "even if a patient would consent to an inferior treatment, it seems to me a violation of competent medical practice, and hence of ethics, to make the offer."!

Practicing physicians still encounter a conflict between the need to observe the autonomy of patients and their moral obligation of beneficence to their patients. Patients, incidentally, who also still expect beneficence to guide their physicians' conduct. Thus physicians attempt to justify paternalism if it contributes to the well-being of a patient, even if it overrides a person's autonomy[51]. Unfortunately, anecdotes all too often are used to justify positions in the controversy between paternalism and autonomy, as many on one side as the other. As explained elsewhere, it should be possible to collect data, and resolve this dispute. Data from another culture revealed that the overwhelming majority of physicians, obviously on the basis of their experience, voted against telling patients that they have cancer: 80% of Japanese doctors when polled in 1987 thought they should not so inform patients[52].

The conflict between a patient's autonomy and a doctor's beneficence most clearly arises when a patient refuses to accept a physician's advice. This can and does eventuate even if the physician has acted to the best of his ability to observe both the principle of autonomy and that of beneficence. In respect to the former, a careful presentation of the choices of treatment available, with the advantages and disadvantages of each, had been made: in other words, informed consent had been satisfied. The physician had satisfied his devotion to beneficence by indicating his preference among the available treatments by stressing the advantages of the medically preferred course and the disadvantages of the alternatives. Despite the time consumed in this presentation the patient chooses a course of action with the least advantages, or greatest disadvantages, or refuses any treatment. We have no data on how often this contingency arises but, in all probability, it is in direct relationship to the frequency of impaired personhood among patients in a doctor's practice.

A decreased ability to reason is recognized as an impairment to personhood and that this disability is increased in illness is recognized by medical ethicists. What data are available indicate that the frequency that impaired autonomy is encountered in medical practice is severely underestimated by ethicists[12,13,14]. Recent evidence of the abysmal lack of knowledge of even college level students and the frightening illiteracy of American students in general[53] should give pause to ethicists in their almost total abandonment of the Hippocratic beneficent tradition in favor of undiluted autonomy for *all* patients. Even academic physicians writing on the interplay in decision making - of scientific data with the interpretation of risk factors by individual patients - possibly can be misled[54]. Without data, they concluded impaired decision-making results from inability of physicians to communicate rather than from any impairment in the ability of patients to make judgments. Also, as late as November 1988 a behavioral scientist, dissatisfied with the achieved degree of observance of patients' autonomy, emphasized (without data) its linkage with the inability of doctors to communicate. The suggested remedy was that medical schools teach all doctors to be expert communicators[55].

While ethicists recommend determining what patients understand and expect and that physicians improve their ability to communicate, they never ask that it be determined what proportion of patients are neither desirous nor capable of exerting their autonomy; nor what damage might be done to some patients by insisting doctors "communicate" more and better so as to obtain complete informed consent. It is assumed by the authors cited, that informed consent based on patients' autonomy is the fundamental ethical principle guiding patient care, and the need for beneficence is nowhere mentioned - indeed it is condemned, as being merely paternalism.

{ The pragmatic physician evaluates the patient's ability to make a rational choice and according to the result tempers his or her degree of recognition of the patient's autonomy with beneficence.} Such a physician will always tell the truth to patients, but will make the all important distinction between brutal frankness and truthful reserve. Ethicists and sociologists interpret the making of this distinction as part of the "widespread tendency for doctors to deceive their patients". It is also not to be denied that the time required to obtain truly informed consent from "unsophisticated" patients is treated blithely by medical ethicists. It is not viewed by them as a compromise of practicing physicians' rights nor an imposition on other patients' time.

It would be thought that there would be general acceptance that severely disturbed psychiatric patients would have their personal autonomy markedly impaired, but even some professionals dispute this[56,57]. However, a thoughtful and experienced clinical psychiatrist examined this question carefully and concluded[58]: "For some ill persons the pure contractual model of the doctor-patient relationship can be employed when treatment decisions must be made. Given the inroads of illness on the effectiveness of this model however, it is likely that the assumption of an absolute autonomy which underlies it is more fictitious than real. Many more, probably most patients, whether medical or psychiatric, will want to be guided by a caring and understanding physician. Patients need to know, however, that their physician will also be prepared to accept the patient's choice even when the physician disagrees with it. But a minimal residue of psychiatric patients seriously ill with judgment-damaging disorders will remain. For these, on some occasions, the physician must take responsibility and bear the onus of deciding what is best for the patient." The use of the phrases "minimal residue" and "on some occasions" in the above quote indicates that even this psychiatrist is subconsciously making his concessions to civil libertarians and those in favor of an overwhelming patient-autonomy, no matter what.

Mill, in "On Liberty"[38], recognized that situations occur in which adult individuals require being taken care of by others. Even rational individuals are made vulnerable and childlike when ill - often physically weakened and frightened. To raise their morale, give confidence, encourage and protect them is paternalism. To abolish this in favor of only patients' autonomy is a sure way to add greatly to the sum total of human suffering, a point philosophers and lawyers are loathe to accept from their points of view. It is a grievous error to assume that the only cause of the failure of patients to exercise their autonomy to their own benefit, is when physicians fail to communicate properly[59].

Clinical research poses another serious conflict to physician investigators. They have to balance the barriers raised by ethicists in the name of proper and full observance of the autonomy of patients when asked for their informed consent to be used as subjects, against the abysmal state of medical knowledge if it were not for clinical trials (see Chapter Seven). The President's Commission for the Study of Ethical Problems in Medicine recommended in 1982 that informed consent remain flexible but nevertheless it "is ethically required of all health care practitioners in their relationship with all patients, not a luxury for a few." This was in answer to the suggestion that informed consent might only be suitable for, and applicable to well-educated, articulate, self-aware individuals. What was meant by flexible cannot be determined from the text, indeed the requirements for informed consent recommended appeared to be inflexible.

The sophistry indulged in by ethicists writing on this subject is illustrated by their suggestion on how informed consent should be obtained when thrombolytic therapy was to be evaluated in patients suffering with an acute heart attack[60]. Such patients need to be treated immediately in the home, or wherever the attack occurs, by paramedics called to the scene. They suggested a "two-step" consent procedure in which the paramedic "reads aloud a brief statement requesting consent to give a loading dose of 20 mg of t-PA only. The paramedic explains that more detailed information will be available when the patient arrives at the hospital and answers any question the patient may have.... If the patient consents, he or she is asked to sign a form...". It is seriously affirmed that a patient in such a crisis possesses sufficient autonomy to give "informed consent" and that the suggested procedure will protect the rights of subjects needed for research projects on emergency situations.

A recent incident illustrated how pervasive the concept of "informed consent" had become. A social-work investigator sent a fictitious article to scientific journals to test their bias. The results of this research were the latest in a series of studies casting doubt on the procedures and objectivity by which journal editors in various disciplines decide which scholarly articles to publish and which to reject. This investigator was faced with charges (in a hearing before the National Association of Social Workers) of being unethical because he conducted his study without the "informed consent" of the journal editors tested[61].

That some physicians' gross transgressions of patients' autonomy has, and does, frequently deserve severe criticism cannot be questioned. However that a minority of doctors misbehave should not be the basis for so belittling beneficence as to make it relatively inconsequential. The original motivation to embark on a medical career added to the educational and licensing requirements assures that, on average, the capabilities and moral standards of physicians will be far above those of the general public. It is manifestly incorrect to approach the doctor-patient relationship as do many ethicists: the patient elevated to the highest common denominator of the sparse elite, and all doctors depressed to the lowest denominator, that of the minority who behave poorly. A more empirical approach should be required before diminishing such a tool for the benefit of patients, as is physicians' beneficence.

The equating of physicians with patients in these discussions, especially the discussions of those advocating a contractual model for the doctor-patient relationship, overlook another item, namely, that the medical profession, from the viewpoint of intellectual ability and educational background, are a relatively homogeneous group as compared with the general public who are their patients.

In some instances of impaired autonomy it is agreed that a physician must proceed without hesitation in a manner that is in the best interests of the patient: as in an emergency, either when time does not permit obtaining proper informed consent or patients are so impaired that their consent is not possible. Other such instances when it is agreed beneficence should guide physicians' actions are: when patients' autonomies are severely impaired by illness or mental aberrations and their lives are in jeopardy and no competent relative is available to act as surrogate (even though there is no emergency in the matter). However, in the latter circumstance in the U.S. it is advisable as of 1989 to obtain consultants to agree in writing with an intended therapy, and to advise the hospital administration of the situation. Sometimes, it even might be wise to obtain a court order.

In the U.K. in 1989, the House of Lords made a final legal decision that allowed a physician to sterilize a severely handicapped 36 year old woman to prevent an unwanted pregnancy without her consent. This judgment, that applies to all types of treatment and not just sterilization, closed a gap in English law under which it was thought doctors could operate only in emergencies and no one, not even the courts, could give consent on behalf of an adult person unable to do so. The law lords confirmed that there is no power in English law for a substitute consent to be given. But they declared that the common law principle of necessity - which allows doctors to treat unconscious patients in casualty - stretches to allow treatment be given to patients unable to consent if the treatment or operation is in their best interests. It was made clear this treatment or operation would not have to be approved by the courts: "If every operation to be performed, or other treatment to be given, required the approval or sanction of the court the whole process of medical care for such patients would grind to a halt."

Instances where ethicists agree that physicians may proceed with treatment in the best interests of a patient who cannot give a fully informed consent are labeled acts of "weak paternalism". "Strong paternalism" consists of overriding the competent wishes and choices of the patient.

Does the principle of patient autonomy require a doctor to comply with the request of the patient for a specific test or treatment? This problem is discussed little, even by those most vocal on behalf of autonomy, although it was being increasingly encountered in the U.S. The problem was increasing because the news media had enhanced the exposure of the public to medical items, and it was a side-effect, of both the increasing emphasis on a patient's right to autonomy and the growth of prepaid insurance plans. The demands for antibiotics, x-rays and special, usually expensive, tests headed the list. An answer given, that the doctor had no obligation to comply with such demands, was too simple. The frequent circumstance of lack of absolute certainty that the demand was invalid (say, even only a 1 to 3% chance the demanded drug would be effective, or that the demanded test would be revealing); the possibility that the taking of the drug or a negative test result would be emotionally helpful to the patient; and the increasing ominous malpractice climate - all complicate the decision of doctors in these situations.

Then again, there is the recent case (reported in 1990) of a child severely impaired from birth, medically as well as neurologically[62]. At two years of age her doctors determined that her insensate state, except for pain, was irreversible and it was against their morality to continue to treat her recurrent pneumonia and sepsis. In the previous two years she had had four cardiopulmonary arrests, along with her recurrent pneumonias. The institutional ethics committee, other chiefs of services, primary care physicians, nurses and hospital counsel unanimously agreed with the position of the attending physicians. Nevertheless, the mother insisted every last possible treatment be administered. The child was stabilized without mechanical ventilation while the hospital staff sought a facility willing to treat the child, as the mother desired. In the meanwhile the mother appealed to the probate court. The judge was inclined to accede to the mother's wishes and asked the hospital and the physicians what they would do if he issued an order to resume mechanical ventilation, should it become necessary to preserve the life of the child. He was told that since the physicians and the hospital believed that it would violate their ethical obligation to the patient, they would refuse to comply with such an order. In the meanwhile, another physician and institution agreed to accept the child in transfer and comply with the mother's desire for whatever treatment necessary to keep the child alive. With the transfer of the child the legal dispute was rendered moot. Two years later the child remained blind, deaf, and quadriplegic and was fed through a gastrostomy. She averaged a seizure a day. Her pulmonary status had improved, but she continued to require intensive home nursing 16 hours a day. Her mental status remained that of a three-month-old infant.

While this case was an unprecedented challenge to the medical team and hospital: a parent's request for aggressive life-prolonging treatment that the staff believed to be futile and inhumane, the reporters of the case (an ethicist, a physician and an attorney) concluded that the primary obligation of health care providers remained "Do no harm."

In 1988 two ethicists, reacting to the emphatic primacy of patient-autonomy established by their colleagues between 1960 and 1980, made an effort to restore an appreciation of doctor-beneficence - but still got it wrong[63]. They recommend a commitment to "beneficence in trust" - a moral principle that allows the doctor and patient to act in each other's mutually negotiated and agreed-upon best interests. Each doctor must negotiate with each patient to act in the best interests of the patient, but within the limits imposed by the patient. That the attitude of these ethicists toward physicians still remained one of distrust was expressed in their doubt of doctors ever being able to ration medical care (detailed in Chapter Eleven).

Another ethicist, reviewing the above book advocating some restoration in the standing of doctor-beneficence, even implied that it had been physicians, not ethicists, who were responsible for the over-emphasis of patient autonomy at the expense of their own beneficence. He thus acknowledged, by implication, that patient autonomy was being over-emphasized[64].

A professor of religious studies and frequent contributor to the bio-ethical literature felt constrained in 1990 to list conditions that would permit overriding or infringing upon the principle of respect for autonomy[65]. These conditions (with each defined) were: Proportionality, Effectiveness, Last Resort and Least Infringement. Presumably a physician would have to have an ethicist at his elbow to sort these matters out, and even then patients presumably would be yielding their "first-order autonomy" (their own decisions on matters) to their "second-order autonomy" (voluntary selection of others to make decisions).

In the controversy on the roles of autonomy and beneficence in medical ethics, the observance of the Aristotelian mean is indicated: physicians need to raise their awareness of patients' autonomy and ethicists and social scientists need to reduce their attacks on beneficence. It should be recognized that elimination (or too great a reduction) of beneficence because it is paternalistic also weakens the doctor-patient relationship. The responsibility felt by physicians for patients is reduced or eliminated when the latter make all the decisions, with a consequent negative impact on the professional ethics of the former. It seems that younger doctors who have been led to believe that they have fulfilled their ethical duty as long as they observe patient autonomy, can act far less caringly in their practices and, in that sense, less "beneficently". Eliminating the need for beneficence by removing decision-making from doctors also impairs the autonomy of the medical profession, and professional autonomy is a requirement for the existence of a professional ethic[8]. Ethicists who view patient autonomy to be uncompromisable, as libertarians see civil rights, do not see that they can at times over-ride justice. Williams clearly states[66]: "The requirements of justice concern, in the first place, what ought to happen."

The theory, presented in Chapter Two, that rights depend upon what is beneficial for the welfare of society, establishes individual autonomy as a fundamental *political* tenet for a contemporary successful society. It is part of individual freedom leading toward equality of opportunity, so necessary for the furthering of civilization. However, it is doctrinaire to extend this observation to make the principle of individual autonomy an over-riding one in all areas of human activity. To do so in a specialized area such as health care, is particularly inapplicable.

Insofar as beneficence is within the concept of altruism, it partakes of the fundamental basis for ethical conduct. Sociobiologists have emphasized, convincingly, that many species, including mankind, have a biologically inherited template (probably sub-cortical) for altruism. Therefore, emphasis on beneficence (which already is part of human nature) to guide doctors' attitude toward patients can only strengthen all other aspects of their professional ethics. Denigration of physician beneficence in favor of patient autonomy (autonomy almost certainly is a cortically recognized principle, and in no way biologically inherited) well may weaken medical ethics, as we now are observing to be the situation.

A final reason to favor preservation of patient dependence on doctor-beneficence, to repeat (v.s. above, this chapter and Chapter Eleven), is its function in the rationing of medical care. It is acknowledged that it is to the advantage of society that all its individuals receive health care - and yet to its intolerable financial disadvantage for each individual to have as much of it as is desired and consumed, when not paid for directly (as when paid for by the state or through open-ended insurance). Consequently health care needs to be rationed[9]. Rationing to be just needs to be carried out by ethical physicians (see under rationing); and for medical ethics truly to be operative, it is required that there be beneficence of physicians for their patients. The extreme position of complete sanctity of patient autonomy at the expense of physician beneficence, demanded by some, is sure to be counter-productive to the doctor-patient relationship, deleterious to the ethics of the former and destructive of their ability to be the instrument for the rationing of medical care. All in all, it might be proper to lower the level of conflict between autonomy and beneficence to the matter of what is the best conduct for physicians in the practice of medicine. This is in recognition that physicians can be overbearing, and not all patients possess the necessary attributes for autonomy. There can be little question that some physicians and investigators require some constraint. This was thought, in the publication of the British Medical Association, to be best accomplished by the profession itself introducing a system for assessing professional competence and ethical standards[67]. Others would consider it only proper that patients have representation on such committees (that is, from the public at large).

Despite these theoretical considerations, deterioration of the doctor-patient relationship, and court decisions in the U.S. establishing patient autonomy and comprehensive informed consent as the law, have settled the conflict in a practical manner, at least for the time being. Any physician in the U.S., especially a surgeon, who favors beneficence over a patient's autonomy in any but the most obviously safe circumstance, does so at his or her own peril. In Britain the law, at the moment, leaves doctors to decide, in the context of their therapeutic relationships, how much information they ought to give patients when obtaining their consent to treatment[68]. The doctor-patient relationship also appears to have remained stronger in England than in the U.S.[9]

2.2 Non-Maleficence

This is a principle that physicians should have the duty to protect their patients from harm. It is a Hippocratic corollary to the principle of beneficence and this, together with its obviousness, makes little comment required. It is when non-maleficence is translated to mean *primum non nocere* - first, or above all, do no harm - and then put forward as a primary tenet of medical ethics, that particularly merits discussion.

This discussion is succinctly presented by Gillon[69] who quickly points out *primum non nocere* as a principal duty for the modern physician is fallacious. It is often necessary for physicians to take the risk of harming a patient in order to achieve an ultimate good result. If avoiding harm is to take precedence over the possibility of doing good, no powerful drug could be used or a major surgical procedure undertaken. There are few, if any, forms of therapy that have no possibility of resulting in more harm than good. The weighing of the odds of doing good against the chances of doing harm is the constant task of physicians in the treatment of patients. Only if such odds are so unfavorable, in consideration of the severity of the illness in question, must the principle of non-maleficence be invoked. This seems to be more a matter of scientific rather than moral judgment.

However Gillon does point out that a moral conflict can arise, as when the patient wishes to take greater risks of harm in pursuit of benefit, contrary to the physician's advise. Arguably, autonomy here should take precedence over non-maleficence, but this seemed far-fetched to Gillon. The patient could pursue treatment elsewhere: perhaps another physician would calculate the odds of harm versus benefit differently.

It must be admitted that in the U.S. all of the discussion on the primacy of patients' autonomy, and the increasing threat of malpractice, has made the above situation most frightening. The physician wishes to recognize such a patient's autonomy, but fears the consequences if all goes wrong, as he suspects it will, no matter how well he documents the case. Even the referral of such a patient elsewhere can backfire: an unhappy patient can always cause great distress by suits for delay in treatment, if nothing else. Even unjustified suits that never come to trial are traumatic and costly to physicians.

Another conflict of moral principles is possible, as when a patient with a contagious or infectious disease refuses identification and/or isolation, yet justice to others requires such "harm" to the patient in question. It would seem no matter how one reasons, either deontologically, consequentially or evolutionarily, justice would take precedence over non-maleficence. This is certainly clear with utilitarian or evolutionary ethical reasoning. Perhaps some extreme deontologist, like a civil libertarian, would consider breaking a patient's confidence or restricting a patient's freedom of movement more harmful than exposing others, unwittingly, to infection? This last conflict may well become the principal one in the current epidemic of the acquired immune deficiency syndrome (AIDS - see Chapter Four).

The moral principle for not doing harm to patients is applicable particularly to the designing of research projects. An ethical dilemma arises from the conflict of exposing some individuals to possible harm and the desire to acquire information for the benefit of all of society. Until recent decades this issue was resolved by the investigators and not always with full disclosure to the subjects, or even the truest calculation of the odds of potential good versus possible harm inflicted. In the contemporary period these practices no longer take place, or at least their occurrence has been reduced to a minimum. The advent of ethics committees for research, and awareness of the increase in exposure to malpractice suits has resulted in research designs being made with more ethical constraint and increased protection for human subjects.

Another view of non-maleficence arising in the course of clinical investigation was expressed by an out-standing English physician and his colleagues, noted for their studies of clinical trials in cancer therapy. In this instance they noted that the principle of non-maleficence conflicts with that of patient autonomy. They believe that therapeutic practice without clinical trials would be in an impossibly abysmal state. Therefore they recommended that, in certain instances - particularly multicentered randomized controlled trials, there should be a national ethics committee that can decide that "the principle of non-maleficence should over-ride that of autonomy". In other words, one should not have to risk upsetting patients for the sake of getting their consent to being used as research subjects[70].

Thus the principle of non-maleficence - not doing harm to one's patients - is a cardinal bioethical principle; while the principle of *primum non nocere* - avoiding even a possibility of doing harm as the consideration superseding all others - is not, in the present era. Veatch[71] made efforts to determine when *primum non nocere* first was enunciated. He decided it was not of ancient origin, but that it had come into vogue relatively recently, perhaps in the Nineteenth or early Twentieth century. Even at that late date it was probably a valid principle since virtually no treatment by a physician could offer even reasonably certain results. At that time it would be ever so much more important not to undertake treatment that possibly could harm the patient. It would have been a justified reaction against bleeding and purging. At a later time, it would have been well if *primum non nocere* had been observed in the procedures of lobotomy, and insulin or metrazole shock, in the treatment of dementia. One can look back only with horror at their own involvement in those tortures! It is interesting to speculate whether heightened ethical awareness and\or better scientific methodology (or neither) would have prevented such wide use of those abominable treatments of dementia, so rampant several decades ago. That those treatments are "abominable" is clear now; it was not so obvious then.

The principle of non-maleficence should compel physicians to be very circumspect about giving treatment without absolute knowledge of its efficacy versus possible harm. It ought to give pause to the use of not only new procedures that are remunerative but also to traditional techniques such as psychoanalysis, or even psychiatric counseling, until sufficient controlled data are available to determine their balance in doing good versus possible harm to patients. "Counseling" is widely, and glibly, recommended in a wide variety of circumstances. Even if no harm is done, and usually data are not available to verify this, it does have an economic cost and if valueless, it should not be done. As an example: it is well known that chronic illness in children causes an increase in emotional disorders, both for the children themselves and often as well as for their parents and siblings. Social-work support and counseling, when evaluated[72], failed to be of benefit in any direction, despite many previous recommendations that it always should be provided. Another example is the lack of value of psychological or psychiatric testimony in the courts, or even that it had a negative influence on the achieving of justice[73].

2.3 Justice

When conflicting claims arise concerning the rights of individuals, either in reference to each other or to the resources of the community, settlement is accomplished by resorting to the principles of justice. Justice is closely related to rights and ethics, and theories for each are sought in similar directions. The attitudes as to what constitutes standards of justice vary according to the political persuasion of the individuals who have proposed the various theories for the origin of this concept. Medical ethicists discuss these various theories *in extenso* and generally side with the theory that suits their personal political preference. Gillon[74], as usual, is most succinct in presenting the various theories of justice.

One theory is derived from a politically conservative approach and emphasizes respect for individual autonomy and, in particular, the right to own possessions[75]. The right to accumulation of possessions is to be protected as long as they are justly acquired: by appropriation of goods not previously possessed, by gift, or by exchange. One should be free to use one's natural endowments to acquire what one can. Possessions should not be taken from one by taxation, to be given to another. With this approach there is no innate right to medical care.

Another conservative approach is that individuals should be rewarded according to their merit. Gillon attributes this view to W. D. Ross and cites in support of this theory: "in all competitions winning is based on skill". Also, "society pays higher wages to the more skilled workmen". This theory of justice, for instance, recommends that physicians should triage patients in their treatment of the multiple injured or sick, according to the likelihood of their responding favorably and/or according to whether they are wage-earners as opposed to being unemployable, etc.

A politically moderate approach to a theory of justice would be a utilitarian one: people deserve to have their welfare maximized or, in other words, the greatest good for the greatest number. According to Gillon this requires an agreement on how to make such a calculation and having society (in view of the conflicting egos) accept the agreed-on calculation, if the latter ever were to be achieved.

A liberal approach is espoused by Rawls[34]. His theory states that all individuals have an equal right to freedom to choose for themselves, and a reasonable person would choose that deliberate inequalities be considered unjust unless they worked to the advantage of the least well off. This latter choice would be made by reasonable persons because at the onset of any situation they could not know into which category they eventually would fall (being "behind a veil of ignorance"). They therefore would opt for the strategy that would assure the least well off persons doing as well as possible, for fear they would be in that category. Justice on such a basis would require increased aid to those most burdened by illness, suffering and inordinate expenses. This theory of justice creates a right to medical care, and a right to affirmative action to repair previous wrongs due to conditions of servitude and/or prejudice.

A still different approach to the theory of justice is propounded by those who believe the ultimate proper form of government is a socialist one. This theory states that people deserve to have their needs met. The corollary to this principle is that all are required to give to the state according to their ability. This principle is believed to be workable because when the needs of each individual are met, individuals will rise up and overcome the contentious, competitive personalities they now possess - created by societies whose economies are based on the principle of competition. Socialists believe, obviously, that nurture is more important than nature. Marxist-Leninists believe that the freedom for the poor to pursue their own desires and freedom to make their own choices (civil rights) are compromised in capitalist societies. Individuals without their economic needs being met, and without rights to equality, find their civil liberties to be useless in obtaining justice.

The possibility that the concept of justice arises in human societies on an evolutionary basis, as proposed for ethics and rights in Chapters One and Two, is not mentioned by medical ethicists. If this possibility were true, it would dictate that the principles for justice be sought in what are the standards for this concept in our most successful communities. The problem of course is to determine which societies will extend their success into the future. (This is a restatement of: "what eventually is to survive in our culture, is what for the welfare of the group ought to survive".) Now, late in the Twentieth century, philosophers and political scientists have a long recorded history to assist them in this evaluation, a circumstance that was less and less available to the brilliant philosophers in the past, the longer ago they existed. Nevertheless, as pointed out in the introduction, the variables in many ethical dilemmas are so numerous that the principle of "chaos" all too often makes the correct solution impossible to predict.

Thus, an evolutionary theory for justice cannot, as yet, settle the debate on what should be all its principles, but hopefully it does channel the debate from attempts to create these principles to efforts to discover them. The most powerful (and in this sense most successful) societies at present have opposing ideologies. There is evidence that the differences in these ideologies are diminishing and perhaps a more agreed upon pattern for justice is within reach. This last statement appears to be obviously correct after the momentous events in eastern Europe in 1989 but, when first written in 1986, it then could only be a hopeful one. While an evolutionary origin for the principles of ethics, rights and justice can, to repeat, be attacked as Panglossian, all alternative approaches appear discouraging. An evolutionary theory would account for our common intuitions for justice and should make it easier for philosophers and political scientists to define the principles of justice for all of us. These undoubtedly would comprehend principles drawn from all other proposed theories described above, particularly those that appear to be universal in all societies and those that conform to the intuitions of the vast majority of rational persons.

2.4 Confidentiality

The right of patients to have their illnesses held in confidence has been recognized from time immemorial and is clearly stated in the ancient codes for the conduct of physicians (q.v.). This right may be looked upon as stemming from the right of an individual to autonomy: to be able to have personal control of one's thoughts, sentiments or emotions and secrets. A right to such privacy has been recognized legally not only for the patient-doctor relationship but perhaps even more bindingly for the relationship of an individual to a clergyman or attorney. Considering the ethical basis for confidentiality even more broadly, it may be viewed as the right of individuals to have promises made to them, kept. This is part of the long Hippocratic tradition of physicians: when patients consult physicians it is done with the assumption physicians promise not to disclose their secrets. Legally, it is looked upon as a contract implicitly having been made between the patient and the doctor, obliging physicians to keep promises and respect the personhood of their patients, a most satisfying Kantian construction.

The principle of confidentiality is helpful to physicians. It permits patients to seek help without stigmatizing themselves and thereby be free to confide more facts than they otherwise would. The more information available to physicians the better their basis for diagnosis and treatment. This provides a consequentialist basis for confidentiality. In fact ethicists when discussing exceptions to the confidentiality principle invariably recommend that utilitarian equations be set up for the conflicting ethical principles and that the solution of the equations will give the correct moral answer[76,77].

The law often dictates that confidentiality does not hold in instances when individual rights conflict with the interests of the community at large. Physicians are required to divulge communicable and venereal diseases, instances of child abuse, and gun shot and stab wounds to the health authorities. Likewise epilepsy is to be reported to the motor vehicle licensing authority in most states (but not, as yet, other potentially disabling conditions). Judicial decisions in several instances have mandated that psychotherapists have the duty to break confidentiality and warn the potential victim whom they believe might be harmed by a patient, and this applies even if the victim is the patient himself or herself. Nevertheless it is also generally held by the courts that a psychiatrist cannot be forced to testify, and can even be enjoined from testifying, against a patient on the grounds that the patient's revelations to the psychiatrist are privileged. The courts in the U.S. and in Britain have held that psychiatrists who become aware, in the course of a confidential relationship, of information indicating a danger to the public on the part of patients, have the duty to communicate the grounds for their concern to the responsible public authorities. Such physicians also are to be protected from suits based on such breaches of confidentiality.

In instances of dilemmas involving confidentiality for which there are no compelling laws, medical ethicists advise, *a priori*, that autonomy should outrank beneficence, but agree the public good should outweigh the obligation to respect individual desire or good. Presently testing for the AIDS virus and the use of illicit and/or addicting drugs are raising these issues and the solution is not yet clear. This will be elaborated upon in Chapters Four and Five.

An issue is made of who employs the physician. If the physician is employed by an insurance company (for medical examination), the state (as in prisons) or industrial firms for examination and treatment of employees, no confidentiality can be presumed by the patient. It may be suggested that the physician in such a situation should warn the applicant for insurance, the prisoner or the employee that the physician is not obligated to keep confidences. This could well impair the physician's ability to obtain the very information for which he or she is being paid to obtain. In practice, no such warnings are issued and it is expected that patients are aware of their exposure to lack of confidentiality in such situations.

Several factors most seriously affect the issue of confidentiality. First is the erosion of doctor-patient relationships generally. The economics of medical practice has markedly diminished the number of family physicians in the United States[9]. Presently, at the most, 12% of physicians in the U.S. regard themselves as family practitioners. Much of medical practice is, and increasingly so, via groups with little personal choice on the part of the patient or continuity of care of one individual by one physician. Confidentiality in such circumstances cannot be as firm a tenet as when there is a long standing one-on-one relationship between patients and primary physicians.

The second factor negatively affecting confidentiality is the increasingly pervasive role of third-party payers. Insurance companies and the government specify their right to review diagnoses and the information leading to the diagnoses and treatment of their beneficiaries. This is put into its clearest perspective in the practice of psychiatry.

Diagnoses in psychiatry are almost always subjective and have the least uniformity of criteria[78]. Opinions as to the amount of disability and the of duration of treatment required, likewise lack firm criteria and are subjective on the part of the psychiatric therapists. Consequently, almost all health policies do not permit, or severely limit, mental health benefits. Insurance carriers wish to reimburse patients only for treatment of diseases or accidental injury. They see their policies, at the most, covering mental disorders but not the problems of living such as foundering marriages, child rearing problems, or "finding the meaning of existence". Nevertheless the public, either as patients or relatives of patients, agitate for such coverage and psychiatric therapists, hoping to increase their incomes, also negotiate with insurance companies for such insurance for their patients[79]. In these circumstances both patients and physicians willingly compromise the principle of confidentiality. This matter has come before a court in a case of mental illness and payment for care by Medicaid. The court ruled that the patient's right to privacy could be invaded but not further than was necessary to protect the integrity of the Medicaid program[79].

Lastly, the widespread collections of data in computer networks have made maintenance of confidentiality more and more difficult. In 1977 the Supreme Court made a unanimous ruling that government had a right to keep a computerized record of the names and addresses of people who had obtained prescription drugs. The Court noted that they were not unaware of the threat to privacy implicit in the accumulation of vast amounts of personal information in computerized data banks. Therefore the right of government to collect and use such data for public purposes must be accompanied by the statutory or regulatory duty to avoid unwarranted disclosures. The supporters of computerized personal medical information cite the inclusion of confidentiality in the physicians' code of ethics as protection for patients[80].

Whether it is because of the factors mentioned above or an increased awareness of ethical issues in one's later years, it does seem that confidentiality presently is treated by physicians in a more cavalier fashion than formerly. We physicians seem to be willing to discuss patients in an identifiable manner in hospital hallways, elevators, waiting rooms and, particularly, in cafeterias. There was a time doctors had private eating facilities and this issue was not even considered when they were abandoned, long ago. Hospital records are available to an enormous number of, even non-medical, hospital employees. Referral slips pursue the hospital rounds with more and more details on them at the insistence of laboratory and radiology departments. Perhaps in the larger referral hospitals the medical records, even if exposed as detailed above, remain confidential because of the lack of familiarity between staff and patients and in the anonymity of large numbers; but certainly the medical records of smaller, local hospitals soon could become available to the entire community.

2.5 Patients' Right to Medical Care

The fact that *Homo sapiens* lives in groups requires that there be individual characteristics that make this possible. The principal such characteristic is altruism. Altruism dictates that the individual should not only desire to preserve his or her own life but also the lives of others. This desire to preserve the life of others comprehends having benevolence and compassion for others and thus it can be easily understood that altruism can extend beyond life-preservation of others, to their quality of life. This extension of altruism makes it readily understandable that the advancing concept of individual rights over the past three hundred years, together with the clear perception in the past 50-75 years that medical care is of value, have raised the concept of equality of access to medical care to the status of an individual right. A Presidential Commission on Health Needs of the Nation stated this as a principle in 1952, and another Presidential Commission for the Study of Ethical Problems in Medicine and in Biomedical and Behavioral Research reaffirmed it in 1982. Still, by 1989 there had not yet been established any legal basis for a right to health care[81].

Some in the U.S. believe that the way to assure all individuals access to health care is to establish such a right by an addition to the Constitutional Bill of Rights. Then the courts could force legislatures to appropriate funds for that purpose[82]. They do not understand that universal access to health care, without rationing, cannot be afforded by any government. The U.S. system of medical care utilizes the market place method of rationing (depriving a portion of its population access to care). Other countries which offer universal access to medical care (i.e. England and Canada) keep down costs by appropriation of funds that are then rationed according to professionally defined criteria (see rationing in this and other chapters).

Physicians agree that patients have a right to medical care and the right of equal access to that care. This attitude is in keeping with their Hippocratic indoctrination and tradition. Doctors and their organizations did oppose proposals for government financial support to assure implementation of these patients' rights, fearing that having to look to government for collection of their fees would impair their (the physicians') autonomy. Events have proven to them that their incomes increased enormously - with government paying for medical care at rates equivalent to what they usually charged, and in addition paying for patients who previously either were treated without recompense or not treated at all. This increase in income, without, as yet, undue intrusion into their autonomy, has allayed most of the fear doctors had 40 years ago.

Nevertheless, in 1989 there were still over 37 million Americans without financial resources for medical care and it was no longer the opposition of physicians or their organizations that prevents extension of government support for their care. It was the extent of the government indebtedness and the prevailing political attitude against further government expenditures that prevented implementation of the right to medical care for the entire population. In order to provide equal and adequate access to a national health system and have it affordable to an economy even as large as ours, the United States would have to adopt a health system analogous to the one in Canada or Great Britain[9]. Neither in Canada nor in Great Britain do the vast majority of doctors find their systems onerous.

The patients without financial resources for medical care in the U.S. either do not receive the medical care they require or do so from physicians and hospitals who are not compensated for their care. I am unaware of any statistics on the total extent of the costs of this care; hospitals do complain bitterly of the cost of the uncompensated care they deliver and make every effort to avoid it. As far as practicing physicians are concerned, it is my personal experience that their contribution to this uncompensated care may not be rare, but it is not continuous for any one patient, and by no means, is it usual. In years past it was an accepted, and in many instances a required, custom for doctors without compensation to staff clinics for patients unable to afford private care. It is true these clinics often served as a training ground for inexperienced physicians, but this ought not obscure the expression of the principle of beneficence involved. Despite the current assault on the Hippocratic tradition, this was another instance of there being much to say for it.

Failure to make medical care available to all is economically short-sighted as well as being immoral. It was said that nearly one third of mothers of babies born in the U.S. never had decent prenatal care, and many even never had seen a doctor. It is well documented that the incidence of premature birth is far higher in pregnant women without prenatal care. The expense of caring for premature infants is severely increased over term births, as is the expense of caring for the increased number of disabled children that are known to result from premature births.

2.6 Patients' Right-to-Know

The right of patients to full disclosure as exemplified by access to their own medical records has received recent emphasis. The problem for physicians has always been an ethical one. The issue to the physician in the Hippocratic (beneficent) tradition has been the patients' right-to-know versus what is good for the patient's peace of mind; in a sense it is the opposition of a legal consideration to an ethical one. Lately, the increasing possibilities of malpractice suits have severely tipped the balance in favor of the autonomy of patients, no matter what be the effect of full disclosure on them.

The disclosure of the diagnosis of multiple sclerosis is an excellent example of this ethical problem. Certainly when the diagnosis is definite the patient ought to be fully informed and they deserve to be informed by the most experienced physician participating in their care. The varied prognoses of their disease with the varied impacts on the course of their lives together with exactly how best to put this disclosure to the particular patient involved, probably requires as much or more knowledge than the purely medical aspects of the disease. However when the diagnosis is uncertain, as when a patient is seen with a single attack of retrobulbar neuritis and only possibly being the first symptom of multiple sclerosis, is every possibility to be discussed? Can a universal answer be given that will produce neither unnecessary alarm nor false reassurance? This is but one of the innumerable circumstances that arise in the normal course of medical practice that have been brought into particular focus by the movement for increased respect for autonomy as extended to full disclosure to patients of their own medical record.

Doctors state that if patients are given full access to their records (by law) then the nature of the records will change: "Physicians will be more circumspect in what they write and this will not benefit the patient and will impair communications between doctors. Tentative diagnoses and plans will be excluded as will be sensitive (and yet possibly vital) information as on sexual or financial problems. Frank and often useful descriptions of patient characteristics will be watered down and the 'thinking out loud' that is an important part of communication between doctors will be restricted to conversations and telephone calls - and so eventually forgotten. Operation notes will be censored to leave out descriptions of the parts of the operation that did not go smoothly, because all that the patient wants to know is that by the end everything was well."[83] This observer goes on to many further cogent points: medical students will be prohibited from writing in the record; the unnecessary alarm to patients and the necessary time to be consumed in alleviating such alarm; etc.

Beyond the argument that respect for autonomy requires that patients have access to their records, it has been suggested it would improve the functioning of the medical care system[84]. Among the problems in the medical care system, since its remarkable expansion following provision for increased access, are maintaining high quality care, ensuring continuity and avoiding excessive bureaucracy. It was proposed that legislation be passed requiring that a complete copy of the medical record, both inpatient and outpatient, be issued routinely and automatically to patients as soon as the services provided are recorded. Present-day practice is often by groups of physicians; consultation, particularly in hospitals, is more and more frequent; and the population has become increasingly mobile. Under these circumstances automatic issuing of the medical record to the patient would insure more continuity of care with more pointed consultations and treatment and avoidance of repetitive tests and patients needing to repeat the history of their illness, *ad nauseam*. It is true that should their records be made available to patients doctors will be more circumspect regarding what they put in them (as discussed above). This is a deficit that will have to be reconciled with the advantages, but it can be anticipated that the record won't be too starved by such a procedural change or else doctors will find other ways to communicate.

While legislation is being introduced mandating access of patients to their records, it is being done more for the purposes of insuring the patients' autonomy than with the intention of improving the functioning of the system. The intention of such laws is: "making patients equal to doctors and no longer subservient to their decisions" and, the adversarial objective of improving the assurance of patients that they have received adequate care and have not suffered from malpractice[85]. Framing the law to work for the purpose of improving the function of doctors in care of their patients could improve the ethics of the doctor-patient relationship. But to make the only purpose of giving patients their medical records a way to increase their adversarial posture can only have a deleterious effect on the doctor-patient relationship and further diminish the perceived need of physicians to maintain their ethical standards.

In England, the Department of Health in 1989 issued a non-statutory code of practice giving patients access to their own medical records. This was following a commitment made during parliamentary debate in 1987 when medical records were deleted from the Access to Personal Files Act. Patients' rights to see records were to apply only to information recorded after the code's starting date and were to be limited to a specified episode of treatment so as to inform patients about their health, "but for no other purpose." Health professionals could withhold information that was likely to cause serious risk of harm to the patient or that would identify another person.

In 1990, a survey of 1036 English general practitioners disclosed that 17% said they gave complete access to their records to all patients, varying in different health districts from 5 to 38%. The majority of GPs (65%) gave limited access to patient's records; for some the limitation applying just when the information might be harmful to the patient, or concerned third parties. Fifteen percent did not give access at all, by patients to their records. Again in 1990, 94% of 1050 men and women aged under 45 responding to a public opinion survey stated that they would want to be told the truth about a serious illness. Eighty percent of 100 male and female doctors of all ages said they would not tell the truth about an illness if the illness was terminal or they thought the patient could not cope with the information[86].

In summary, it is the avoidance of extreme positions again, even in the "patient's right to know", that will serve the community's interest best. Increased recognition of patients' right-to-know and increased access to records are not bad things, and good physicians don't mind. However, complete "leveling" with patients and their access to every last item in their records are not always in their best medical interests. Should increased access to their medical record be granted patients, beneficent doctors would find a way to exclude information harmful to the patient and yet communicate with each other. The present climate of distrust of physicians, at least in the U.S., has been fostered by attacks on all paternalistic practices and demands in favor of patient autonomy, no matter what the consequences. *Complete disclosure* is sponsored by ethicists and demanded by lawyers, and has already demonstrated its harmful effect on patients, and on their relationship to doctors.

3. Summary and Conclusions

The origin of medical ethics is traced, and in all societies the strength of the doctor-patient relationship was found to have been based on the beneficence of physicians. The factors causing a weakening of the doctor-patient relationship in the U.S. over the past several decades are reviewed. The principal ones were economic changes in the system of the delivery of medical care, and a moral philosophical change demanding that patient-autonomy take precedence over doctor-beneficence.

The second portion of this chapter is devoted to the various rights of patients and their influence on patient care. It is from this perspective, that the controversy between autonomy and beneficence is again discussed and the conclusion reached that there should be a restoration of previous dependence on doctor-beneficence as a, if not *the*, principal tenet for the ethical practice of medicine. Society would benefit if the focus of attention be returned to beneficence as the principal criterion in the evaluation of physicians' ethics; and for physicians to recognize, that for them to be thoroughly beneficent requires that they be constantly aware of the importance to individuals that their autonomy be observed - within the limits of their (the patients') capabilities and desires. From an evolutionary ethical point of view, the *a priori* pronouncements in favor of patient-autonomy over doctor-beneficence (which in recent years has been offered on a *prima facie* basis in discussion of bio-ethical dilemmas) can only be validated if proven to be to the benefit of the majority of patients, and for society as a whole.

With the scientific progress in medicine constantly introducing new techniques, patients face increasing possibilities of harm as well as benefits. This increases the responsibility of physicians in the modern era to calculate properly the solution of the equation - possible benefit versus possible damage - for each treatment, in order to observe the beneficent principle of protecting their patients from harm (non-maleficence). The impact of new epidemics (AIDS and drugs) most strikingly re-enforces an evolutionary ethical conclusion on the invalidity of the principle of *primum non nocere*: avoiding even the possibility of harm to one's patient above all other considerations, even at the expense of others.

The increasing costs of medical care require that society be protected from this burden by the proper allotment of that care. This factor, and the increasing complexities of medical care and of modern communities, add new meaning to patients' rights to justice, confidentiality, to medical-care and "to-know". Evolutionary ethics dictates that justice (particularly as it is concerned with access to the resources of the community), as well as the latter mentioned patient rights, are not absolute - but that the extent to which they will be observed will be governed by what is to the greatest advantage of society.

SUMMARY and CONCLUSIONS TO PART ONE

The first part of this book deals primarily with theoretical considerations. Both philosophical and biological arguments are offered in favor of an evolutionary basis for ethics. The recently introduced concept of a "dual evolutionary" origin of culture is particularly favorable for such a conclusion. It is suggested also, that the evolutionary approach furthers a reconciliation of utilitarianism with the deontological concept of ethics.

The rights of the individual and of society play important roles in bioethical discussions. It is contended that rights, too, arise from what is in the best interests and welfare of society, and therefore have an evolutionary purpose.

Finally, the origin of the doctor-patient relationship is traced and the factors affecting this relationship are presented and discussed. Evolutionary ethics dictates that there is validity to the restoration of a goodly measure of physician beneficence in the doctor-patient relationship, with physicians maintaining a proper regard for patients' autonomy. "Proper" refers to the true amount of autonomy each patient possesses in a particular circumstance, and as it relates to the physician's beneficent duty.

The balance between doctor-beneficence and patient-autonomy should be regulated by empirical studies, and not by *a priori* reasoning. In any event, cultural evolution is ongoing and, while patient-autonomy for the moment seems to have almost obliterated doctor-beneficence as a determinant of medical ethics, the present balance well might not persist into the future.

Traditional patients' rights (not to be harmed, to justice, confidentiality, to have medical care) are re-examined from an evolutionary ethical point of view.

PART TWO

A PHYSICIAN'S PERSPECTIVE ON PROBLEMS
IN MEDICAL ETHICS
(From an Evolutionary Ethical Point of View)

INTRODUCTION

The second part of this book deals with leading issues in contemporary biomedical ethics. The accent is upon empirical observations and/or pragmatic considerations, as opposed to the theoretical emphasis of Part One.

In Chapters Four through Six the principal considerations are the rights of the individual as opposed to those of the community as a whole. The establishment of policy for public health often requires the resolution of this dilemma. If the dilemma is not resolvable on the facts of the situation, then a choice must be made between the opposing principles: the public welfare as opposed to that of the individual. Presently, this specific moral discussion has been heightened by the appearance of new scourges of epidemic proportions - AIDS and drugs - and its intensity would have astounded previous generations. It is the current climate of increased concern with the rights of the individual, together with the severity of the epidemics, that accounts for the force of the controversy.

The discussion, on the right of the community to be protected as opposed to the right of an individual to privacy and protection from discrimination (for social and economic reasons), is all to the good when the effort is to arrive at a solution of a problem in which the data are incomplete. The promise of solution resides in the expectation that sufficient data will accumulate as the dimension of the problem unfolds.

Often a conflict even arises in a disagreement on how much individuals may be imposed upon to collect data. The forces delaying solutions reside in zealots taking an uncompromising position, *a priori*, and maintaining it regardless of the importance to accumulate data, or the import of any data accumulated.

Chapters Seven through Eleven, for the most part, are concerned with problems resulting from innovations created by the scientific advances of modern medicine. Very often it is the concept of rationing that is involved but, in any event, the objective is to analyze the problems from an evolutionary ethical approach. This implies, as explained in the introduction to Part One of this book, that it is not always possible to predict solutions at any given time. It does mean that dilemmas eventually will be settled in ways that prove to be best for society and that a factor which early does not appear to be too important often later, with the accumulation of experience, develops into being the determining one. Therefore, in many current problems (such as those created by new technology), since the correct solutions often are not apparent with certainty, all that can be done now, is to present their parameters and denote the adverse effects of extremists striving for premature and possibly incorrect answers. Thus this part of the book represents a relatively simple task for the author as, for instance, when compared with that of many biologic and social scientists who strive to make evolution a *predictive* science for denoting the behavioral traits of the individual.

CHAPTER FOUR
PUBLIC HEALTH POLICY AND RIGHTS (AIDS)

1. Introduction to the Problem

"Microbes...remain our competitors...for domination of the planet. The bacteria and viruses know nothing of national sovereignties. In that natural evolutionary competition, there is no guarantee that we will find ourselves the survivor."[1] This is the introduction in an article by Joshua Lederberg on the seriousness of viral epidemics such as AIDS and the need for intensified research not only on its virus, but also a systemic watch for new viruses before they become irrevocably lodged in the human race. He emphasizes that recombinant DNA technology (see Chapter Seven) "...still a scare word in some quarters, is our most potent means of analyzing viruses and developing vaccines."

AIDS is the acronym for the disease whose name is the *a*cquired *i*mmune *d*eficiency *s*yndrome. The term HIV refers to an individual who is not yet ill with AIDS but whose blood tests are positive for, and must be harboring, the *h*uman *i*mmunodeficiency *v*irus and can transmit it. From its very nature AIDS poses particular ethical dilemmas. In the first place those infected, outside Africa and Haiti, are principally homosexuals and drug users (a large proportion of whom are black or hispanic), already the objects of social prejudice and in need of protection as to their rights.

Secondly, the incubation period (interval between infection and onset of disease) is extraordinarily long, 4 to 15 years, and infected persons feel well and can transmit the disease all during this time. The most extensive survey, done on homosexual men in San Francisco and reported in 1989, determined the mean period of incubation to be 9.8 years. In this connection it should be remarked that there is also a delay in individuals between acquiring the virus and their blood tests revealing the presence of the infection (usually by the finding of antibodies to the virus). In most people this is a matter of at least several weeks (a median estimate is 2.1 months) and 90 to 95% of those infected will have positive blood tests within 5.8 months, but delays up to a year or more are possible. These latter delays can be explained by a finding that the virus can "hide" in some blood white cells, monocytes or macrophages, for these lengths of time without producing a detectable antibody response in the blood.

Thirdly, at least up to 1990, once the disease became manifest, it could not be prevented from being fatal. Data from New York City in 1987[2] indicated this last statement might have to be amended in the future. In this study of 5833 AIDS victims about a half had died within one year of diagnosis of the disease becoming active, but 15% had a chance of surviving at least 5 years. It would appear the ethnic background and/or the mode of transmission influenced length of survival. Black and hispanic intravenous drug users had the worst prognosis, surviving an average of less than a year. Gay white men whose primary symptom was Kaposi's sarcoma, and without other complications, lived over two years on average, and had a 30% chance of surviving 5 years. Therefore it may be too soon to say that AIDS is invariably fatal, although others, and the authors themselves, questioned the reliability of this data[3].

A fourth feature of AIDS, adding to the ethical dilemmas encountered in its control, is that although not contagious (*not* transmitted by casual contact) it is feared to be so by much of the public. It is communicated, actually, through sexual relations (largely heterosexual in Africa and Haiti and, so far, principally homosexual elsewhere), or directly into the bloodstream from the sharing of contaminated needles and syringes by drug addicts, or in relatively small numbers, from receiving transfusions of infected blood or blood products.

Lastly, the AIDS epidemic, so far (1989), has had a highly focal geographic nature. It was overwhelmingly present in large cities and, in the U.S., only five cities in five states (New York, New Jersey, California, Florida, Texas) had more than two thirds of all cases. Five other states (Vermont, Idaho, Montana, North and South Dakota) have had, as of 1989, fewer than 10 cases each. All this makes it politically difficult to mount the massiveness of national response the epidemic deserves. However, by 1988 an increasing proportion of cases reported in the U.S. were coming from smaller cities and rural area. Metropolitan statistical areas with populations less than or equal to 500,000 reported 10% of all cases before 1985, compared with 19% in 1988.

Since its identification in 1981, AIDS was estimated by 1987 to have about 200,000 known carriers in the U.S. and between 1,000,000 and 1,500,000 probable carriers. Most persons in the latter category were thought to be ignorant of their exposure to the AIDS virus. It was believed in 1987 that one in 30 men between the ages of 20 and 50 carried the AIDS virus, a shocking statistic even though this estimate varied widely[4]. Most surveys of homosexual and bisexual men found that by 1988 between 20% to 50% carried the AIDS virus, but the rate of new infections in this group had dropped remarkably since 1982[5]. Homosexual and bisexual men were said to constitute between 50% to 70% of AIDS victims in the U.S. and they accounted for 56% of the new cases reported during 1989. The rate of those with the AIDS virus among intravenous drug users was believed to be from 50% to 60% in the New York City area but lower elsewhere; overall in the U.S. they accounted for 30% of AIDS patients in 1989. Twenty percent to 60% of the sex partners of drug users carried the AIDS virus. Four percent of the infected heterosexual population were people with no risk factors other than heterosexual contacts. These estimated figures were not at all reliable, but any effort to obtain more dependable statistics were resisted by minority group advocates[6]. Late in 1989 the estimate for the numbers infected at that time (HIV positive) was lowered to between 700,000 to 1,310,000. The lowering of the number of estimated cases was due to a further slowing of spread of HIV among homosexual and bisexual men who were not illegal drug users, and the availability of new surveillance data.

It had been found that the rapid transmission of HIV in homosexual men had been strongly associated with anoreceptive intercourse with multiple partners. In one study, such men reported an average of 279 different sexual partners over a 5 year period, and a mean of 24 partners in the 6 months preceding the survey[7]. By contrast, anopenetrative intercourse was not associated with HIV infection. The remarkable drop in the number of new HIV infections among homosexuals, alluded to above, was accounted for, not only, by the use of condoms, but also by the changing of sexual habits with a reduction in the number of sexual partners and an avoidance of anoreceptive intercourse.

Homosexual activity has been reported among many other mammalian species, but in unusual circumstances and exclusive homosexual preference is a uniquely human phenomenon. The development of human homosexuality appears to be multifactorial, with early hormonal effects possibly contributing but being neither necessary nor necessarily sufficient in itself. The fact that human homosexuality occurs at a fairly constant rate (5-7%) in all societies studied, supports the view that exclusive homosexuality has a biological basis. It must be noted here that accurate data on homosexuality is extraordinarily difficult to obtain, and to be certain of the data collected[8]. Social factors are likely to be important and the available evidence, while not conclusive, is that homosexuality is more likely in those societies that strongly reinforce sex role stereotypes (i.e. machismo) with exploitation of women by men, rather than in those that condone the practice[9]. Therefore a society seeking to reduce homosexuality would be most likely to succeed by fostering sexual equality. Sexuality, in a large measure, is a function of the brain; the more complex the brain becomes in a species the more varied will be its behavioral patterns.

The extent of the prejudice against homosexuality in the U.S. can be illustrated by the successful attachment to the Health and Human Services Appropriations Bill for 1988 of an amendment stipulating that "none of the funds made available under this Act to the Center for Disease Control shall be used to provide AIDS education, information, or prevention materials and activities that promote or encourage, directly or indirectly, homosexual activities."[10] The amendment also stated that any materials funded by the government "shall emphasize abstinence from sexual activity outside a sexually monogamous marriage (including abstinence from homosexual activities)." This amendment passed the senate by a 94-2 vote, despite it giving support to the well-known ultra-conservative sponsor of the bill. Nonetheless, the homosexual community and their sympathizers had no hesitancy in sponsoring large demonstrations in Washington and London as well as in San Francisco and New York for more public spending on AIDS research and care, anti-discrimination laws and even for free AIDS drugs.

By April 13, 1989, 90,990 people suffering with AIDS had been reported in the U.S. (over 30,000 more than in the report of April 1988), and 58% of whom were already dead. Twenty percent of reported cases occurred in heterosexual IV drug abusers, and 4.4% were ascribed solely to heterosexual contact, with the majority having had sex partners who were IV drug addicts. Nine percent of all reported cases were in women (up from 7% of reported cases before 1985), with half believed to have acquired AIDS from sharing needles and 30% through heterosexual intercourse - in most instances with men who were drug users. By 1989, in all AIDS cases reported since the onset of the epidemic 21% were in IV-drug users, and 7% of such patients were both homosexual or bisexual males *and* IV-drug abusers. However, in the single year 1988 AIDS associated with intravenous-drug use accounted for 33.3% of the 32,311 cases reported in the U.S. It took from 1981 to 1987 for the first 50,000 cases of AIDS to be reported in the U.S.; the second 50,000 were reported between December 1987 and July 1989.

It was projected (1987) by the Center for Disease Control in Atlanta that more than 270,000 cases (range: 185,000 to 320,000) of symptomatic AIDS will have been diagnosed by 1991 and more than 140,000 will have died[11]. Three years later (1990), subsequent accumulated data confirmed this estimate as being a reasonable one[12]. AIDS was already by 1987 the leading cause of death in men ages 25 to 34, greater in this age group than the combined total of deaths due to traffic accidents, suicide, heart disease and cancer. The greatest variation in surveys of HIV infection was among IV drug addicts (0 to 70%), while surveys of homosexual men revealed infection rates of 20 to 50%[13]. Infection with HIV ranged from 0 to 2.6% in limited surveys of sexually transmitted disease clinics made up of heterosexual men and women without a history of IV drug abuse or known sexual contact with persons at increased risk. It was estimated that by the summer of 1988 more than 5000 women in the U.S. were suffering with AIDS. It was projected this number could increase to 30,000 by 1991[14].

By the summer of 1989 the forecast for the number of AIDS cases in the U.S. by the end of 1991 was raised to range between

300,000 and 480,000. The changing of this prediction in just a two year period and the inability to project more exact estimates reflected the problems in collecting data, to be elaborated upon below. As a matter of fact at the end of 1989 the estimated number of AIDS cases that will have occurred by 1993 in the U.S. was lowered by 15% from the 1987 estimate given above[15].

U.S. AIDS patients are disproportionately black (27%) and hispanic (15%), compared with the proportions of blacks (12%) and hispanics (6%) in the U.S. population. The proportion of AIDS cases in which the mode of HIV exposure was homosexual activity among men was lower for U.S. blacks and hispanics than for U.S. whites or Asians. These data reflected the higher proportional number of IV drug abusers in the black and hispanic minority populations[16]. However, there was evidence that blacks and hispanics were disproportionately susceptible to acquiring HIV infection and developing AIDS[17]. In the U.S., of the 13,008 drug users reported with AIDS as of August 1, 1988, 51% were black and 29% were hispanic, percentages that were disproportionately high, even considering that more of these minority groups were exposed to drug abuse. In a previous study (1985) the HIV infection rate in heterosexual drug addicts in San Francisco was two and a half times greater in blacks and hispanics than in whites. There was some correlation to the fact that racial minorities among IV addicts use cocaine, and share needles and syringes in "shooting galleries", disproportionately. However, from the data analyses, these items could not be the whole explanation. In more recent years, evidence from sexually-transmitted-disease clinics revealed that many who smoke cocaine in the form of crack were acquiring HIV in heterosexual transmission (mostly through ulcers caused by other venereal diseases). Crack, unlike heroin, causes an increase in libido which leads to more sexual activity with resulting increase in venereal diseases. Also, it was thought that young minority peoples, in particular, rush into commercial sex to raise money for their addiction to crack.

According to the World Health Organization (WHO) by January 1, 1989, 143 nations had reported nearly 133,000 cases of AIDS, 49,000 (37%) more than reported in March 1988, and the latter was double the number of cases that had been reported in March 1987.

It was estimated that there were at least one and a half times as many cases unreported, mostly in undeveloped countries. After the U.S., France reported the largest number of patients with AIDS - 3073 of a total of 10,177 in all of Europe by March 1988.

The WHO estimated that by 1987 there had been 150,000 cases of AIDS worldwide (less than half having been reported) and that by 1990 there would be, conservatively, a cumulative total of 1,000,000 cases. By the end of 1988 25,000 new cases of AIDS were expected in Europe. Most of the cases were occurring among homosexuals and intravenous drug users, but the proportion of cases acquired heterosexually in America, Europe and Australia had increased from 1% in the early 1980's to 4% in 1987. WHO estimated that up to 10 million persons worldwide were infected with HIV by the summer of 1988, and that another 1 million persons would become infected each year for the subsequent five years. By the year 2000, perhaps 50 to 100 million persons worldwide could be infected with the virus[18].

In the United Kingdom over 600 cases of symptomatic AIDS cases had been reported by December 1986, increasing to 2049 by the end of January 1989, with 1089 known deaths; 7007 persons were reported to be HIV positive (with 100,000 estimated to be unreported); the number of deaths from AIDS in the U.K. by 1990 was projected to be 5500, if the rate of increase noted in 1987 was maintained[19]. Since the mean age of death from AIDS was 35, the loss of potential working life for the British would total more than 165,000 years. Despite this data, and much advice to the contrary, the British Government's policy on testing for AIDS was announced in May 1988 as being unchanged from that of screening only blood donors. However, in November 1988 the British Secretary of State for Health announced the institution of a major program to anonymously test without consent for the prevalence of HIV in the population. Blood taken for other purposes was to be stripped of all identification and then tested for the presence of HIV.

AIDS was on the increase in central Africa, where it was believed to have originated. Five percent of the 2,000,000 people of the Congo were estimated to be infected with the AIDS virus by 1988, and it was projected that 100,000 Congolese, men and women, would die in the next decade[20]. A similar rate of infection in the U.S. would mean 12,000,000 American deaths in the next 10 years. Surveys in the capital cities of seven other central African countries disclosed similar infection rates (5%) as in the Congo. No segment of the population was escaping the epidemic, and transmission was confirmed to be principally heterosexual, and from mothers to newborn infants. Blood transfusions also accounted for large numbers of AIDS infections because they had not yet purged their banks of infected blood. Transfusions are widely used in central Africa to combat the anemia due to malaria (mostly done in children) and it was judged this was the number two source of AIDS infections there. Even in Zimbabwe, richer than central African nations and with a safe blood transfusion service since 1985, it was estimated in 1989 that one million persons (one-quarter of the adult population) were infected with HIV[21].

The World Health Organization said that by July 1988, 14,000 AIDS cases had been officially reported in Africa. It was estimated that this represented less than 10% of AIDS patients on that continent. This 90% rate of under-reporting in Africa should be compared with the estimated 20% of under-reporting in the U.S. By the end of 1988 African nations were improving in their reporting of AIDS cases.

Various reasons have been offered to explain the predominance of heterosexual transmission in sub-Saharan Africa and Haiti. High rates of sexual partner exchange and/or frequent exposure by men to a relatively small number of infected prostitutes (who constitute an important reservoir for HIV) were contributing factors. It was also suspected that the high rates of other sexually transmitted diseases as exists in Africa, particularly those with genital ulcerations such as syphilis and chancroid, were associated with increased risks of HIV transmission. The latter fact was thought to explain the predominance of heterosexual transmission of HIV in Africa as opposed to what was occurring in industrialized nations. Other possible contributing factors to the high rate of heterosexual transmission of HIV were the dearth of male circumcisions and the tendency to circumcise females in Africa. In the U.S. 85% of white males are circumcised.

The human immunodeficiency virus is the same in Central and East Africa and the rest of the world and is now labeled type 1 (HIV-1). A second such virus, HIV-2, was identified in West Africa in 1985 and antibodies to it were present in about 5% of that population. All evidence in 1988 indicated it was transmitted heterosexually, it too was pathogenic, and it was endemic in Gambia[22]. By 1989, seven cases of HIV-2 infection had been identified in the U.S., all in individuals who had originally been from West Africa.

The Pan-American Health Organization reported that by December 1988 9,453 cases of AIDS had been recorded in Latin America and 1,146 in the Caribbean. It was believed that the real number of cases was much higher and that half of the known victims had died. Brazil had the highest number of cases, 4,439, with there being 11 men to every woman reported. In the Dominican Republic and Haiti a third of all cases were women, but in Venezuela there was only one woman to every 30 men reported. There are very few I-V drug users in this region so that AIDS is, for all practical purposes, a wholly sexually transmitted disease. It was thought at least a half million people were HIV positive in Latin America and the Caribbean. Data, in early 1989, indicated that there was a potential for a massive AIDS epidemic in South America and the Caribbean that could parallel the situation in Africa, where many cases, too, remained unrecognized and unreported[23]. This ominous potential was possible because of the number of bisexual men found involved, in addition to IV drug users, spreading HIV heterosexually to females, especially prostitutes. While the total numbers were still below those reported in North America, the rate of increase in AIDS cases between 1986 and 1987 was 95% for South America and 113% in the Caribbean as compared with 40% for North America.

The incidence of AIDS in Asia had been lower than elsewhere, but in April 1988 the incidence of intravenous drug users in Bangkok testing positive to HIV was 16% but only 10 cases of AIDS had been reported. There are 100,000 such drug users in Bangkok and in 1987 only 1% had tested positive to HIV. By early 1989, the WHO reckoned there were 25,000 people HIV positive in Thailand, and if so, this would account for one half of HIV infection in all of Asia. With 5 million tourists a year (including thousands of U.S. sailors on shore leave) and a thriving sex trade, the Thai government discouraged public discussion of the problem. Only 1% of AIDS cases reported world-wide were from Asia and, other than in Thailand, most cases were said to be foreigners, or Asians infected elsewhere and who returned home. Still, in March 1990, 146 cases of AIDS were reported in Yunnan Province on China's southwest border resulting from the use of dirty drug needles. This shocked Chinese officials who previously had asserted that almost all AIDS cases had involved foreigners, and deflated their notion that Communist China had no AIDS problem and totally had overcome the drug one of the preceding era.

In 1990 the new director of the United Nations' Global Program on AIDS said that about half of the known HIV infections in 1985 were in developed countries, and mostly in the U.S. By 1990, two-thirds were in the less-developed countries and by 2000 three-quarters of HIV infections will have occurred in developing countries, including those in Asia. In the early years of the epidemic most cases were among homosexual men. By 1990, 60% of the infections world wide were believed to have been spread by heterosexual acts. That proportion was expected to increase to 80% by 2000. "The selective impact on young and middle-aged adults, who include business and government workers as well as members of social, economic and political elites, could lead to economic and even political destabilization in some developing countries," he said[24].

Drug addicts, as previously mentioned, comprised 30% of current AIDS victims in the U.S. in 1989 and, of these, blacks and hispanics formed the largest group, by far. It was said, in 1988, that there were 900,000 regular IV drug users in the U.S. and at least 200,000 more who occasionally used drugs intravenously. In New York City, 200,000 people injected themselves with heroin or cocaine at least once a week, and it was estimated at least half were infected with HIV. In one N.Y. methadone clinic 70% of the patients tested positively for HIV; infection rates in surveys of other cities with sizable drug- abusing populations ran from 2.9% (New Orleans) to 59% (Caguas, Puerto Rico). Once infection appears among IV drug users it spreads rapidly and it was predicted that where infection rates were currently low (1988), within two to three years, they would rival New York. Similar rapid spreads of HIV infection among users had been documented in Edinburgh and Milan. Drug users were aware of AIDS but the cost of using clean needles and syringes, and the ritual of "sharing" the habit, prevented educational programs from being effective[25].

Intravenous drug abusers constituted the major potential reservoir for transmission of HIV by heterosexual intercourse, outside of Africa and Haiti. 78% of pediatric AIDS cases were children of intravenous drug-abusing women or sex partners of drug abusers (other children acquired AIDS from blood products). It was estimated that by 1991 there would be over 10,000 infants and children with AIDS in the U.S. While the number of intravenous heroin users had stabilized and could decrease as use of cocaine replaced heroin, increased sexual activity accompanying the use of cocaine (with "crack houses" replacing "bath houses") would maintain, or even increase, the window through which AIDS could enter the heterosexual population[26]. It was believed a resurgence in the number of syphilis cases and other sexually transmitted diseases in certain areas could be explained on this basis. These sexually transmitted diseases cause genital ulcers which greatly increase the likelihood of transmitting HIV, especially heterosexually. In 1989, an increase in the number of syphilis cases had been documented to accompany all drug usage[27].

The taking of cocaine intravenously also had been spreading, so that the number of intravenous drug users was being maintained, despite the fall-off of the users of heroin. The duration of the effect of cocaine is shorter than that of heroin and consequently those using cocaine take many more injections per day than do heroin users, with their chances of spreading HIV being that much greater. Studies have shown that cocaine injection was more closely linked to HIV exposure than heroin injection[28]. As was to be expected, since drug abuse is greater among socially deprived, minority racial groups, heterosexual spread and transmission of HIV to children was found to be a more serious problem among blacks and hispanics.

A study in late 1987[29] revealed that the number of intravenous drug users dying from AIDS in 1982 through 1986 in New York City had been grossly under-reported. The investigation showed that 2520 AIDS-related deaths had not been included in the city's official register. Including these cases meant that the percentage of intravenous drug users in AIDS-related deaths was actually 53% of the total and that the AIDS epidemic was more rampant among drug users than had been believed. Previously it had been reported that drug users were only 31% of the total AIDS-related deaths. As a result of these new statistics it was stated that to control the epidemic it would be necessary to broaden the effort to control the spread of drug addiction. It would be insufficient to rely on educating drug addicts to use clean needles and syringes and condoms. The frightening aspect of this study, especially if found to be true for other communities, was that the "window" for heterosexual spread, which the drug addicts represent, was far larger than previously believed, and that the AIDS threat to the entire community was greater than had been feared.

Another possibility was that AIDS in drug addicts was more promptly fatal than in homosexuals, because their habit impaired their general health, and therefore their percentage of the total number of AIDS cases was as previously estimated. It was also possible that the racial minorities, who compose a large percentage of IV drug abusers, were less resistant to the AIDS virus. Further data over the years, or experimental testing programs for exposure to the AIDS virus are necessary to verify or disprove these conjectures.

An avenue for heterosexual spread in Europe was through the sizable numbers of European advisers and expatriates in Africa. In a voluntary testing program in Belgium 1.1% of 1401 Belgian advisers working in Africa and 0.9% of 4564 European expatriates living in Africa tested positive for HIV[30]. Of the 56 persons HIV-positive one third were women, none were IV drug users and only one was homosexual. Analysis of case data indicated transmission from women to men by vaginal intercourse seemed the most probable route for the infection. In Brazil and the Honduras it was reported that probably the activity of bisexual men, rather than that of intravenous drug users, was the principal transmission factor by which HIV was being introduced into the heterosexual population[31].

Prior to the introduction of tests for detecting infection (1985), individuals requiring transfusions of blood were exposed to the possibility of contracting AIDS. This was particularly true of people requiring frequent transfusions, such as hemophiliacs, or were transfused in areas where AIDS was rife. Approximately 2.5% of the cases of AIDS reported to the U. S. Centers for Disease Control were related to transfusions; an estimated 12,000 transfusion recipients in the U.S. had been infected with HIV before HIV-antibody testing of that nation's blood supply was begun in 1985. The blood supply in the U.S. is protected not only by testing for antibodies to HIV in all donated blood but also, since the blood test is only 99.9% accurate, by using a questionnaire to exclude as donors all those who could be identified as at particular risk to be HIV positive. Such risk prone individuals are homosexuals, I-V drug users and individuals from Haiti or sub-Saharan Africa. However, in 1990 because of protests that the latter query was racist in origin, a Food and Drug Administration Advisory Panel voted it be deleted. Should the questioning as to Haitian origin be omitted, the FDA estimated this could expose an estimated additional 36 patients a year to HIV as the result of a blood transfusion[32]. "Preventing discrimination is a high priority. Keeping the blood supply free of a deadly disease and insuring adequate supplies surely ranks even higher."?

Blood transfusions, thus, are another window for heterosexual spread of AIDS, albeit since 1985 almost infinitesimally small. Even in 1988 there was a very small chance, one in 40,000, of contracting HIV from a blood transfusion. This was due to individuals becoming donors who did not admit to an identifiable risk factor and/or harbored HIV before their blood was reactive[33]. No one needing a blood transfusion should be deprived of it because of this minute added risk, yet the circumspection always required prior to ordering a blood transfusion needed to be reinforced.

A single sexual contact can cause infection but seldom seemed to, particularly if it was heterosexual. However, there seemed to be a heterogeneity in heterosexual infectivity: some couples experienced a transmission after only a few contacts, whereas other women remained uninfected after many, even thousands, of exposures. This is a distinction from other sexually transmitted diseases. A study in Edinburgh[34] showed that of 123 subjects without any risk factor for HIV infection other than having had heterosexual intercourse with an infected person, only seven were found to be infected. However, in 41 regular partnerships (sex partners of IV drug abusers for more than 18 months) where the test statuses were known for both partners, there was a 15% rate of transmission.

The fear was that heterosexual transmission would increase in the West and the epidemic would become universal in the population. In the United States the proportion of women acquiring AIDS via heterosexual contact rose from 12% in 1982 to 26% in 1986 in the total of 1819 women with AIDS reported between 1981 and 1986[35]. In 1985, 1.7% of adult cases of AIDS reported to the Center for Disease Control were acquired through heterosexual contact, rising to 4% in 1987. It was projected by 1991 heterosexual transmission would account for at least 5% of adult cases (3700 patients). This estimate could be raised to 10% if patients born in areas outside the U.S. (where heterosexual transmission was predominant) and other patients in no identifiable risk group were to be added to the estimated total. Of all the women in New York City identified to have AIDS (1364), 60% were IV drug users and 22% were the sexual partners of drug users. The large number of pediatric cases in that city was also associated with IV drug use.

Statistics up to 1989 indicated that, in the West, heterosexual transmission of HIV was predominantly male to female, in the ratio of 3.5 to one. The data suggested that in industrial societies transmission was less efficient from female to male, than from men to women. A British reviewer concluded that: "The future of the heterosexual epidemic in Europe and the United States will depend on the rates of partner change in the heterosexual population. Thus we must collect information on sexual behavior in representative samples of the population; monitor behavior change in response to educational programs; and continue research on transmission. Since heterosexuals far outnumber male homosexuals, heterosexually acquired HIV may eventually account for a higher proportion of cases than at present.... Untempered optimism, such as delayed our public health response to the homosexual epidemic, should not colour our response to a potentially devastating epidemic."[36]

There really was no data by 1989 on sexual attitudes and actions. Epidemiologists, in evaluating heterosexual spread of HIV, had to rely on the Kinsey reports of 30 to 50 years before, and which were skewed by being collected from a limited segment of the population. Several more recent studies indicated that sexual practices among modern Americans were quite different from what the older surveys revealed. They suggested that an unexpectedly high percentage of American women regularly engaged in anal intercourse, and that an unexpected number of gay men and women had intercourse with members of the opposite sex. Such findings, if confirmed, could have a profound effect on estimates for spread of HIV among heterosexuals[37]. Both the U.S. Congress and the British Government in 1989 vetoed proposed studies on sexual behavior. The impetus for the survey in the U.S. was a 1987 recommendation of the National Academy of Sciences that it be done as an aid for devising strategies to deal with AIDS.

Whether or not the spread of AIDS into the heterosexual population is a real danger depends on the "basic reproductive rate": the average number of secondary infections produced by one infected subject in the early stages of an epidemic[38]. An infection will spread in a population only if this variable exceeds 1.0. For a sexually transmitted disease the basic reproductive rate depends on the product of three other variables; (a) the average duration of the infectiousness; (b) the average probability that the infection will be transmitted from an infected person to a susceptible partner (during each partnership); and (c) the effective average rate at which new partners are acquired. If the rate is just below one, the infection will continue to spill over into the heterosexual community but will not propagate widely. If it is just above one (even 1.1), the doubling time of the heterosexual epidemic during the early stages might be about 8-14 years. Thus, even with the present proportion of people infected with HIV being a fraction of 1%, the potential for a slowly developing, but eventually catastrophic, heterosexual epidemic would be possible. Little of the critical data necessary to truly evaluate the situation were available, as of early 1989.

2. Testing for HIV

Limited mandatory testing for exposure to the AIDS virus had been recommended in early 1987 by some public health officials who feared the disease was spreading into the general population unrecognized, because of its prolonged incubation period. Another fear was that education alone would not be sufficient to change life styles of the at-risk groups nor influence everyone to use protective measures (as condoms and spermicides), and control the spread of the epidemic. Nevertheless, control of the AIDS epidemic does depend, for the most part, on reducing the risk of transmission by modifying behavior, and therefore testing, at least select groups, is necessary to delineate epidemiological parameters. The problem was to persuade a representative sample of volunteers to cooperate in screening programs. Some recommended, as a first step, that testing for exposure to the AIDS virus be mandatory for all those entering hospitals or applying for marriage licenses. It was anticipated the resulting data would give better insight into the dimensions of the problem than previously available. Two states of the U.S., by late

1987, did have laws making testing for exposure to the AIDS virus mandatory for couples wishing to obtain marriage licenses.

In 1989 Illinois ended their law requiring premarital testing for HIV. In the one year it was in effect, 1988, only 26 of the 155,458 people tested were positive, a rate of about 1 in each 6500 persons tested (6 of the 26 positive results were estimated to be possibly falsely so). The cost ranged from $25 to $125 per test, averaging $35, and the cost of finding each of the 26 infected people was said to be $209,000, totaling $5.4 million. The costs of the tests had driven couples to neighboring states to marry, there being a 22% drop in marriages in Illinois during 1988. One law-maker, opposed repeal, stating the law was reassuring couples that they were not infected, and it was unlikely couples would demand the test of each other if the state did not. Also to repeal the law would give the message that Illinois no longer regarded AIDS as a serious problem. Louisiana, the only other state to have required premarital AIDS testing, repealed its law in early 1988, after an experience similar to that of Illinois.

In response to the call by some for routine, anonymous testing of all patients entering hospitals, in 1987, the Federal Centers for Disease Control issued guidelines for hospitals testing for the AIDS virus and these were endorsed by the American Hospital Association. The guidelines called for explaining the test to patients and getting their consent for it; counseling them before the test and again after it, if the result were positive; and making every effort to keep the result confidential. These guidelines were still in effect in 1990 and only a small minority of hospitals were routinely testing for AIDS, mostly for the purpose of protecting their personnel and then without strict observance of the guidelines.

The U.S. Department of Defense decided in the fall of 1985 to test all applicants to the armed forces and all personnel on duty for exposure to the AIDS virus, citing the need to protect military blood supplies. By 1988 it was reported that 5,890 were identified to carry the virus in the 3.96 million people tested; that is a rate of 1.5 positive reactors in every 1,000 tested. The total cost of the program was $43.1 million up to the time of the report. A surprising observation was that the infection rate had remained constant over the two-year period. It was believed these results did not give an accurate picture of the rate of infection among the population at large. On the one hand homosexuals and drug addicts, the two groups at risk for infection, are discouraged from applying to the armed forces, but on the other hand, those that do apply are in the age group that is sexually active. All applicants who tested positive were denied admission to the armed services; those already on active duty were allowed to remain, but they were to be closely monitored for any sign that the disease had become active.

Statisticians and epidemiologists in 1986 decried the fact, that although six years into the epidemic, so little was known about the crucial aspects of the spread of AIDS[39]. In particular there was a desperate need to know about heterosexual spread and the transmission rate of infection by vaginal intercourse. This led to the call for anonymous testing of blood samples routinely obtained from pregnant women and for widespread anonymous testing of the general public. It was believed such data was essential for the constructing of mathematical models of the spread of AIDS: models are useful to identify which risk factors for spread are most important. For instance, data on patterns of sexual activity were needed - as rates of changing sexual partners and the effects of using "safe sex" - not only for high risk groups but also for heterosexuals. Even as late as July 1988 the number of individuals harboring the AIDS virus in the U.S. could not be estimated, with any degree of certainty, to less than 50%[40]. In 1989 the National Research Council of the U.S. continued to state that there still was the same lack of data necessary to begin to control the AIDS epidemic.

Mandatory testing for AIDS was opposed by many as an invasion of the right to privacy of the minority groups who were at greatest risk. The right of an individual not to be tested is based on the Fourth Amendment to the Constitution of the United States. This Amendment protects an individual from unlawful search or seizure, stating there must be a reasonable presumption of guilt, certified by a warrant from a judge, before either practice can be carried out. Civil libertarians were adamant that this constitutional right did not only apply to the criminal law but also applied to testing for contagious or infectious disease. More importantly perhaps, to control the AIDS epidemic by testing and then quarantine (the practice in controlling other epidemic diseases} would require: first, universal testing of the population, almost impossible tactically; and secondly, confining the infected people in concentration camps, also an Herculean task, as well as being a politically unacceptable solution in the U.S. in 1989.

Another objection to mandatory testing was offered by an analysis of compulsory premarital screening for AIDS which revealed it to be a relatively ineffective and inefficient use of resources[41]. In this low prevalence portion of the population it would cost more than $100 million to detect fewer than one tenth of 1% of individuals infected with the human immunodeficiency virus (as proven in the Illinois experience during 1988, see above). In addition more than 100 infected individuals would be told they were not infected with the AIDS virus (false-negative results) and more than 350 people would be told incorrectly that they had antibodies to the AIDS virus in their blood (false-positive results).

Others disputed these projections and believed premarital screening was indicated[42]. It seemed rational to them that because a baby has a 20 to 60% chance of contracting AIDS from an HIV positive mother (v.i.). To the contrary, an ethicist said that to prevent an HIV positive woman from conceiving is an "extraordinary invasion of privacy" in view of the "50 to 75% chance the baby will be born healthy"[43].

The extent of the opposition to any form of mandatory testing was revealed in the discussion of a report of the Working Group on the Monitoring and Surveillance of HIV Infection and AIDS (of the British government)[44]. It recommended, in the spring of 1988, that antenatal testing for HIV infection be on a voluntary named basis (with provision for voluntary unnamed testing) as a first step in the surveillance of the general population. The Group concluded that making HIV infection and AIDS notifiable under the Control of Disease Act of 1984 would "understandably hold people back from testing, advice, and treatment." Doctors, opposed to this group's recommendation, pointed out that those most likely to be exposed to infection were most apt to decline to be tested and make meaningless this most important insight into heterosexual spread of the disease. The doctors also stated blood was being taken from pregnant women anyway, making HIV testing less expensive, and that they would be satisfied with totally anonymous, but mandatory, testing of all pregnant women. In this discussion preceding the report, the College of Midwives took the position that pregnant women were a captive audience and to use them in a new monitoring and surveillance exercise for AIDS would be morally wrong. The Faculty of Community Medicine responded that they were convinced that the ethical worry on mandatory testing was "a quibble" compared with the much larger problem of the lack of information about the spread of the epidemic.

The British Medical Association supported those physicians opposed to testing prenatally for HIV only on a voluntary basis, but stated that testing, when done without specific consent, should be absolutely anonymous[45]. It was recognized "absolutely anonymous" screening lost much of the epidemiological value of mass testing but at least it would supply the overall prevalence of HIV seropositivity and its rate of change over time. Since the blood taken was consented to for other tests, there could be no legal objection to testing on an anonymous basis. The claim of ethical violation because the donor of the blood is deprived of the right to consent is countered by the fact that the strict anonymity of the sample detaches it from the source. Many doctors, nevertheless, believe that testing should be mandatory, as is done for other sexual diseases and hepatitis B.

The continued opposition of some of the public to anonymous testing (or sometimes called "blind testing") for HIV was illustrated by a suit in Pennsylvania as late as in 1990. A pregnant woman sued to prevent the anonymous testing of her prospective infant for HIV, after delivery, on the ground that it was an invasion of their constitutional rights if done without consent. It was claimed this was so even if the test was done on blood drawn routinely for other purposes and the laboratory testing for HIV had no means of identifying from whom the blood had been obtained.

Many officials opposed to mandatory testing stated it would be self-defeating. It would drive underground those at the greatest risk for fear that disclosure of their life-style would make them objects of discrimination in their work, housing, etc. On the other hand, it had been found that those who refuse testing for HIV in a sexually-transmitted-disease clinic were 5.3 times more likely to be infected than men who accepted testing[46]. Male homosexuals and black and hispanic who refused testing were 7.3 and 8.8 times, respectively, more likely to be infected with HIV than their counterparts who accepted testing.

It was further argued by those opposed to mandatory testing that, as proposed, so few cases would be detected it would be a waste of money. A more valid criticism of any mandatory testing program was a statistical one: even highly accurate tests, such as for AIDS, err in identifying healthy persons to be infected in a percentage of tests done - the "false positive rate". The screening test for AIDS is the enzyme-linked immunosorbent assay (ELISA) which has a false positive rate of 7%. The Public Health Service had emphasized that an individual be considered to have serologic evidence of HIV infection only after an ELISA screening test was repeatedly positive and another test, such as the western blot test or immunofluorescence assay, had been performed to validate the results. This procedure reduced the false positive rate to 0.005%, or one person erroneously identified as a carrier in every 20,000 tested, but markedly increased the costs.

These tests detect circulating antibodies that are created by individuals infected with HIV. They really are splendid tests and work well when testing high risk populations such as homosexual men or drug addicts. However testing a low risk population, such as expected to have one in 10,000 persons testing positive (women in general), the situation is different. Then even such excellent antibody detecting tests as done for AIDS will erroneously accuse one healthy person of harboring the AIDS virus (a false-positive result) for each two persons rightfully detected. This statistical fact widens the conflict over all mandatory testing, but especially for drugs where tests are much less accurate than for AIDS. The critics of mandatory testing for AIDS favored greater efforts to persuade individuals at greatest risk to take the test voluntarily, and this greater effort should include making the results of tests more certainly confidential. Strengthening the position of those *in favor* of mandatory testing for HIV were reports of constant improvement in the confirmatory tests - giving no false positive results and reducing the inconclusive results to less than 1% (from 12%)[47]. In December 1987, it was reported that testing more than 250,000 low-risk people for AIDS was done in Minnesota without giving a single false positive result[48]. Confirmation of this high degree of accuracy was contained in a 1988 report on the U.S. military program of testing 1.2 million applicants from 1985 to 1987[49]. The ELISA test backed up by a western blot test (on positive ELISA results) gave only one false positive out of 15 positive obtained from a subset of 135,187 recruits tested (0.00074%); or a specificity for the diagnosis by these tests of 99.9993%. This can be contrasted to the 93% of results that were truly positive (14 of 15) in this group of 135,187 men aged 17 or 18, and who had resided in a rural county in a state with a known low incidence of AIDS.

There was reported, in 1987, that a few individuals with sexually transmitted infections of HIV-1 could harbor the virus in certain white blood cells (monocytes, or macrophages) for months or years without having antibodies in their blood[50]. Consequently the standard tests for HIV were reported to be negative in these individuals; but a new test, the polymerase chain reaction (PCR or macrophage test) could identify the virus in the cell directly. A subsequent study indicated that the number of such infected individuals without an antibody response to HIV for prolonged periods of time (up to at least 36 months) was much larger than originally believed, as many as 23% of all seronegative homosexual males who continued to engage in high-risk activity were proven to harbor the virus anyway[51]. An implication of these studies was that the number of infected people had been seriously underestimated and that the screening tests for protecting the blood supply and organ donations were less reliable than previously presumed. This new test, each costing $145 as opposed to $10 to $50 for antibody tests, will surely add to the already severe expense of testing for AIDS and to protect the blood supply and transplant recipients.

The new polymerase chain reaction test was also valuable in detecting which infants of seropositive mothers really were infected with HIV. This was important because for them, the ordinary antibody tests were known to be unreliable. Newborn infants of HIV positive mothers, without actually being infected, could have HIV antibodies in their blood from still having their mothers' blood in their circulation.

Some physicians would deem it wise, as a public health policy, to test some of their ill patients for AIDS even if a patient refused. Legally this would be ill-advised. At the present time (1989) doctors, almost certainly, would risk civil or even criminal proceedings if they tested for the AIDS virus without the patient's consent. Even if HIV infection was likely, and the motivation for testing was to protect personnel caring for the patient, it probably would be illegal to test without permission. The reasoning offered for this was: if a patient is suspected to be HIV positive and refused testing, then infection could be assumed to be present and precautions taken as though the infection had been proven, and thus it would be to no one's detriment *not* to test without permission.

On the other hand, in January 1988, the first successful AIDS-based medical negligence case had been decided in favor of the patient[52]. A Boston women, aged 32, with two sons, was awarded over $600,000 by a jury who agreed her doctor had been negligent for not recognizing she had AIDS (and not testing for it). This problem could be avoided if routine testing of patients for AIDS were permitted, as has been condoned for syphilis for decades. The rational for routine testing of patients for syphilis certainly exists for AIDS - the manifestations of the disease being so variable (including the lack of them) that the diagnosis can be overlooked. Also it is incongruous to health workers that the restraints on testing are limited to HIV. For instance, the U.S. Centers for Disease Control recommend that all pregnant women be routinely tested for the hepatitis B virus without any admonishing constraints. The epidemiology of the Hepatitis B virus closely parallels that of HIV: it is transmitted sexually (though heterosexual almost equals homosexual transmission) and by the sharing of unsterile syringes and needles. The differing approach to the testing for these two viruses can only be explained by there being an effective vaccine against the hepatitis virus, the wider publicity given the AIDS epidemic, and that AIDS more clearly involved minority groups.

The American Medical Association, in October 1987, recommended that testing for the AIDS virus should be mandatory for donors of blood and organs and other tissues intended for transplantation; donors of semen or ova collected for artificial insemination or in vitro fertilization; immigrants to the U.S.; inmates in federal and state prisons; and military personal. They justified mandatory testing of prisoners because they have a greater incidence of high-risk individuals than the general population and were confined, thus requiring special protection; of military personal because traditionally they had been subjected to mandatory immunizations; and of immigrants because the nation had the right to protect itself from having its communicable disease problems increased. The AMA went on to suggest that at-risk persons may not respond to educational programs and it may be necessary to penalize them if they knowingly exposed others to AIDS.

The Royal College of Physicians of Edinburgh in late 1987 also issued their recommendations to physicians for AIDS testing. Testing must be done on all individuals about to undergo treatment that might exacerbate infection such as giving of steroids or drugs necessary for transplantation. It should be done to confirm a diagnosis of suspected AIDS and in high risk groups: people seeking treatment for sexual diseases; intravenous drug users; people who considered themselves at risk; and females who had indulged in high risk activity prior to pregnancy or when they first presented in a pregnancy. It was appropriate to offer testing: to adults or children who were victims of sexual abuse or rape; to mentally handicapped patients whose habits posed a risk to staff or others about them; mothers who offered their babies for adoption and, if they were positive, their babies should be tested; such children in care should be tested, if the mothers were unavailable. Testing was not recommended for health care workers, routinely on inpatients, or as a condition for employment. They stressed, as did the AMA, that the permission of the patient must be obtained and that confidentiality must be maintained. Other health workers could not be informed of test results without permission and it was inferred that not even a negative-testing sex partner of a positive-tested patient could be informed without permission.

The U.S. Congress passed a comprehensive AIDS bill in October 1988, but without a $400 million three year provision for guaranteed completely confidential testing. The majority of legislators were reported[53] to favor the confidentiality amendment but could not overcome the parliamentary maneuvering of a few conservative senators. The conservative senators contended that a physician ought to be required to inform the spouse when a patient tested positive for HIV. A compromise was reached to drop the entire testing provision so that larger sums could be provided for research ($900 million over 3 years), home health care ($200 million over 2 years), and AIDS education ($ 900 million over 3 years).

It was interesting that the basis for their dissent against mandatory testing for AIDS by the American Civil Liberties Union[54] rested chiefly upon its probable lack of success in controlling the epidemic, and less upon the matter of any perceived abridgment of individual rights. Was it because the AIDS epidemic was exerting such fear that even our liberal society was on the verge of being willing to suppress their preference for individual rights in favor of the public right in this matter?

Probably another important factor that limited dissent against mandatory testing was that the public continued to have serious prejudice against homosexuals. While progress in the liberal point of view, and in science, had begun to convince society that homosexuality was a statistical fact and a natural event of our species, neither to be praised nor to be condemned, it still was not acceptable to the majority of the population and remained a matter of their prejudice. A prejudice certainly heightened by the prevalence of AIDS among homosexuals and by the erroneous fear that it might be contracted by ordinary contact.

The heightened prejudice against homosexuals and the unjustifiable fear of contracting the disease by ordinary contact increased the need for confidentiality in testing for AIDS. This, in order to protect the rights of those who tested positive. However, the objectives of those testing positive for *only exposure* to the disease are diametrically opposed to those of public health officials. Positive testers wanted absolutely anonymous tests of which they and no one else, not even their doctors, knew the results. They wanted to be sure their employers, landlords and insurers would have no basis to discriminate against them. Their point of view was heightened by the knowledge that there was no cure for the disease, should they develop it. However public health officers need names, for an important way to prevent spread of AIDS is to trace infected people's sexual partners and inform them. Nevertheless, even in mid-1987 a leading medical ethicist[55], after reviewing the above and other factors still concluded that a physician should not reveal the result (especially positive) of a patient's AIDS testing, not even to other doctors, without consent of the patient.

The objective of liberals in sponsoring confidentiality and anti-discrimination laws was to protect the rights of individuals, while the purpose of conservatives was to encourage the minorities involved not to be afraid of being tested or coming forth for what treatment was available. Ultra-conservatives were against any confidentiality and/or anti-discriminatory legislation.

Insurance companies believed it was necessary for them to test individuals in the high risk categories before issuing policies to them. This was being resisted by civil-rights and gay-rights groups. So far (early 1988) the companies were winning more battles than they had lost; test bans were in effect only in California and the District of Columbia. In many areas insurance companies stopped underwriting (in D.C.), or used "red-line" tactics: refusing policies to those in high risk groups or to those living in areas of high incidence[56]. The insurance companies stated if forced to issue policies ignoring the AIDS epidemic, they would have to radically increase rates. They argued it would be wrong to make their other policy holders subsidize those who develop AIDS; that should be a government responsibility. Insurance executives suggested people with HIV should get health insurance through state established "high-risk insurance pools" subsidized by state governments. The decision of the majority of courts not to ban testing for AIDS by insurance companies, of those seeking their policies, seemed fair to the vast majority of moderate-minded people.

A Presidential Commission on AIDS was appointed in 1987 and reported in November of that year that there was a lack of valid data on how the disease was spreading[57]. It was stated that the disease "was not spreading like wildfire, but it's not under control either". It seemed unlikely that the public would cooperate with a national survey of testing so that the spread of the disease could be charted. In fact a survey by the National Center for Health Statistics did find that 31% of the public said they would not allow their blood to be tested for exposure to AIDS, even if assured of complete privacy. Therefore the commission proposed to encourage and expand a "family of surveys" (a collection of small epidemiological studies to be done by state and local health departments) in the 20 top metropolitan areas containing 25% of the nations population and 75% of the reported AIDS cases, and in 10 other cities with moderate to low prevalence of AIDS. Blood samples were to be collected anonymously at selected hospitals and at clinics for sexually transmitted diseases, drug addiction, tuberculosis, pregnant women and family planning. Blood is always taken for testing in these locales, and after routine examinations were done, the blood samples, without the name identification, was to be turned over for HIV tests. This plan was to be operational by May 1988 and 1.6 million people were to be tested annually in this survey costing $40 million a year. While the blood samples would not be identified by name - the age, sex, race and area of residence would be known. If a sample were found to be infected, it would be impossible to notify the donor of his or her infection. Nevertheless, health experts feared the individuals most likely to be infected would refuse to cooperate and thereby cause a large underestimate of the infection rate. It was believed some results would be available by the end of 1988 and while they could not be definitive at that early date, it was expected there would be enough data to at least see some patterns.

In accordance with the recommendation of the Presidential Commission, the Centers for Disease Control first encouraged the attempt to do a pilot survey of households in Washington D.C. during the summer of 1988. Demographic information and blood samples were to be gathered, with the objective to find out how many Americans carry the AIDS virus, while carefully preserving the anonymity of those surveyed. The opposition of gay and minority groups caused failure of the project. Still in 1989, according to the report of the National Research Council: "Without better information on the prevalence of [the AIDS] infection, the nation will be unable to prepare adequately for future demands for hospital beds and other health services.... Without better data scientists and the American public can anticipate endless debates about whether the disease is spreading 'rapidly' or 'slowly'."

The first survey (a Household Seroprevalence Study) was finally done in Dallas, Texas in the fall of 1989, but proved to be relatively inconclusive[58]. Investigators visited random households and took blood samples and found 0.4% of those tested were HIV positive. Applied to the general population of Dallas County that would mean 2200 to 7500 people were infected, considerably lower than the 5600 to 16000 estimated previously by health officials. However, the sample obtained in the random door-to-door survey was only from those who agreed to have their blood tested. When those who refused were interviewed again, those who ultimately agreed to the test were found to have a higher rate of infection. Various groups had advised a boycott of the study, and the final figures were considered "statistically insignificant". Nevertheless, officials said the results of the

Dallas investigation encouraged them to continue with plans for a nationwide survey.

The President's Commission on AIDS also endorsed the National Academy of Sciences recommendation of the previous year (1987) that a study of sexual habits of Americans be done. Despite this endorsement, in 1989 both houses of Congress turned down the request of the Department of Health and Human Services for funds ($11 million) for such a study.

3. Problems in AIDS Control

It was unlikely voluntary testing would catch enough carriers to be effective and the problem would remain: how to contain an epidemic the parameters of which, including its very extent, were unknown. In addition, the very special characteristics of AIDS set it apart from other infectious diseases and, of themselves, make uncertain what measures for the control of this epidemic are correct. In 1986, in a review of the AIDS problem in the U.S., it was concluded that restraints on the freedom of persons who are sources of infection (other than AIDS) imposed by previous law should not apply to AIDS: "because the restraints on individual liberty and privacy imposed outweigh the social costs of the disease being controlled"[59].

It remains to be seen if these authorities are of the same opinion in 1993. For instance, a year after the above observation was made, it was reported that prison inmates in New York manifesting the symptoms of AIDS were being paroled early, "for humanitarian reasons"[60]. However, this policy raised fears that these paroled AIDS victims would endanger their families and associates, since prison officials are barred by federal and state laws from disclosing the medical condition of an inmate. In the two years prior to March 1987, 50 inmates with AIDS were paroled early from N.Y. prisons.

AIDS was the leading cause of death among the 37,000 inmates of N.Y. prisons, rising from 3 deaths in 1982 to 124 in 1986. In 1988, there still was opposition to an obvious public health measure taken by N.Y. authorities to segregate HIV-positive prisoners not yet ill. Lawyers of the Prisoners' Legal Services of New York sued to end the practice as a violation of prisoners' rights to confidentiality[61]. Nevertheless, by 1989 14 states were testing all incoming prisoners for HIV; a total of 20 states were segregating all prisoners with

AIDS; 6 states segregated patients even if only HIV positive; and the federal prisons were testing a randomly selected 10% of incoming prisoners (but were not segregating those testing positive or those with AIDS), and were testing all of those leaving the system. Released prisoners could well be another way for HIV to reach the heterosexual community.

That there was a modicum of change in the thinking on the matter of segregation of AIDS patients was evidenced by an editorial in the New York Times for June 6, 1987. This newspaper, generally regarded as liberal, remarked on discussing testing for AIDS: "Once all carriers are identified they will somehow have to be put in detention. That's a shocking idea but it's not foolish. Conceivably it might one day be seen as brave." Also in discussing the possible confining of people with false-positive tests the editorial goes on to say: "If that were the only way to protect public health, maybe even that should be thinkable." This latter was an expression of "statistical morality" that requires the sacrifice of a few individuals for the least harm to most people. Undoubtedly, as the AIDS problem remains uncontrollable, forcible confinement and segregation will be more and more discussed. In 1988, only the evangelical Christians (including Pat Robertson, the 1988 fundamentalist Republican presidential candidate) openly advocated national measures for quarantine and segregation of those infected with HIV[62] (see below for segregation policies in other countries).

"Statistical morality" is opposed by many groups, as for instance those in opposition to vaccination against whooping cough. Their opposition to vaccination is based on the premise that society cannot be responsible for the large numbers who die from nature's scourges, but are guilty for causing the deaths of the very few from the vaccine.

The rising concern caused by the epidemic had begun already by mid-1987 to infringe on the perceived right of privacy for AIDS victims. Reports were beginning to appear of physicians and health authorities notifying spouses and sexual partners of individuals testing positive for AIDS[63]. Ethicists were publicly supporting this action on the basis that the right to privacy is absolute until it infringes on other peoples' right to safety. In June 1988 the AMA, in a radical shift from the traditional oath of physicians to confidentiality, recommended to physicians that they warn the sexual partners of their HIV positive patients if there was no other way (as through the patient or local health department) to alert them to their danger. It also recommended that physicians sponsor legislation making it legal to do so in those locales where such a breech in confidentiality (especially in regard to AIDS) was illegal. The only opposition to this position of the AMA was expressed by gay rights advocates who called it "crude and thoughtless" - "it would undermine the physician-patient relationship and undermine the effort to control the epidemic" because patients, either homosexual or heterosexual, won't go to doctors!

In early 1989 a leading U.S. medical journal published an article calling for, at least voluntary, routine testing of everyone entering the health care system[64]. It was pointed out that such routine testing was not only of benefit to public health but also for the individual testing positive. The contention was that most of those who were HIV positive were unaware of it: thus 0.043% of first time blood donors and 0.15% of applicants for the military were HIV positive. When detected, such individuals should be treated to prevent other infections. They should be tested for tuberculosis (before a loss of immune reaction would turn negative those tuberculin-positive) and if positive be given prophylactic treatment. They should be vaccinated against influenza and pneumonia. Secondly, AIDS in its early stages had become treatable so as to delay the ravages of the disease. Also, it would alert those found to be positive to modify their behavior so as to protect their loved ones. Data was cited that hemophiliacs, despite their risks to becoming HIV positive, still engaged in unprotected sex. As for public health benefits, in addition to aiding collection of epidemiological data, it was stated that it would help undercut the divisive we-they mentality that isolated much of the public from the problem. These authors mentioned that improvement in testing had reduced the incidence of false-positives, and anyway went on to cite the principle of "statistical morality" (sacrifice of a few for the benefit of the vast majority) to support their position.

On the other hand, the California electorate defeated by a 2-1 margin a referendum on AIDS in the November 1988 election. The referendum, if it had been successful, would have required that anyone testing positive for HIV be reported to the state health department and if not done, the doctor (or blood bank) was to be fined $250. Secondly, it demanded that anyone known, or reasonably believed by doctors or the health department, to be infected with

HIV must divulge a list of intimate partners or be charged with a misdemeanor. It would have permitted the use of AIDS tests by insurers and employers and would have allowed doctors to do HIV tests on a patient's blood without written consent. Lastly, it would have made transmission of the virus a crime. At that time all states required AIDS cases be reported to state and federal health agencies, but only a quarter of them required reporting of patients who were only HIV positive. Ten states previously had declared willful transmission of AIDS to be a felony. Californians did approve a referendum that requires HIV testing of suspects in sex crimes and in assaults on police and emergency workers.

In September 1988 the three major television networks reversed their position, of many years standing, by agreeing to accept advertisements for the use of condoms. These advertisements were to be directed particularly to the prevention of acquiring AIDS. However, no such advertising had appeared on national television by February 1989, though it was being carried by some local stations. That a more intense campaign for the use of condoms should be undertaken was recommended in the report of the National Research Council in February 1989.

Also by 1988, a growing trend to wider testing across the U.S. could be detected, as illustrated by the testing of newborns and pregnant women. Every infant was tested (anonymously) that was born in a 12 months period in New York State: of the 276,609 infants born, 1816 (0.66%) had positive tests. One of every 80 babies (1.25%) born in New York City tested positively, while only 0.16% were positive in upper New York State[65]. Rates of seropositivity were distinctly higher among blacks and hispanics than among whites, reflecting the greater percentage of drug usage among those minority groups. Babies were tested even though at birth they temporarily retain the antibodies of the mother. It was estimated 20 to 60% of babies born to infected mothers will inherit the disease itself (test positive for HIV permanently). A separate study was done in New York City: testing 4000 women anonymously, after delivery of a child or undergoing abortion, and it revealed 1.37% were positive. This confirmed the above infant study that 1.25% of babies born in New York City tested positively for HIV.

Another program for testing new-born babies in Massachusetts revealed, in a seven month period, that one out of 476 mothers were infected with HIV, or 2.1 per thousand[66]. This extraordinary high HIV infection rate (in Massachusetts the incidence of AIDS cases among women is 0.02 per 1000 and only 0.25 per 1000 among men) was unexplained, or it could mean that the disease was more widely spread in the population than previously suspected. Massachusetts had reported only about 2% of AIDS cases in the U.S., a distant sixth among all the states.

The grave possibility of an HIV-positive mother transmitting AIDS to her infant demands that HIV-negative women co-habiting with men at risk for HIV be certain to use contraceptives. The most reliable contraceptive to prevent transmission of HIV is the condom; its use however requires the cooperation of the male, who too often is unreliable. Indeed the whole problem of contraception in the female population at greatest risk is beset with "unreliability". The obvious solution for HIV-positive women is sterilization. But this is often unacceptable to the woman (and many others), and in addition, is unacceptable to her because of the implication that there is no hope of a cure for her HIV infection.

Some epidemiologists[59] noted that AIDS already by 1988 was a major source of morbidity and mortality in the U.S. and would continue to increase in the ensuing few years. While more specific information, particularly at local levels, would be useful - they concluded the major modes of HIV transmission for the present and the future were known. Epidemiological principles should provide the basis for directing the considerable resources needed to prevent sexual, perinatal, and IV drug abuse transmission of HIV. Progress in prevention efforts and control of HIV infection would require a long term commitment of both science and society. They did not mention the epidemiological principles they had in mind and one may speculate on why they did not. Did they believe mandated testing of some groups would be necessary, and/or some people should be segregated to contain the epidemic?

In mid-1987, in an effort to resolve the dilemma in testing for AIDS, some recommended that strong laws be passed that guaranteed medical records would be confidential - inaccessible to employers, insurers or anyone else. Also it was proposed there be laws to guarantee protection against discrimination in housing, employment, etc. on the basis of AIDS. It was hoped this would make voluntary testing more attractive. Advocates of these laws, insuring the rights of those exposed to AIDS, gave as their reason for being against mandatory testing the "slippery slope" argument: that legislating mandatory testing for AIDS would lead to other medical conditions, at some time, being used to persecute other Americans.

Some pointed out that there were sufficient laws already extant to prevent discrimination against the handicapped, and AIDS in their opinion was a form of impairment and came under the laws for the handicapped. Others disagreed that the definition of handicap in these laws - "a physical or mental impairment that substantially limits one or more of such person's life activities" - included AIDS victims[67].

The Supreme Court ruled (March 3, 1987) that the 1973 law protecting the rights of handicapped people barred discrimination against those suffering contagious diseases unless they posed a real risk of infection to others, or they could not do their work[68]. The case in question, a school teacher infected with pulmonary tuberculosis, was remanded to a lower court to determine if, in fact, she was infectious and posed the threat of spread of disease to her pupils and others about her. In effect, the decision as to infectiousness or ability to work was to be decided on a case by case basis.

Although the decision on the tuberculosis victim did not directly involve the problem of AIDS, it was hailed as a major victory by homosexual rights advocates and others concerned about discrimination against victims of AIDS. They reasoned that since AIDS was not acquired by casual contact, it was not contagious, and therefore, the Supreme Court decision placed those carrying the AIDS virus under the protection of the law forbidding discrimination against the handicapped. It gave legal recourse to children excluded from public schools because they have AIDS and to infected adults who are dismissed from jobs - both, because of an irrational fear of contagion. The majority opinion in a footnote, however, explicitly declined to decide whether the 1973 law (on handicapped rights) protects carriers of the AIDS virus who do not suffer physical symptoms, but who can transmit the disease. A California Federal Court ruled in July 1988 that the Federal law barring discrimination against the handicapped does protect healthy HIV carriers as well as those who actually develop the disease, since they are not contagious. This confirmed that interpretation of the Supreme court decision as being protective to those with AIDS under the anti-discrimination law.

The Justice Department in October 1988 issued an opinion that the protection of the Federal Anti-discrimination law extended to those infected with the AIDS virus and that they should be treated like all others in the federal workplace, unless they posed health or safety risks. This opinion reversed a previous one of the Justice department and re-enforced an existing executive order of President Reagan to this effect. This latest Justice Department opinion and previous Administrative order were recognition of the fact that the Supreme Court decision of 1987 gave anti-discrimination protection to AIDS victims, because AIDS is not contagious.

The first real evidence of pharmacological progress in the treatment of AIDS was a report in August 1989 that the drug azidothymidine (AZT) actually could prevent (or markedly delay) development of the AIDS disease in a sizable percentage of those who were HIV-positive but had not yet had symptoms. Symptomless HIV-positive individuals who were beginning to have impairment of their immune system as revealed by a drop in the number of certain circulating white blood cells were the ones who now could be treated. AZT previously had been reported to slow down the progress of symptoms in those who had already developed AIDS, and had been the first drug approved by the FDA for the treatment of AIDS. Later reports indicated that AZT began to lose its power to protect against development of AIDS after 6 months of use, and by 18 months its clinical value was sharply reduced. Another problem was that the drug cost $7000 to $8000 per patient per year and many patients had inadequate medical insurance. Government financing for AZT treatment was limited, the Medicaid system had been designed for only those already disabled and not for preventing disability, and the Federal program to pay for AIDS drugs for those unable to afford them was due to expire with no immediate prospect that it would be renewed. As many as 600,000 symptomless HIV-positive persons would need AZT treatment and therefore the cost for the drug alone would be as much as $3 to $4 billion yearly.

An important side-effect of this progress in treatment was the undermining of one position of those against programs for increased testing for HIV, especially any form that made it mandatory. Where previously advocates of widened HIV testing programs only could have epidemiological purposes in mind, now their objective could also comprehend meaningful treatment for the individuals tested.

A month after AZT had been approved for distribution, another anti-AIDS drug, dideoxyinosine (DDI), was approved for early distribution. DDI was approved before determining its safety and effectiveness through establishment of an FDA "parallel tract" program, in response to lobbying by AIDS advocates who argued that standard FDA procedures were allowing thousands of desperate patients to die who would be eager to take chances with unproven drugs that showed some promise of slowing their disease. DDI was approved for distribution without charge to those patients with AIDS (or HIV) who found AZT too toxic or ineffective. The FDA usual evaluation of the safety and effectiveness of drugs is via the method of clinical trials that, of necessity, are prolonged if carefully done.

Scientists and public health officials expressed concern that the policy of early distribution of new drugs would make it difficult to get patients to volunteer for clinical trials - in which only half the patients get the new drugs and the other half get other drugs for comparison. All AIDS victims opting for the "parallel track" were sure to obtain the new drugs. If refusal to enter clinical trials became commonplace, the whole structure for testing and evaluating drugs could collapse. As an example, by 1990 some 8,000 patients were being treated with DDI in the parallel track, but only 700 of the 1500 needed for the clinical trials had signed up for them. Emphasizing the dilemma created by the parallel track policy was an early report that the death rate among parallel-track patients taking DDI was more than 10 times the rate among patients in the clinical trials. One plausible explanation offered was that the parallel-track patients were sicker to start with, than the clinical-trial ones. Yet, several patients taking DDI in the parallel tract program apparently did die from one of the drug's toxic side effects. The deaths were related to pancreatitis, a previously discovered problem with DDI[69].

Previously, in August 1988, the commissioner of the Food and Drug Administration had decided to allow individuals to import small quantities of unapproved drugs for personal use. His motive was "not to go down in history as the heartless bureaucrat who robbed AIDS patients of hope"[70]. Apparently large amounts of such drugs had been coming into the U.S. illicitly for years - from Mexico and Europe and, in particular, dextran sulfate from Japan (which nearly 10,000 people were taking). Investigators expressed grave concern that a freer flow of such drugs would make rigorous testing of them far more difficult. They feared if patients were allowed to take a variety of unproven drugs in a variety of combinations, it would be impossible to untangle the subtle signs of either efficacy or toxicity. "It would only prolong the time needed to develop new AIDS drugs and open the door for charlatans selling snake oil".

In some countries where AIDS had not yet become a widespread problem, AIDS victims were being isolated. Sweden, despite its politically liberal stance, had legislated (1985) compulsory detention of AIDS victims and prison sentences for individuals convicted of spreading the disease. Cuba, was reported by 1989 to have 259 HIV positive individuals, all of whom had been confined for life to a guarded sanitarium[71]. Cuba was testing its entire population starting with all soldiers returning from Africa and all entering foreigners. By January 1989 Cuba had tested 3.2 million of its 10 million people (46% of its sexually active population, and 246 were HIV-positive). Egypt, with at least 40 cases of AIDS, stated that after isolation of all known cases, there was no spread of AIDS[72].

In August 1987 the Soviet Union adopted measures authorizing mandatory testing of selected Russian (suspected of carrying HIV) and foreign citizens (who planned to remain in the Soviet Union for longer than 3 months) and stateless residents, with liability to expulsion for non-Russian citizens who evaded testing. Up to five years of incarceration could be imposed on those who knowingly exposed others to the risk of infection, and up to 8 years if infection was actually transmitted. As of late 1988, 17 million persons had been tested in the Soviet Union, and 334 foreigners and 112 Soviet citizens had been found to be carriers. Most of the foreigners had since left the country. In all, 5 foreigners and 3 Soviet citizens had shown symptoms of AIDS and one (a Leningrad female prostitute) had died[73].

Nevertheless in February 1989, 27 babies and 6 of their mothers were reported to have contracted HIV in a small city on the Caspian

Sea (Elistra) 750 miles south of Moscow, and where few foreigners ever go. Wider testing in that area was immediately undertaken to determine the origin and scope of the problem. It then was reported that a man after working in Africa, returned in 1982 and infected his wife who gave birth to an infected child. HIV was then spread to the other children by the use of contaminated syringes and needles in the hospital. It was determined that the mothers became infected through nursing the infected babies, it being customary in that region to nurse babies until long after they acquired teeth[74]. All infected children and some of their mothers (if they also were infected) were isolated in a special hospital in Moscow. The hospital was described as a derelict school building that hurriedly had been transformed into an epidemiological clinic[75].

By May 1988 25 other countries had mandated HIV testing for some categories of individuals, usually those desiring to enter for an extended length of time or arriving from certain designated parts of the world[76]. The World Health Organization opposed mandatory testing and requirements of certificates from international travelers. W.H.O. considered such measures to be counterproductive, because they would have little effect in slowing the spread of disease and they could lead to cheating by people who feared they might be infected. Also, such certificates can easily be forged[73].

The above procedures may appear Draconian, but they are only in line with previous public health measures to combat infectious, especially sexually transmitted diseases. A method previously thought vital in controlling sexually transmitted diseases is "contact-tracing", which requires mandatory testing, treatment, and notification of potential partners to break the chain of disease transmission. Heretofore isolation had been viewed as justifiable, especially when the disease had no specific treatment, as is the situation with AIDS. Therefore in societies with a low prevalence of infection the above procedures are viewed as not only justified, but also necessary - because their inhabitants do not perceive themselves as at-risk and will not respond to educational efforts directing them to "safe sex".

While contact-tracing has proven of value in AIDS in small populations, the inherent delays both in diagnosis and the manifestations of AIDS, together with the high costs of contact-tracing in large populations with high incidences of infection, make it a less promising technique in the latter circumstances[77]. Nevertheless, the U.S. Centers for Disease Control (CDC) has required states, having AIDS prevention and surveillance projects supported by the CDC, to implement procedures for confidential notification of sex and needle-sharing partners of AIDS patients and HIV-positive individuals[78]. State Health departments were making every effort to comply, but the success of these programs were hampered by the differences of the HIV infection from other sexually transmitted diseases in which partner-notification had been so successful in the past. The prolonged incubation period for HIV and the hopeless prognosis once AIDS developed (reducing cooperation of victims), of themselves, made success for contact- tracing unlikely.

Further, the legal issues surrounding "confidentiality" and "protection from discrimination", not previously encountered in combating other sexually transmitted diseases, were hurdles that probably contact-tracing in AIDS could not overcome, at least as appeared to be the situation in late 1988. An illustration of one such hurdle was the decision of a New York State Supreme Court Justice, in November 1988, that refused a petition of groups of various physicians, as well as the Medical Society of the State of New York, to force the listing of AIDS as a communicable and sexually transmitted disease (as it obviously is). The physicians argued that mandatory testing and tracing of contacts (which would be required if AIDS were officially listed to be communicable and sexually transmitted) was necessary to control the spread of AIDS and to allow health professionals to protect themselves against infection. The State Health Commissioner previously had refused to list AIDS, explaining such a listing would be counter-productive, for all the reasons mentioned in previous portions of this chapter. The Health Commissioner, undoubtedly, believed his decision was also a politically expedient one, at that time.

In 1989 both Houses of the British Parliament did reject an amendment to the Employment Bill that would have made it an offense to discriminate, in employment, against people who are HIV-antibody positive.

Searching for a vaccine against the AIDS virus raises an ethical problem common to this type of research (see Chapter Seven). Testing a vaccine requires exposing healthy volunteers to the possibility of harm as a side-effect of the vaccine, or even infection with the disease. Some ethicists have proclaimed such use of healthy individuals, no matter what the purpose, to be unethical. Another ethicist, recently addressing this issue, implied testing of vaccines must go forward and it is justified, if the autonomy of the participants be respected by adequately warning them of the risks, and they be compensated for any disability[79].

A circumstance that distinguishes AIDS vaccine research from all others is the likelihood that volunteers could test HIV-positive by the ELISA (antibody) test after being inoculated with the vaccine, and yet not be infected. Other tests could distinguish the volunteers as not being infected, but they nevertheless could be subjected to social stigma and discrimination, as in donating blood, obtaining insurance, traveling internationally or entering government service. Therefore extreme efforts to confidentiality are required in testing vaccines in volunteers. Advanced trials require such confidentiality anyway, since the volunteers would have to be uninfected members of the minority groups known to be at-risk to acquiring AIDS.

Another serious dilemma arises when the volunteers are required to be from high-risk groups. Their being in the high-risk group obligates physicians to counsel them against behavior that would place them at risk to becoming infected with AIDS. On the other hand, such counseling could diminish the exposure of the vaccinated volunteers and reduce the value of the data on the adequacy of the vaccine. The proper answer is to use a sufficient number of volunteers so as to have vaccinated and control groups, provide both groups with proper education and counseling and still be able to make a determination on the efficacy of the vaccine.

The difficulties in vaccine testing continued to mount. In the first place, the spread in the homosexual population had abated to the point where infections in any such study group were so few, even if its members volunteered to take the vaccine, that the efficacy of the vaccine cannot be tested. Secondly, although the virus was still spreading rapidly among drug-using populations, they had been ruled out for initial vaccine tests because such people are difficult to keep under surveillance during the many years required to test a vaccine.

U.S. health officials suggested if ever a vaccine became promising, the required large scale trials would have to be done in Africa where the disease was still spreading rapidly. This, of course, would raise many socio-political problems, especially because the tests would require many thousands of volunteers and at least eight years to follow them. There were shortages of trained personal in Africa through whom informed consent could be obtained and counseling for subjects be provided. Moreover, African health officials had been quoted as stating they do not wish their populations to be used as "guinea pigs". Other demands were that any vaccine go through several stages of testing in the country of origin, and that African scientists be brought up to the level of American and European scientists so that they could participate in any trials as equal partners[80].

A final problem was the decrease in the U.S. of the number of companies willing to manufacture vaccines, because of their exposure to liability suits[81]. AIDS vaccines would likely be even more contentious than other vaccines, because of the added problem of making individuals HIV-positive, alluded to above, and the inability to actuarially define their risk of acquiring AIDS, because of the long incubation period between HIV infection and the development of AIDS. There was no legislation yet in place to protect experimenters and manufacturers of AIDS vaccines. Even without all these problems, by the summer of 1988 scientific difficulties were making the chances of obtaining an effective vaccine seem rather less, than more.

As the epidemic and the fear of it had spread, isolated reports appeared of health workers, including one doctor, becoming infected. The chance for infection usually occurred after accidental pricks by hypodermic needles that had been used on AIDS patients (80% of exposures), or from inadvertent spilling of contaminated blood over breaks in the skin caused by cuts with sharp instruments (8% of exposures) or through a skin disease such as eczema (7%). The Centers for Disease Control reported 1,600 such incidents in doctors, nurses and hospital workers (accidentally so exposed over a period of five years) with only four (0.42%) of 963 cases adequately tested subsequently developing a positive reaction for HIV[82]. No health worker exposed to fluids other than blood (106 cases of contamination with saliva, urine or an unspecified fluid) became infected. Nevertheless, following upon these reports, some health workers (including doctors) refused to care for AIDS victims. In their defense, a computation can be cited that placed the numerical risk for a member of a surgical team becoming infected, over a professional lifetime, at 2.5% if working in an area where HIV infection was endemic with a seroprevalence rate of 10 to 15% (not uncommon in central city areas)[83]. Early in 1990 the American Society of Law and Medicine, based in Boston, claimed the actual number of health workers that had become infected on the job could be as many as 100 (the Centers for Disease Control having reported 19 such cases in the U.S. at that time).

Actually, The Centers For Disease Control gave the chances of becoming sero-positive for HIV by health care workers who suffer documented work-site exposure to HIV to be only 0.42% (about 1 in 250). Although this ought to provide reassurance that "the risk for nosocomial HIV transmission is small, it is clear that the emotional impact of work-site HIV exposure is profound."[84] Certainly, the fear of contracting HIV seemed to far outweigh the fear of becoming infected with the even more dangerous hepatitis B virus. There is a vaccine to protect against the latter, and yet as of 1990, less than 40% of health workers had availed themselves of that safeguard against the hepatitis B virus.

Could the serious disregard of fundamental duty by some physicians (not to attend AIDS victims) have been abetted by the attack of ethicists and sociologists on the Hippocratic tradition of doctor beneficence in favor of patient autonomy? Without doubt, all the other factors weakening the doctor-patient relationship in the U.S. (previously noted in Chapter Three) did contribute to physicians daring publicly to announce their intention not to attend AIDS victims. That such announcements were only isolated incidents, and were deprecated so widely by the profession, speaks well for doctors continuing to perceive their role as a beneficent one.

That the AIDS epidemic was placing a further strain on the doctor-patient relationship cannot be denied, especially in emergency rooms. Young people, especially young males, are looked upon with special caution: no longer does a physician rush to give mouth-to-mouth resuscitation, and the rush to stop bleeding is interrupted to put on a gown and gloves. Surgeons are beginning to demand that their patients be tested for HIV before they agree to operate[85]. They further pointed out that testing in the hospital protects against lawsuits by patients who later contend they became HIV positive from exposure while in the hospital.

Perhaps one area in which physicians should be more vocal, and prove their beneficence has not been irretrievably impaired, is in the terminal care of the victims of AIDS. The agony of these patients must be excruciating, and probably is exacerbated by the prejudice against, and the fear of, them by hospital attendants. In all the discussion of the cost of AIDS there should be a plea for provision for hospice care, where trained attendants and the surroundings would ameliorate the anguish of their last days.

The general practitioners of Great Britain were being mobilized (or possibly better expressed as mobilizing themselves) to educate their patients against AIDS[86]. It will be interesting to monitor their results for comparison with those of the medical delivery system in the U.S. that has such a small remaining cadre of that breed. U.S. general practitioners are particularly few in areas where the epidemic is most rampant. It is said that drug abusers (or their parents) in Britain turn first to their general practitioners for help[87] and 18% of addicts tested positively to HIV (in Edinburgh the figure was 50%). Therefore British general practitioner organizations were mobilizing to educate their members: to reverse the prejudice against the treating of addicts; on the techniques in the treatment of addiction; and how to counsel on the risks of AIDS and hepatitis B.

A random survey of general practitioners in London reported by 1989 that they were quickly becoming involved in the care of patients with HIV infection and their relatives and friends. They were counseling patients and testing for antibodies themselves and regarded this as an integral part of their work. A considerable part of their workload in primary care consisted of patients who obsessively feared contracting HIV infection[88].

Dentists were most reluctant to treat patients with AIDS: a survey by the American Dental Association released in November 1987 reported 4 out of 5 dentists would not knowingly do so[89]. Dentists more regularly than medical doctors (other than surgeons) encounter the blood of their patients. They also stated that they do not want to be known as treating AIDS patients for fear that would hurt their practices. Most dentists now wear rubber gloves routinely and this also was recommended by the Center for Disease Control - not only to protect dentists but also their patients. Not treating AIDS patients was more a matter of ignorance or prejudice on the part of the dentists because 64% of the dentists surveyed (2181 replied of the 5711 sent questionnaires) unhesitatingly would treat patients with hepatitis, which is very much more contagious than HIV.

By 1990, testing for the AIDS virus still could only be done with the informed consent of the patient or next-of-kin, no matter what the circumstance. Health workers would often desire to test for HIV so as to determine when precautions should be taken to avoid the exposure that accompany many procedures. In view of the constraints on testing, and the known long delay in tests becoming positive after an HIV infection occurs, it was widely recommended by many authoritative groups that all precautions be taken with every patient, an expensive and time consuming process. This recommendation for universal precautions means treating all body fluids, from each and every patient, as if they were vehicles for transmission of HIV[90]. Despite the legal restraints, nurses were demanding HIV testing of patients if an accidental needle puncture did occur. To repeat, it seemed incongruous to many health workers that these restraints on testing were limited to the HIV infection, and indeed a few hospitals were routinely testing for HIV without observing the restrictive guidelines for such a practice (see this chapter above).

The fear of health workers that they may acquire AIDS from contact with patients or their body fluids had caused a severe shortage in the availability of rubber gloves, early in 1988. Health workers, including dentists, felt constrained to use rubber gloves at all times, and often two pairs at once. Surgeons, because of the shortage, often had to settle for wearing rubber gloves of the wrong size, and hospitals had to scramble to renew their supplies of gloves. Some suggested the increased use of condoms contributed to the shortage of rubber for gloves. Innumerable accidental needle sticks suffered by all health workers and inadvertent knife injuries to surgeons were causing a race to create methods to circumvent needle sticks, and gloves impermeable to knives or needles.

The obverse of the problem under discussion is whether health workers who have acquired AIDS should be permitted to attend patients? As of September 1988, 3,182 health workers with AIDS, including 356 physicians, had been reported to the U.S. Centers for Disease Control[91]. How many health workers are HIV positive was unknown. Actually, barring an accident in which a doctor or nurse is cut during an invasive procedure on a patient and their blood drips into an open wound or onto a mucous membrane, there is no chance of transmission of HIV. However, the majority of the public (1987 Gallup poll) are against being treated by an infected health worker. Lawyers state that the doctrine of informed consent should be interpreted as "what a reasonable patient would want to know, and not what a reasonable physician would disclose". On this basis hospitals and other organizations were advised to disclose those workers with AIDS. The result was that many patients refused to accept attenders who were infected. One physician infected with AIDS, bitter about being driven out of his profession, advised other physicians who contract AIDS not to disclose their illness[91].

A further dilemma created by the AIDS epidemic was the problem of how much money the U.S. government should spend for research on prevention from acquiring the disease, and its cure. In late 1986 a special committee of the Institute of Medicine recommended a standing Presidential Committee or a joint Presidential-Congressional Commission that would give continuing advice on the problem for at least 5 years and that federal funding for AIDS research be quadrupled to $ 1 billion annually by 1990[92]. Federal spending on AIDS prevention and research was $1.3 billion in 1988, overshadowing the money spent on heart disease that year. In 1989 the money spent on AIDS by the U.S. government was to exceed the money spent on cancer. It was surprising to many that these expenditures on AIDS should exceed those on the two chief causes of death; and secondly that so much money was to be spent on a disease predominantly afflicting homosexuals and intravenous drug users, two groups scorned by numerous people, including legislators. The probable reason for such spending was the fear of AIDS spreading into the general population.

The economic costs of just treating AIDS patients also was proving to be a serious concern. The cost for one patient in the U.S. ranged from $50,000 to $150,000, and it was estimated that $5 billion yearly was being spent on treating AIDS patients by 1989. It was believed that the National Health Service in Britain would spend 80 million pounds ($140,000,000) to treat 3000 patients in 1988-89. These costs needed to be added to the severe one due to loss of the productivity of the victims, almost all in the age group of 25 to 45.

The cost of treating AIDS in New York City in 1987 was $385 million and it was estimated it would be more than a $1 billion annually by 1991. It was projected that the lifetime care for the 270,000 victims in the U.S. from 1981 to 1991 will be about $22 billion[93].

These costs were said to be comparable to the costs of caring for other serious illnesses, except, in the same article, the authors stated "the treatment of AIDS patients is more expensive than most other patients,". It was also to be noted that individuals suffering with AIDS were younger and the loss in productivity was consequently higher than with other illnesses. The cost in terms of lost output per AIDS patient was estimated to be from $541,000 to $623,000. The economic effects of AIDS will be felt far heavier by the citizens of San Francisco and New York than the rest of the country.

The total amount to be spent on the care of AIDS patients in 1991 in the U.S. was estimated to be 1.5% of total national health care; this was considered by some to be a small amount[93]. Moreover an ethicist[79] believed this was an area where "the principle of respect for autonomy must take second place, as those of us who are financially well off are called upon to share in meeting the needs of the less well off, presumably through the payment of increased premiums and taxes."

Some health officials decried the disproportionate amounts being expended on AIDS when other sexually transmitted diseases were increasing in even greater numbers and, certainly, were also of epidemic dimensions[94]. The infections cited were gonorrhea, chlamydia, human papilloma virus, hepatitis B virus, herpes simplex viruses and syphilis. Only about $60 million annually was allocated by the U.S. government to all these diseases, in toto. The rising number of cases of pelvic inflammatory disease and other changes wrought by these diseases suggested that the fertility of the next generation might be severely compromised. The rise in sexual promiscuity and the failure of "just saying no" campaigns were ascribed as reasons for the sexually transmitted diseases epidemics.

In early 1988, the eighth year of the AIDS epidemic, the Secretary of Health and Human Services announced, in a striking shift of view, that the much feared explosion into the general population was not occurring and it seemed unlikely it ever would.

The basis for this optimism was not clear, except that the spread into the heterosexual population remained, for the most part, confined to the partners and children of IV drug addicts, and the epidemic among homosexuals (those most severely affected in its early years) was abating. AIDS was still spreading among drug users and their sexual partners, which always posed the most serious threat to the heterosexual population. In the first quarter of 1988, the number of new patients reported to have AIDS in New York city for the first time consisted of more drug abusers than homosexuals, 386 to 385. It may be that the epidemic among addicts was less worrisome because they are not mobile (far less so than homosexual men). Addicts are chiefly in the inner cities, and while it is true once the virus appears in a group of drug users it spreads rapidly, the spread to distant cities is slow. There were estimated to be 1.2 million intravenous drug abusers in the U.S. and only 148,000 in treatment programs at any one time. Another emerging fact that was slightly encouraging was that it was beginning to appear that not all of those testing positive for HIV would necessarily develop AIDS. It was reported that 20% would still be free of the disease seven years after contracting the infection[95].

For the most part, by 1988, those who were to develop AIDS in the ensuing five years were already infected and nothing would alter the course of the epidemic in the near term. The educational program was being effective for the homosexual population, but whether it was sufficient to control the epidemic in that population remained to be ascertained. Education alone was patently insufficient to control the spread among drug addicts. The President's Commission on AIDS (v.i.) recommended, in February 1988, that an extra $2 billion per year be spent to the setting up 3,300 drug treatment centers and to employ 32,000 drug treatment specialists. The funds were to be half supplied by the Federal Government and half by state and local governments[96].

Seventeen to twenty-five percent of AIDS victims were drug addicts, most having acquired the disease from sharing needles and syringes. In some localities, as in the Netherlands, addicts could obtain a supply of sterile syringes and needles from authorized centers, hoping this would reduce the spread of HIV. Other areas testing the effect of supplying clean needles in preventing the spread of AIDS were parts of England, Scotland, Denmark, Sweden,

Australia and Tacoma, Wash. This creates a moral dilemma -
encouraging one epidemic (drugs) in an effort to contain another
(AIDS). There is some analogy to the methadone treatment of heroin
addiction - which some object to on that basis (substituting one
addiction for another). Methadone taken orally has the virtue of
blocking the desire for intravenous heroin (but not cocaine).
Experience in those areas where clean needles were freely distributed
was insufficient by 1988 to be certain of the effect of such a program
on the spread of AIDS, but preliminary reports indicated it produced
a marked decline in the seroprevalence rate[97]. The experiences *were*
sufficient to allay the fear that it would promote drug abuse.

In August 1988 New York City announced that it would test the
effect of giving free needles to 200 addicts on the spread of the
AIDS virus in that group[98]. The obvious intention was to broaden
such a program, if successful. Opposition to this experiment was
expressed by law enforcement officials who argued that it condoned
and facilitated drug abuse. Some government officials said that drug
abusers should be viewed as criminals needing to be punished rather
than as sick people needing help. Representatives of the black and
hispanic communities appeared to be particularly offended by the
intended free needle program, claiming the program had racist
implications.

Even as early as 1989 it seemed that the seriousness of the
AIDS problem, as opposed to the limited influence of distributing
free syringes and needles on the encouragement of the use of drugs,
resolved the dilemma in favor of free distribution of clean needles
and syringes. The same utilitarian reasoning justifies the free
distribution of methadone via clinics that can control the heroin
addicts and regulate its issuance. The National Research Council of
the U.S. in their February 1989 report endorsed free needle exchange
programs, as well as the distributing of disinfectants for cleaning
needles. The fact that drug addicts with AIDS are the largest
"window" for spread into the general (heterosexual) population and
undoubtedly they are least amenable to AIDS education, well could
lead to the eventual most drastic conclusion, that they must be
quarantined.

The single most important message to prevent heterosexual
spread was said to be that individuals should have sex only with
partners who are known to be at a low risk of carrying HIV

infection[99]. Admittedly, it is difficult to judge whether a potential partner is at low risk to HIV infection unless one knows that person very well. Therefore "condoms with spermicide should be used whenever people are uncertain of the risk status of a sexual partner. Even when they have chosen a partner they believe is at low risk, some people may choose to use condoms and/or spermicides to reduce further their risk of becoming infected".

The problem, in the view of one ethicist, is how to control the epidemic without unjustly discriminating against particular social groups and without unnecessarily infringing on the freedom of individuals[79]. The answer offered is that educational efforts must be expanded, the treatment of drug addicts widened and public programs for exchange of sterile needles and syringes introduced, and, if need be, IV drug users be given controlled access to injectable drugs. Prostitution should be decriminalized and be licensed and regulated, which would be helpful in controlling the epidemic, and "At the same time displays...a greater respect for the autonomy of adult persons to perform acts that affect chiefly the persons themselves, especially if the transmission of disease is prevented through the use of condoms and through regular health examinations." On the same ethical basis, private homosexual acts should be decriminalized and there should be legal prohibition of discrimination against people who engage in private consentual homosexual acts. This should encourage such individuals to disclose their pattern of sexual activity and also open them to discuss use of condoms or the avoidance of anal intercourse. This ethicist could find no moral justification for mandatory testing at this time (1988).

An international conference on AIDS sponsored by the London School of Hygiene and Tropical Medicine in March 1988 continued to reflect the above point of view. The conference themes were "that there should be no mandatory testing either of the general public or "high-risk" groups, and that attempts to eradicate AIDS should focus on behaviours and practices, not individuals or groups of individual"[100]. To do otherwise, it was believed, could cause comparison with the Nazis' "final solution" and only would add to the already severe burden of illness by causing stigmatization, shame and discrimination. The course of recommended action continued to be to increase educational efforts to change behavior, and not to do screening "but to trust and to base that trust on preventive health measures." What those "preventive health measures" were to be, was not spelled out. It was reported to the conference that while stabilization of the rate of spread appears to be occurring in those groups known, for years, to be at high risk (homosexuals in San Francisco and intravenous drug addicts in New York and Edinburgh), the AIDS virus was spreading rapidly among intravenous drug abusers in Bangkok, female prostitutes in some African cities, and among prison inmates in North America and Europe[101].

The President's Commission on AIDS, appointed in 1987, in its final report in June 1988, in general, upheld the above points of view. The chairman emphasized that a national law barring discrimination against those who carry the AIDS virus should be enacted. This could be accomplished by broadening and extending (to the private sector) the anti-discrimination provisions of the 1973 Rehabilitation for the Disabled Act. The vote of the Commission on this proposition, however, was narrow - seven in favor and five against. Those against the proposal complained that it would force businesses to hire people HIV-positive, thus driving up insurance rates, and it would expose business owners and landlords to possible litigation by infected people.

The Commission recommended that there be firm guarantees of confidentiality of test results. It explained that current health strategies for gaining epidemiological data and fighting the spread of AIDS were entirely dependent on voluntary cooperation, which cannot be obtained without such laws. It recommended mandatory testing only for donors of blood, tissue, and organs. The Commission suggested that sexual offenders "submit to an HIV test at the earliest possible juncture in the criminal justice system", a move the American Civil Liberties Union opposed[102]. The Commission recognized that uninfected persons in danger of being exposed to HIV need to be protected and that this should be the responsibility of state health departments. Virus carriers as well as AIDS patients, therefore, need to be reported to the state health departments by doctors and other health-care personnel. The majority of the Commission believed that it should be a criminal offense to knowingly transmit the AIDS virus.

The Commission further advised that there be larger expenditures (about $3 billion more in fiscal 1988) for programs for the treatment of drug addicts, for expanded educational efforts, and for the licensing of all medical testing laboratories. Upon receiving the Commission's report the President appointed his special assistant for drug policy to review its over 600 recommendations and chart a future course to deal with the AIDS epidemic. This was an acknowledgment of a major message of the report: that control of the spread of the AIDS virus was related to drug abuse.

Opposing educational efforts on AIDS are the opinions of many theologians and most religious fundamentalists. For instance, they believe educational programs recommending safer sex, by the use of condoms or reducing the number of sex partners, promote licentiousness. The use of condoms is a sin in the eyes of the Pope and the Roman Catholic Church, since they are an artificial barrier to conception. They all urge the focus be on the restriction of sexual activity to within heterosexual, monogamous marriage. These same people oppose, as do many officials, the distribution of clean needles and syringes. Probably a goodly number of people whose views generally are more moderate would also oppose these and/or some of the other "liberal" measures proposed by the ethicist[79] quoted above.

Nonetheless, others believe it is worth noting that the majority of people in the U.S. approve the advertising of the use of condoms for safer sex and sex education - just as there are majorities in favor of abortion, contraception, indifference about school prayer, and accept that evolution has occurred[103]. It was observed that, so far, the U.S. Government because of the protests of the squeamish and moralistic minority portion of its population had not pursued with sufficient vigor an educational program for safe sex that is necessary to contain the AIDS epidemic (as is being done in Europe). It was stated by still others that an obsession with the red herring of compulsory testing had diverted the debate away from public education[104].

AIDS and HIV infections are more prevalent in prisons than in the general public[105]. This is because a high proportion of the inmates are drug users and homosexual activity is rife in prisons, even among men that are normally heterosexual. Most prisoners eventually are released, so to protect society it is important to reduce the spread of HIV in prisons. Measures advocated are to test all prisoners, segregate those testing positive, distribute condoms (with counseling) to inmates, and supply clean needle and syringes to addicts. Varying groups oppose each of these measures, and few if any prisons had a coordinated policy to address this problem by the end of 1988.

Some believe, in addition to other efforts, that social scientists should collect data to determine if it is true that the ethics of recent generations permit increased freedom in sexual activities and also weaken their matrimonial bonds (providing for more single parent families and its consequences). If so, it could account for the rise in drug usage and spread of sexually transmitted diseases, including AIDS. If the many opinions that such relationships do exist were confirmed, then educational campaigns to restore previous ethical standards in these areas would be justified in the long-term effort to combat the drug and AIDS epidemics. Adding to this point of view were the data on the increased chances of acquiring or transmitting HIV with increasing the number of different sexual partners[106].

The panel of the U.S. National Research Council, reporting in February 1989, stated flatly that many traditional approaches to changing behavior, such as messages based on moral dictates, do not work. They went on to say that efforts to prevent AIDS will be most effective if they are explicit and offer choices, rather than prescribing a single behavior, such as abstinence. AIDS messages had to be realistic and diverse to reach different audiences. As an example, some studies indicated three-fourths of all girls had sex during their teen years and 15% had had four or more partners. "A message that simply says, 'say no to sex', will be unacceptable to many of them". They should be told that a condom with spermicide will markedly reduce the chances of getting AIDS. Since one of the fastest growth areas for AIDS is among IV drug users, their sex partners and children, the Council recommended giving them clean needles and syringes and disinfectants for needles[107]. Fears that such programs, as well as increasing methadone clinics, would encourage or condone drug addiction were unsupported by any data. In fact, studies from extant syringe and needle exchange and other "safer injection" programs had found no increases in IV drug use[28].

4. Conclusions

It is to be presumed that it will be "moral" to pursue other solutions only if all present measures to confine the epidemic fail. Yet, because the religious fundamentalists and more conservative elements of Western societies already favor mandatory testing and segregation, the liberal sentiment against these measures is especially resistant. However, if all of society perceives itself sufficiently threatened, there can be no doubt that it will do what is necessary to preserve itself and its well-being.

Unquestionably, as the data accumulate a consensus will be achieved for the correct solution of the utilitarian equation: balancing the welfare of the entire community against the rights of individuals and minority groups, in the control of the AIDS epidemic. It should be emphasized that as late as by the end of 1989 the effort to protect individual, and particularly minority, rights still had precluded mandatory testing in most meaningful situations, so that not even the number of people infected with the AIDS virus could be estimated with any degree of certainty. Notifying those at risk by exposure to HIV positive individuals (such as sexual partners) was still *verboten*, so that "contact tracing" was impossible. Also, it still was considered unethical to notify medical personnel caring for an HIV-positive patient of that fact without the patient's consent, unless it was necessary for the patient's care, or that the health team would otherwise be placed at serious risk - and then the doctor must be prepared to justify his or her action[108].

If evolutionary ethics has any predictability value at all, it would be safe to say that some of the myriad of ethical constraints voiced in our liberal society will have to be compromised to deal with this deadly epidemic. Even if it is to be only those moral compunctions in the testing of vaccines that will be overlooked, that will be the very least of concessions required. In 1989, vaccines and curative treatment appeared to be many years away, so, as the epidemic worsens in that interim, more serious ethical compromises and invasions of individual rights will be demanded. In all probability mandatory testing in many situations with reporting of positive results to public health authorities will be an early step deemed necessary, and demanded by the vast majority of the public.

Emphasizing the political ideologic aspect of the AIDS problem were the reactions to proposals by one of France's best known and respected physicians, appointed French Minister of Health late in June 1988. He proposed that all pregnant women and patients scheduled for surgery be tested for HIV and that the government distribute drugs to addicts as part of a treatment program. The Socialist Party and civil libertarian groups protested the call for mandatory testing for AIDS, and political parties to the right attacked the call for the partial legalization of drugs. The Health Minister, who was a non-Socialist appointed by the Socialist Premier, was forced to resign nine days after taking office, a record for briefness of service by a French cabinet minister.

CHAPTER FIVE. PUBLIC HEALTH POLICY AND INDIVIDUAL RIGHTS (DRUGS)

1. Drug Addictions (and Alcoholism)

1.1 Introduction

Drug addiction is of epidemic proportions in the U.S. and elsewhere, but the problem of its control is obviously different from that of AIDS. It is more akin to the problem of alcoholism than to infectious disease: there are social and cultural elements and perhaps an inheritable tendency to addiction; drugs, like alcohol, support business enterprises (legal or illegal); drug addiction is treatable, though it is a chronic, relapsing condition.

While it is generally agreed that drug addictions are more frequent in individuals of lower socio-economic and minority status, a recent study casts a modifying light on this conclusion[1]. A study in 1989 which tested the urine of all pregnant women enrolled for prenatal care at any of the five public health clinics in a Florida county, or at any of 12 private obstetrical offices in the same county, reached the conclusion that there was little difference in the prevalence of positive results between the two groups (16.3% in the public clinics versus 13.1% in private offices). The frequency of positive results was also similar among white women (15.4%) and black women (14.1%). However, black women more frequently had evidence of cocaine use, whereas white women more frequently had evidence of the use of marijuana. Despite the similar rates of substance abuse among black and white women, black women were reported at approximately 10 times the rate for white women, and poor women were more likely than others to be reported (mandatory to county health authorities).

The treatability of drug addiction generally is overestimated and even more difficult and more unpredictable than that of addiction to alcohol, the treatability of which is also exaggerated in the minds of most[2,3,4]. The association of AIDS and drug addiction has generated demand for more methadone programs (substitution of an oral drug addiction to relieve the cravings of an intravenous heroin habit) and residential treatment centers that aim for drug-free rehabilitation. These are expensive programs, especially the latter, and data on their success rate were desperately needed - as late as 1989 their usefulness was, at best, controversial.

It was estimated (by the National Institute on Drug Abuse) in 1987 that 37 million Americans took illicit drugs at an annual cost, mostly in lost productivity, of $34 billion[5]. Another calculation by a federally sponsored study in 1989 increased the estimate of this drain on the nation to $60 billion a year, and medical costs for crack addicts and drug-addicted AIDS patients represented a significant portion of the rising expense[6]. It was not known how many people were severely addicted and entirely dependent on drugs, and the estimates varied from 2 to 6.5 million. It was believed the use of heroin had stabilized by 1987 at about 500,000 aging individuals, and the regular users of cocaine (mostly in its potent, smokeable form called "crack" which gives a more potent "high") had increased, by 1988, to a stable number of 5 to 6 million. Marijuana users were estimated to total 18 million. The illicit drug trade worldwide was estimated in 1990 to be worth as much as $500 billion a year. If this estimate be true, the drug trade was larger than that in oil and only exceeded in value by armaments[7]. The UN Secretary General remarked at an international conference in April 1990: "It is a sad commentary on the state of mankind at the end of the twentieth century that the bulk of our vast productive energies is devoted to manufacturing our own destruction".

"Crack" is cocaine that has been separated from its hydrochloride salt and occasionally is called the freebase, referring to the freeing of the cocaine base from its salt. Crack is vaporized by heat and therefore it can be smoked. When smoked it can produce a "high" within less than a minute, only equaled by cocaine if taken intravenously. In the 1980's cocaine, in one form or another, replaced heroin as the major national concern because cocaine had become more plentiful and cheaper: in 1981 a gram of cocaine cost $600 and by 1986 it was down to $200 and said to be even cheaper in 1988[8]. In 1981 5.8% of high school seniors reported taking cocaine sometime in the previous month and in 1986 this figure was 6.2%; however in 1987, for the first time since 1981 there was a decrease in this rate, down to 4.3%. Similarly, there was a drop in the proportion of seniors who had "ever used" cocaine from 16.9% in 1986 to 15.2% in 1987[9]. These decreases in the use of cocaine (as well as "crack" and other illicit drugs - even marijuana) by high school students were continued into 1988 and 1989. It was hoped this was an indication that the drug epidemic was beginning to wane. A report in the summer of 1989 stated that the use of heroin was making a comeback[10]. It was being smoked in a pipe in combination with crack, lengthening the crack high (which by itself lasts only about a half hour) and reducing the intensity of the depression that follows it. Smoking this mixture was considered to be particularly dangerous because it combined the physical addiction of heroin with the intense high of crack. An interview with 100 drug abusers in New York City disclosed that 37 had used the mixture.

At first glance it might seem that smoking crack (or crack and heroin) at least was safer, in regard to the transmission of HIV, than taking drugs intravenously. But this is not so, because the association between crack and increased sexual activity, including more sex-for-drug transactions, increases the possibilities for the spread of the AIDS virus. The 200,000 intravenous drug (heroin and cocaine) addicts in New York City, who frequently shared needles and syringes, posed a greater AIDS danger in that locale than did homosexual activity.

1.2 Alcoholism

Alcohol abuse involves even larger numbers: 56 million people in the U.S. and costing $117 billion a year (1987), again mostly in lost productivity[11]. At least 10% of those who use alcohol regularly can be classified as alcoholic addicts (consuming amounts that damage their health and society), and the threat of alcoholism to their health and lives is awesome. Average daily consumption of more than, or equal to, 1 ounce of pure alcohol a day (approximately two drinks of wine, beer, or spirits) is regarded as "heavy drinking". The risk of dying from cirrhosis is seven times higher in heavy drinkers than non-heavy drinkers[12]. Cirrhosis of the liver kills at least 14,000 alcoholics each year; alcoholic drivers are implicated in at least half of the 46,000 annual automobile fatalities; 70% of the nations 4000 drownings and a third of the 30,000 suicides each year are believed to be associated with alcoholism. It is said that 20 to 40% of adult admissions to hospitals are alcohol related.

A report from the Institute of Medicine said that light-to-moderate drinkers actually cause more trouble than alcoholics[13]. Even though 10% of the adult population has serious drinking problems, the committee said: "the 60% of the population that consumes light or moderate amounts of alcohol, by the sheer weight of their numbers, is responsible for the greatest proportion of personal and societal alcohol-related problems." Although alcoholics and alcohol abusers have the most severe disorders, moderate drinkers are also vulnerable to a wide range of physical and social problems, including medical diseases, accidental and intentional violence, unemployment, and family discord.

Alcoholism devastates families and contributes to mental illnesses, birth defects, other drug usage and homelessness. Just as drug addicts, alcoholics account for a large percentage (perhaps a third) of burglaries, assaults and rapes. The cost of alcohol abuse and its creation of health problems, both of which are rising steadily, already are greater than those of smoking[14] (although the number of deaths directly due to smoking exceed those directly attributable to alcohol).

The National Institute on Alcohol Abuse and Alcoholism were only getting round in 1987 to comparing the treatment results of various research centers, and distinguishing between the effectiveness of inpatient and outpatient care. They admitted that no one knew what one got for expenditures of $3,000 to $20,000 a month for the inpatient treatment of alcoholism[15].A study reported, in early 1989, that outpatient treatment costing $175 to $388 was as efficient as inpatient care costing $3,316 to $3,665 in having alcoholics (with mild-to-moderate withdrawal symptoms) refrain from drinking for at least six months after completing a program[16]. The majority of the 400,000 people who undergo alcohol detoxification in the U.S. annually, do so as inpatients.

An important pharmacological difference between alcohol or tobacco and cannabis, heroin and cocaine is that the latter three in even small amounts impair cerebral neurotransmission and prevent the brain from functioning normally. Also, the addictive power of the latter two are far more potent: while only 9% of users of alcohol become addicted, 95% of those using heroin and cocaine are compelled to use the drugs on a daily basis. There is evidence that the use of drugs such as cocaine and amphetamines (dopamine agonists) can trigger schizophreniform psychoses even after only a single large dose[17]. It is suspected psychotic attacks after hallucinogen (lysergide and psilocybin) usage, as well as after the use of dopamine agonists, can be long-lasting. There appears to be a clear relationship between cannabis abuse and psychoses. It is not known if incipient psychotic states predispose to drug usage, or the relationship is actually vice-versa.

In contrast to alcohol, smoking has come under considerable public condemnation and is beginning to be viewed, not just as something that is unhealthy or irrational, but as a deviant behavior. In great measure this is so since the wide publicity given the evidence that smoking tobacco can not only be dangerous to its practitioners, but also to those in the vicinity of the smokers. More and more public places are being declared off limits for smoking. Nonetheless, there are a modicum of civil libertarians who aver such bans are abortive of a group's prerogatives. In the 24 years since the Surgeon-General first declared smoking to be dangerous the number of smokers had declined by 1988 from 42% to 26% of the people in the U.S., and the decline was most notable in the last years. As could be expected, the poor, less educated portion of the population continued to have a higher rate of smoking, just as in the use of alcohol and drugs.

Despite its great cost, the public has a seeming indifference to alcohol abuse which causes a hundred times more premature deaths than hard drugs. It is also recognized that alcohol may act as a "gateway" to other drugs. Alcohol does considerable damage to the public - through car accidents and hooliganism as examples. Yet governments do not sponsor anti-alcohol campaigns to match their anti-smoking and anti-drug campaigns. Probably it is that the use of alcohol has been so widespread in so many communities throughout history that it is not politically feasible to attack such a tradition. This attitude is re-enforced by the perceived failure of the prohibition of the use of alcohol in the U.S. over 60 years ago. Some libertarians believe that to seek to influence the nation's health by legislating the price of alcohol curtails individual freedom; also, increasing the cost of alcoholic beverages is certainly not a vote winner. Perhaps society's amused tolerance of alcohol abuse would change if it were realized that such an attitude makes it more difficult to persuade abusers of other drugs to desist.

The prohibition of alcohol by the 18th Amendment and the Volstead Act did not prohibit the use of alcohol or its production for one's own consumption, but it is argued that they did reduce its consumption dramatically[18]. The death rate from cirrhosis was reduced by almost two-thirds, the admission rate for alcoholic psychosis was more than halved and arrests for public drunkenness declined by 50%. There was no recorded increase in violent crimes during Prohibition, despite the publicity on criminal syndicates, gang wars and corruption. Further evidence of the value of restricting alcohol consumption by law was in the Swedish experience: after such laws were scrapped in 1955, there was an instant 50% rise in per caput consumption, followed by a fourfold increase in cirrhosis[19]. Nevertheless, it was argued, by those urging its repeal, that Prohibition was an imposition of the will of a minority upon the wishes of the majority (that used alcohol). That Prohibition was a success, as demonstrated by the above remarks, was contested by others[20].

Recently, stronger laws against driving after drinking alcohol had been enacted in many states. This was reported to reflect a major shift in the attitude of the American public on this particular facet of alcoholism[21]. It was further reported that some object to the strengthening of the drunk-driving laws as an infringement on constitutional rights, such as due process or, as in the case of roadside checkpoints, the absence of probable cause. Despite these questions, their was little opposition to these new laws because their intent, to save lives, was unassailable. Also, campaigns against drunken driving are attacks against individual behavior rather than against the use of alcohol.

That there was some shift in the public attitude to the use of alcohol is reflected in the U.S. Anti-Drug Act of 1988 - it did contain an amendment that required a health warning be placed on all alcoholic drinks. It was to read: "GOVERNMENT WARNING: (1) According to the Surgeon General, women should not drink alcoholic beverages during pregnancy because of the risks of birth defects. (2) Consumption of alcoholic beverages impairs your ability to drive a car or operate machinery, and may cause health problems." The sponsors of this amendment desired a broader and more forceful statement, but they had to compromise for the above watered-down one. In addition, it would be well if the medical profession would lead a campaign to counteract the widespread opinion that alcohol in moderation is healthful. Physicians themselves have supported this erroneous opinion, based on evidence that has been controverted since first reported[22].

France had the highest annual per capita consumption of alcohol in 1988, 13.9 liters; the Soviet Union rate was about 10 liters; the U.S. was 19th on the list at 7.7 liters, followed by the U.K. with 7.1 liters; Japan was next to last at 4.4 liters and Norway last with an annual 4.1 liters per capita.

The Soviet Union in recent years, in efforts to restructure their economic system, observed that alcoholism was exacting a severe toll on their productivity, probably a more serious one than is true of alcoholism in the West. The per capita consumption of alcohol in the Soviet Union was estimated to be one third more than in the U.S.[23] They began a serious government-sponsored campaign against alcoholism with a consensus opinion that abstinence was the only alternative to societal alcoholic problems. It was admitted that total prohibition of alcohol was contemplated even though it was recognized that the use of alcohol is part of the traditional customs of their population. The production of alcohol and the number of retail outlets for its sale were drastically cut back. However, in early 1988 the anti-alcohol measures were substantially modified. The reasons offered were that there was evidence of much illicit distilling and that the long queues at the State liquor stores provoked much anger. Also, the money saved by the populace in the reduction in the use of alcohol was being spent to empty the shelves of other products. This caused unexpected inflation and further strained the government's efforts for peristroika. The failure of the 1985-88 Soviet anti-alcohol campaign reiterated the American experience, and previous Russian ones, with Prohibition. It would seem Prohibition simply does not work, even though statistics appear to show that the amount of alcohol consumed is reduced and health data improved.

Great Britain, of course, also has a severe problem with alcoholism: half of the violent crimes are related to alcohol; a third of the drivers killed in car crashes had more than the legal limit of alcohol in their blood; 10 million work-days are lost annually, and the social cost of alcohol abuse amounts to over $3.75 billion[24]. At least 28,000 excess deaths per year are caused by alcohol in England and Wales. Besides the force of tradition, the anti-alcohol campaign in Britain is blunted by the alcohol industry, as in the U.S.

Another problem in attacking alcoholism in the U.S. is whether it should be regarded as a disease, and thus without moral significance, or is it the result of willful behavior? Even addiction, apparently, is believed by the majority to involve at least an element of personal choice and willful misconduct, and thus raises the issues of values and morality.

The matter came before the Supreme Court in a case regarding the provision of certain benefits to veterans who claimed to be recovered alcoholics. On April 19, 1988 the Supreme Court in a 4 to 3 decision ruled that the Veteran's Administration can continue to deny disability and other benefits to veterans on the basis of alcoholism. This involved the educational benefits under the G.I. Bill, but was not expected to affect benefits for medical disability, to which alcoholic veterans are entitled. The Court made clear, in both the majority opinion and the dissent, that the issue they addressed was not whether alcoholism is a disease whose course its victims cannot control. The key issue to them was what Congress had intended: as to who is eligible for veterans' benefits and what was to be prohibited by the law on discrimination against handicapped people. Nevertheless, the majority opinion did contain the statement: "Even among many who consider alcoholism a 'disease' to which its victims are genetically predisposed the consumption of alcohol is not regarded as wholly involuntary." Also, the majority opinion said that the government's long-standing policy of denying disability compensation to veterans disabled by "primary alcoholism", which was not directly involved in the case, was also valid.

The extent to which alcoholism is the result of willful behavior had not been resolved as of 1989. The National Council on Alcoholism had taken the position that whether any particular individual who drinks will become an alcoholic is largely the results of forces beyond his or her control. Yet, the data (as to how many potential alcoholics abstained before their drinking got out of control and what factors made the difference) still was missing that could indicate how much volition truly was involved. A corollary problem was whether public drunkenness should come under the criminal law and such individuals taken to jail or should they be taken into care. As of 1989, it was the former procedure that was being followed, but, in all probability, most physicians would recommend decriminalization of public drunkenness. For reasons that are not at all clear, similar controversies do not exist with the use of drugs. Drug usage generally has not been regarded as a disease, even if users generally were being treated leniently by enforcers of the law (as compared with drug dealers).

The reasons that alcoholism has been questioned as willful behavior is that an hereditary factor had been demonstrated in some addicted alcoholics, and a difference in its metabolism had been noted in others (including many of those with evidence for inheritance to its addiction). A decreased sensitivity to alcohol due to a difference in metabolism may make it more difficult for such persons to learn to stop drinking before harming themselves. No one believed there was a single gene that caused all forms of alcoholism; rather it was that some people were more predisposed to addictions because of the vulnerability of their nervous systems, which could be genetically inherited. Recently two subtypes of alcoholics have been identified and provided a new viewpoint on the inheritability of alcoholism[25]. Type 1 is characterized by onset after age 25 in either sex, with relatively mild antisocial behavior or occupational problems. Type 2 alcoholics are typically biologic sons of alcoholic fathers and have an earlier onset of social problems, a history of violence with and without alcohol, and a greater chance of drug use.

Studies on twins revealed that identical ones were approximately twice as likely to be in concordance for alcoholism as fraternal twins. Similarly, young children adopted away from alcoholic biological parents and raised in a non-alcoholic family developed many more alcoholic problems as adults than similar adoptees whose biological parents were not alcoholic. Also, several physiological markers have been associated with alcoholism or the risk for it: diminished platelet adenylate cyclase response to a variety of stimulants; diminished lymphocyte adenylate cyclase to adenosine; difference in the pattern of evoked electroencephalogram responses in children born to alcoholic fathers from children of non-alcoholic parents[26].

A possibility that has been regarded as enhancing the argument for alcoholism being "willful behavior" is that the relief from anxiety by alcohol is the basic cause for its addiction. This could be a cogent explanation for its greater prevalence in the poor and disadvantaged minorities, and among those more prone to emotional disorders.

Although the observations on heredity and metabolic factors in alcoholism are undoubtedly true, it should be obvious that these same factors apply to all addictions. Albeit that alcoholism is much more prevalent throughout society than is drug addiction, it still has similar demographic characteristics: it is far more prevalent in the poor, in disadvantaged minorities, and among those more prone to emotional disturbance. Therefore, it is incongruous that it should be sorted out from other addictive states to be viewed differently, on medical grounds, by the courts.

From the point of view of a physician, while many factors leading to any addiction clearly can be regarded as "willful behavior", the addictive state, per se, is a bodily alteration and therefore a disease. Whatever the legal implications of this fact, it does provide a reasonable basis for planning efforts to control the epidemic of substance usage (elaborated upon below).

A consideration that limits viewing alcoholism (and other addictions) as a disease is that, in the liberal atmosphere of present day societies, it would place an enormous burden on the state. If addictions are diseases, then its victims would be eligible for support under the various laws for aid to the disabled and "handicapped". These laws are abused already in the view of many doctors required to review these cases (q.v. Chapter Six); and if alcoholics and drug users were eligible for support, it could be said addictions were being encouraged.

Early in 1988 a company with a large number of employees and providing health care on a self-insured basis decided to deny health-care benefits for ailments resulting from certain "life-style decisions"[27]. These were specified as drug and alcohol abuse, self-inflicted wounds and AIDS proven not to have been contracted from blood transfusions. This decision by the company (a large retailer) was criticized by civil libertarians and advocates for homosexual rights as illegal discrimination against some of its employees. The resulting publicity caused the company to suspend its decision for "review", within a few months after announcing it. The company said it wished to clarify the language and some of the conditional exclusions in its decision, and that it was "extremely concerned about containing the costs of medical insurance for employees." It intended to issue a revised policy on the issue.

1.3 Testing for Drugs

A principal moral dilemma in the problem of drug addiction is the conflict between the public right to test individuals for the use of illicit drugs in an effort to control the epidemic, and the right of individuals not to have their privacy invaded. It is averred that to force or coerce individuals to be tested is in violation of the Fourth Amendment of The Bill of Rights: protecting against illegal search and seizure.

A specific problem was that the urine tests used to screen for drugs were not always reliable, certainly far less than the blood tests for exposure to the AIDS virus. The urine screening tests for drug-use determined only whether an individual had used drugs in the past and did not give any information of any impairment produced, or even if the individual was intoxicated. Moreover, the screening test could be positive for smoking marijuana only once in the 1 to 2 weeks previous to the test and as long as 3 to 5 weeks for chronic users, even if no exposure had occurred in the interim. A heavy intake of poppy seeds, as on rolls, could cause a positive urine test for opium the next morning. Opiates could generally be detected 2 to 4 days after use; but a urine test could not distinguish marijuana from analgesics. Heroin and cocaine disappear within 72 hours of use and the test could not differentiate cocaine from codeine. There were between 10 and 30% of results that were false-positive, many because of individuals having taken medication for upper respiratory infections or allergies. Perhaps more importantly, even as late as 1989, laboratory error in drug testing was rampant: laboratories operating without guidelines, certification or surveillance. The high false-positive rate in drug testing made the statistical objection to its use in low-risk populations particularly objectionable (vide supra under AIDS).

By 1987 improvement in the techniques and use of testing for illicit drugs had taken place, reducing the false-positive rate but markedly increasing the cost and complexity of testing[28]. It was reported the new screening test based on recombinant DNA technology (the EMIT test) was 98% accurate with the error biased toward false-negatives[29]. "Samples that come up positive on the EMIT test are retested with gas chromatography-mass spectrometry for confirmation, a process that renders 100% accuracy".

False-negative reactions always have plagued drug screening tests. These tests are done on urine samples and it was reported up to 10% of samples collected by the military were false samples, and that guaranteed-drug-free urine could be purchased from a number of commercial sources[30]. Many professional athletes are adept at substituting false urine samples, even under direct witnessing of the act of urination. Direct observation of urination is not practical for widespread use and may represent an invasion of privacy. The federal guidelines for drug testing programs do require that the temperature of the urine specimen be measured at the time of voiding to document freshness.

The President's Commission on Organized Crime in 1986 recommended widened testing for drugs. It was pointed out that it is more feasible to cut off the demand for drugs than its supply, because only about 10% of drugs were intercepted on their way to U.S. cities. The Commission suggested that the federal departments should demonstrate the "utter unacceptability of drug abuse" by formulating suitable drug testing programs for their employees and that government contracts be awarded only to companies that similarly test their workers. This recommendation had been opposed by many people including some members of the Commission[31].

Despite extremely vocal opposition, the Reagan Administration through the Office of Personal Management issued guidelines subjecting one million federal workers in "sensitive" jobs to random testing for drug usage. The order covered workers with access to classified information, presidential appointees, law enforcement officers and others in jobs "requiring a high degree of trust and confidence." A worker with only a single positive urine test could be fired and a second offender must be, though the rules stated that the employee who tested positively should have the illicit use of drugs confirmed before being let go. Members of the armed forces regularly had been tested for drugs and, after testing started, a marked reduction in the use of drugs by the military was noted[32]. Results of federal testing programs showed that one in six members of the federal work force had used illicit drugs on a regular basis, and 44% of all new employees had used drugs such as marijuana and cocaine in 1986[33].

The Administration's random screening program was only one part of providing a "comprehensive drug-free workplace" which included education, supervisor training, and employee assistance programs. The increased use of urine drug testing frequently resulted in dramatic reduction in employee drug use. By 1988 the prevalence in the government work force had dropped to between 5 and 10%[34], and in the navy program the indicated use level in enlisted personnel under 25 dropped from 48% in 1981 to less than 5% after 1984[35].

About a quarter of the 500 largest companies in the U.S. required drug testing of job applicants by 1985 and this number were said to be increasing steadily. These companies also tested current employees: workers in high risk jobs, if there was an accident on the job, or if a supervisor reports a suspicion of drug use. The Insurance Institute for Highway Safety found 18% of three hundred truck drivers, who had agreed to drug testing, to have some amounts of illegal drugs in their system, mostly marijuana[36].

In the year between the summers of 1987 to 1988, only 3% of all establishments had a program for random drug testing and less than 1% of the workers in the U.S. had been tested[37]. This was because it was only the largest employers that had programs, and the vast majority of firms are small employers. 7,502 non-government and non-agricultural firms were randomly testing their total of four and a half million workers. Of the 953,100 employees tested, 8.8% tested positively for illegal drugs. This was a lower percentage than had been expected from previous smaller surveys, but was not thought to be conclusive. This report showed that job applicants were more likely to be tested than those already employed. A total of 3.9 million applicants were tested with 11.9% testing positive.

Particular controversy surrounded mandatory testing of individuals in sensitive jobs by the government. For instance, the Federal Aviation Administration in 1986 and early 1987 pondered the advisability of ordering mandatory random tests of airline pilots for drug and alcohol abuse. This was opposed by the pilots' union, and civil libertarians, as being intrusive into the privacy and dignity of the pilots. Testing was agreed to by the union only when there was "reasonable suspicion" of drug or alcohol impairment on the job. No matter how rational it would appear to have mandatory testing of such responsible persons as pilots, it was pointed out that there never has been a fatal accident involving an airliner attributable to drug or alcohol abuse. The slippery slope argument was also invoked: if mandatory testing is legislated for pilots to protect passengers, why not test bus drivers, train engineers, ferry boat captains? Why not truckers? Why not all drivers? Why not then test all employees whose employers cite dangers to others? Thus the apparent "common sense" exception to the principle of respecting civil liberties and individual rights such as mandatory testing of pilots for the protection of their passengers can set a precedent for broad government intrusion on everyone. "Is this not McCarthyism?", asked the libertarians[38].

Other objections to mandatory drug testing programs were that their costs would exceed any possible benefits and the substantial number of false-positive results that would be encountered[33]. A further criticism of the federal drug testing program was that it did not cover barbiturates, alcohol, or any of the thousands of "designer drugs" that had come into use. This latter objection was countered by the statement that the government wished to avoid stigmatizing those on therapeutic drugs and that testing for alcohol would involve major additional costs and catch too many persons. The program would test for the use of marijuana, cocaine, opiates, amphetamines and phencyclidine (PCP).

Mandatory, random drug testing on government employees and American workers was a violation of the Fourth Amendment to the Constitution against unreasonable search and seizure and this right is not limited to the criminal law, according to the Civil Liberties Union[39]. An opposing argument was that mandatory testing is for the good of the person tested, because if drug use is detected the individual then can be treated. This was rejected as paternalism. Apparently in the present climate of medical ethics, paternalism can be cited as being obviously wrong and no further explanation is necessary[40].

The Federal Appeals Court in April, 1987 ruled that mandatory drug testing of applicants for jobs with the U.S. Customs Service was *not* a violation of the Fourth Amendment to the Constitution. For the government to wish to employ individuals free of drug use in a department concerned with drug enforcement "is reasonable and not unconstitutional"[41]. Three other Federal Appeals Courts had reversed lower court decisions that random testing for drugs was illegal: one case involved prison guards in Iowa, another concerned jockeys in New Jersey and a fourth approved random testing for Chicago Transit Authority drivers. A Federal District Judge ordered the army to stop random testing on 9,400 civilian employees in March 1988. He believed the army had failed to prove that random drug testing was necessary to assure safety and security and, therefore, it was an excessively intrusive search prohibited by the Fourth Amendment. He thought it appropriate that his decision be appealed to higher courts[42]. These decisions also seemed to reflect a hardening of public opinion on the subject.

A Federal Appeals Court in California had another view of the problem. It declared, early in 1988, that Federal regulations requiring railroads to test the blood and urine of workers whose trains were involved in specific types of accidents to be unconstitutional. In August 1988 a random drug testing program for the Justice Department was blocked by the Federal District Court of Washington D.C. The Administration had taken this decision to the Federal Appeals Court for review. The Supreme Court agreed to rule on Appeal Court Decisions in the railroad employees and Customs Service cases, and arguments were heard in November 1988.

In March, 1989, by a 7 to 2 vote, the Supreme Court overturned the ruling of the U.S. Court of Appeals for California in the railroad case. The Supreme Court opinion agreed that the tests were "searches" within the meaning of the Fourth Amendment to the Constitution. But their conclusion was that they were reasonable because, on balance, the privacy interests of the workers was diminished against the Government's compelling interest in detecting and determining drug use on the rails, without the need of a showing of "individualized suspicion". For one thing, the opinion went on, a railroad worker can be impaired by drugs, with "disastrous consequences," before any impairment is evident to a supervisor.

In the same session, the Supreme Court upheld the ruling of the Federal Appeals Court that the Customs Service could make drug testing a condition of employment in, or transfer to, certain job categories. The Court, apparently, had more difficulty with this case, their ruling having only a 5 to 4 majority. The Customs Service program, involving a urine test on 5 days' notice, applied to

employees who work directly in intercepting drugs, who are required
to carry firearms, or who are required to handle classified material.
Again, the majority opinion stated the Government did not need
"individualized suspicion" before testing front-line interdiction
personnel or those who carry firearms. These employees, too, have
a "diminished expectation of privacy" .... "because successful
performance of their duties depends uniquely on their judgment and
dexterity." Also, the Governments interest in safeguarding the borders
and the public safety was compelling and outweighed the privacy
interests of these two categories of workers. The Justices did not see
the reasonableness of these principles extending to those employees
of the Customs Service dealing with classified materials, and sent this
part of the testing program back to the Court of Appeals for further
examination.

   An additional argument offered by the union against the U.S.
Customs Service testing program was that its in-service applicant
screening portion would be ineffective (!), since five days notice was
to be given. Workers could abstain or else arrange to adulterate their
urine. Evidence was offered that abstention for five days would
permit light and moderate users of marijuana, cocaine, opiates,
phencyclidine (angel dust) and amphetamines to escape detection by
urinalysis. Justice Kennedy replied, in his majority opinion, that it
would catch the heavy users and furthermore, it was unlikely that
addicts could abstain for even a limited period of time.

   On November 14, 1988 the Department of Transportation had
ordered 4 million non-government workers be randomly tested for
drug abuse. This included about 3 million interstate truck and bus
drivers. Also covered by this order were airline pilots, navigators,
flight attendants and mechanics; railroad engineers, brakemen and
conductors; subway engineers and bus drivers in mass transit systems;
seamen with coast guard licenses, and pipeline workers. A
transportation worker would have a 50% chance of being selected
each year, at random, for a urine test to detect the presence of
marijuana, cocaine, opiates, amphetamines and phencyclidine (PCP).
An initial positive test would have to be confirmed by a second test,
virtually eliminating a possible error.

   This was the first attempt of a government agency to require
random drug testing of non-government employees. The program was
to be started in December, 1989, and the cost was projected to be $2

billion over 10 years, and was to be borne by private industry and local mass transit authorities. However, it was estimated that $8.7 billion would be recovered by a reduction in accidents, decreased absenteeism, and lower costs for sick leave, medical insurance and workmen's compensation. A Federal District Court Judge in San Francisco already by December 1988 had issued an injunction against this random drug testing program at the request of an organization of independent truck drivers. The new Bush Administration, thereafter, voiced their support for the program, and added the tests should not be just for drugs, but for alcohol as well.

In May, 1990, New York State's highest court voted 4 to 3 to uphold random drug testing of jail guards of New York City. This was a shift in the attitude of that court which in earlier decisions appeared to be antagonistic to random drug testing programs that embraced whole classes of workers. The dissenting opinion accused the majority of making an important constitutional right a casualty in the war on drugs. The majority opined that the 10,000 jail guards, by joining a paramilitary force, voluntarily gave up certain cherished freedoms. They pointed out that drug testing was a reasonable addition to a long list of searches the 10,000 jail guards were already subject to because of their jobs, and, furthermore, drug-related disciplinary actions already had been brought against 149 of them in a 32-month period. The decision of this New York court was decried by the Legal Action Center, a public interest group based in Washington, D.C., and the Civil Liberties Union.

Sweden, viewed as a progressive society, nevertheless legislated selective mandatory testing of high school students and routine testing of military conscripts and had halved the addiction rate in their teen-age population[43]. There, it is legal to take babies from mothers who are addicts and jail drug abusers who refuse confinement to treatment centers. These measures, plus a national media campaign, was being more successful in dealing with the problem than was the U.S.

Another example of a conflict between observance of individual liberty and public good is the random breath testing for alcohol in automobile drivers. The English Government rejected such a recommendation by the Department of Transport in 1976 as an infringement on civil liberties. Finland in 1977 legislated a program for random breath-testing of drivers,and over the next five years the drinking and driving rate was more than halved. In this same period, while Finland was having a marked reduction in deaths and injuries from road accidents associated with drinking, Britain had only the slightest decline in these statistics[44]. In the same time period, laws had been passed in the U.S. and abroad mandating helmets for motorcyclists and seat belts for car drivers. These were a comparable infringement on individual rights, but had the general approval of the public, undoubtedly because the number and costs of deaths and injuries prevented were viewed to far outweigh the slight curtailment of individual liberties.

The National Institute of Justice, a research arm of the U.S. Department of Justice, reported in early 1988 that projects which tested and treated drug addicts caught up in the criminal justice system reduced recidivism[45]. A New York State program, which identified drug addicts in voluntary testing of prisoners and then placed them in a residential treatment program for 9 to 12 months before parole, reported 78% had no re-arrests or parole violations over the ensuing three years. By contrast, of a comparable group of prisoners who did not go through the program, only 40.5% avoided violations or arrest.

A pilot program was started in Washington, D.C. in 1984 to try to identify drug users among the 35,000 people arrested each year. After the arrest, each person was asked voluntarily to give urine samples for drug tests. If defendants tested positively, the judge often offered to release them before trial if they would agree to stay off drugs and be tested regularly. In some instances defendants were referred to treatment programs. Only 16% of those who were tested regularly and found to be drug free were re-arrested on new charges, as compared with 32% of those who did not reappear for testing or were found to be continuing on drugs. A great advantage seen for this program was that it reduced prison crowding. The Justice Department had funded similar programs in Indianapolis, Tucson and Portland, Oregon. Spokesmen for the Civil Liberties Union and the Legal Aid Society condemned these programs for violating the rights of the defendants. Even if the tests were voluntary, in their view it amounted to coercion, and possibly was unconstitutional. Moreover, "the results could be computerized and follow these people around for the rest of their lives."

The National Institute of Justice further reported[46] that drug tests obtained voluntarily from 2000 men arrested over a two month period (June and November, 1987) in 12 scattered U.S. cities revealed an average of 70% positive results (range 53 to 77%). This compared with a previous estimate, based on interviews, that 20% of those arrested used drugs. The results of tests on women were not yet available, but preliminary data indicated that drug use was even higher among them. The new finding, based on urine tests on men accused of serious street crimes such as burglary, grand larceny and assault, was taken as overwhelming evidence that drugs were related in a major way to criminal activity. Therefore it was recommended that more money and efforts needed to be allocated to the former, if the latter is to be better controlled.

It appeared, as late as 1989, that the settling of moral problems related to the testing for use of drugs, alcohol and AIDS in efforts to control these epidemics would have to await the arrival of a consensus on the solution of the utilitarian equation involved: the balance between the damage done to society by alcohol and drug abuse and AIDS versus a precedent created by the abridgment of the civil rights of individuals perceived as being necessary to test. Perhaps wider testing for drugs, together with sharper penalties for even occasional use, might discourage those whose only sporadic forays into drugs were said to be the source of the truly enormous profits in this illicit traffic. In the U.S., mandatory random drug testing of urine in the workplace already had been proven to lower the number of positive-testing urine samples, and frequently the drop had been dramatic.

1.4 Controlling the Use of Drugs

Most informed persons seemed to agree that attack on the demand for drugs was the only feasible approach to control their use. Efforts to reduce the supply of drugs, on the whole, had been unsuccessful. Even if the supply were reduced it would only increase the price, and higher prices would increase the amount of crime. By contrast, reducing the demand for drugs would simultaneously reduce consumption, criminality and blunt the threat of the heterosexual transmission of HIV. In an effort to reduce demand, the fundamentalist Islamic government of Iran in the summer of 1989 announced it had rounded up 50,000 drug addicts and confined them to labor camps[47]. It was planned to confine another 150,000 registered drug addicts, and to identify the estimated 800,000 unregistered addicts (in the total population of 55 million). This segregation of addicts followed upon the execution of about 700 drug traffickers in the previous six months. The ultimate effects of these draconian measures should be of interest to the entire world.

The U. S. Federal Government in 1988 estimated there were 1.2 to 1.3 million intravenous drug users, but treatment programs for only 148,000 with a six month wait for anyone wanting to enter a program[48]. The yearly cost in 1988 for treatment ranged from $2,300 per person for drug-free outpatient treatment to $3,000 each for methadone maintenance programs. Long-term residential programs, or therapeutic communities meant to keep addicts in treatment for 18 months, cost up to $14,600 per year per patient. These costs were to be contrasted to those of $100,000, per year per person, to temporarily alleviate the health effects of AIDS, or $14,500 per year to imprison an individual. The report, however, repeated that there was no hard data on the success rate of treatment programs. After 23 years of experience, even the value of methadone maintenance treatment programs was controversial, with the principal data indicating it was mostly ineffective[49]. It should also be clear that methadone does not affect the addictive state: it simply substitutes for heroin a weaker, cheaper, non-AIDS transmitting, and, therefore, a more socially acceptable, addiction. Moreover, methadone is not a substitute for cocaine (or crack), and none is known. Some worried that methadone would "leak" into a black market and, in reaction, the U.S. Government, which supported the methadone clinics, insisted that the clinics include large numbers of counselors and other staff. Such costs limited the number the clinics could serve, and many had to turn addicts away.

The likelihood of discovering the precise mechanism of addiction and then developing drugs for breaking addictions immediately is very real. Advances in neuroscience give promise of finding what changes in brain cells are caused by drugs that arouse the cravings of addiction[50]. Then biotechnology, in all probability, would permit the construction of substances to reverse those changes permanently. It is likely that the control of the drug epidemic will have to await such scientific developments. Many scientists plead that more resources be allocated for these research projects.

It was occasionally suggested that an abridgment of rights, even more drastic than would be required by mandatory testing, may have to be countenanced[51]. Such a proposal was that the isolation or confinement of addicts, especially if infected with HIV, might be necessary, even in the U.S., to control the two epidemics. Communities with, as yet, limited exposure to AIDS and drugs already had decided it was more feasible to proceed in that direction, than to await the widening of the problem.

Despite the opinion of most informed individuals that reducing demand is the most promising way to control the drug problem, it is repeatedly proposed that the supply of drugs be interdicted before it ever reaches the U.S. Some members of the U.S. Congress (over the strenuous objection of the military commanders) suggested that the entire armed forces be used to prevent the importation of drugs. This was being advocated despite the preponderance of evidence indicating (at that time) that it was hopeless to attempt to control the use of drugs by attacks on their supply. Other efforts were directed to dissuading foreign countries from producing or processing drugs. By 1988 the economies of four South American countries (Peru, Bolivia, Colombia, Ecuador) were dependent upon the raising of cocoa and the processing of cocaine. Also, the economies of several Asiatic countries (Burma, Laos, Afghanistan - especially the American-supported rebel zone, Iran, Pakistan, Bekaa region of Lebanon controlled by Syria) were similarly dependent upon the raising and processing of crops for illegal drugs, principally poppies for heroin and other opiates. The U.S. State department said that to make a difference in drugs supplied from these countries, massive infusions of economic assistance to that region would be required[52]. It was estimated that the international trade in illegal narcotics in 1989 amounted to $500 billion, more than the world trade in oil and second only to the arms trade[53].

The attempt to get the producer countries to desist raising crops for the drug trade precipitated confrontations between the third-world and the industrialized nations. The third-world leaders demanded adequate financial support to reduce production (a form of blackmail?) and insisted, bitterly, that the focus of industrialized nations be on the curbing of demand. They also pointed out that the industrialized nations were responsible for the supply of chemicals used in drug manufacturing and of modern arms to drug-smuggling cartels. Speakers for the third-world stated it was an infringement on their autonomy and unacceptable for the U.S. to station warships off their coasts to interdict smugglers.

Some suggested that the only way to control the use of illegal drugs might be to legalize them and divert the enormous profits from the criminal distributors to the state via taxation. The perceived, but disputed, poor experience with the prohibition of alcohol in the U.S. was cited as pointing to this course, and the least that would be achieved is that the criminal distributors would be eliminated. Educational programs enhanced by the money gained from drug taxes might reduce their use in general (as is being effective with tobacco), and the hard core of insane, weak-willed, or young and foolish would remain. Then drug addiction would be clearly one of mental health and not complicated by the criminal aspect which aggravates the problem with these users at present. Yet, would the legalization of drugs permit companies to be formed that could advertise and promote addiction to drugs, just as do manufacturers and distributors of alcoholic products?

Other reasons advanced to legalize the use of drugs were that the criminal justice system, including prisons, was overwhelmed by drug cases and were unable to function effectively (drug cases were said to represent 50% of the workload), and it would sharply cut the annual $8 billion cost of the U.S. drug enforcement effort. A few people with extreme views on the rights of individuals believed laws against drug use (or even drug trafficking) were prohibitions against personal choice and/or conduct, and that they were an imposition of society's moral values on the individual.

Others believed legalizations of drugs should be done on a one by one basis. For instance PCP (phencyclidine) has extremely destructive chemical effects and induces violent behavior and should never be legalized, yet it might make sense to decriminalize marijuana.

A middle ground would combine legal availability of some or all illicit drugs with vigorous efforts to restrict consumption by means other than resort to criminal sanctions[54]. The best model for this view of drug legalization is the tobacco control model advocated by those who want to do everything possible to discourage tobacco consumption short of criminalizing the production, sale, and use of tobacco. Consumption taxes have proven effective in limiting consumption rates of alcohol and tobacco, as has negative advertising.

Most people believed that legalization of drugs would only increase their use and the number of addicts, as was said to be the experience in Great Britain two decades ago, and in Iran from 1968 to 1979[55]. On the other hand, in the 1900's heroin was legal in the U.S. and the proportion of addicts in the population was no higher than it is today. The Netherlands noted a decrease in the percentage of users after legalization of cannabis (marijuana, hashish, etc.)[54].

Another view on the legalization of drugs was that it would be plausible for heroin, but that it would aggravate the problem with cocaine[56]. Heroin is not destructive to the personality of the addict and they can get along for years on regulated daily small doses. Crack addicts go on uncontrolled "binges" that destroy their ability to function in society, even to the point of violent behavior, and, therefore, to legalize it would not reduce crime. Moreover, heroin is expensive - $150 or more per day, and legalizing it could drive down its cost and reduce illegal profits as well as criminal activity of the addicts. Crack was already so plentiful in 1989 that its price was much reduced, costing no more than $50 for a full day's smoking.

Some in favor of legalization of drugs view addicts as self-indulgent and irresponsible, but that they injure no one but themselves. If they die of an overdose, that is their affair and it should be a matter of indifference to the rest of us. The criminal consequences of addiction are largely due to the illegality of drugs, and, therefore, the making of drugs illegal can be viewed as a triumph of moral fervor over common sense, which is helping to produce a disastrous corrosion of law and order throughout the civilized world.

One interesting sidelight of the move to legalize drug usage was the recommendation that, if legalization took place, the drug problem then should be turned over to physicians[57]. The goal of the liberalization of drug laws would be to help users create as little social harm as possible and it was believed physicians "would be likely to make more humane and individually correct decisions." Really this recommendation, unintentionally, was a recognition of physicians role in rationing (see Chapters Three and Eleven).

If legalization of hard drug-use was to be justified by reasoning on its analogy to the failure of prohibition to control and discourage the use of alcohol, then an analogy to the legalization of crime in order to deter criminality, was used by some who were against legalization of drugs. However, this was merely another example of the pitfalls of reasoning by analogy (slippery-slope): it being a truism that it is rare that two circumstances are so precisely identical as to justify the verification of the one, by an experience with the other. The legalization of drug-usage and its supply might well be condoned as a necessary experiment when all other measures for control and deterrence had been given a fair trial and failed, as already might be the circumstance. From an evolutionary ethical point of view there can be no objection to the legalization of drugs when the goal is to obtain control of the epidemic of their use.

Another moral issue that was being debated, increasingly, was whether clean needles and syringes should be supplied to intravenous drug users in an effort to prevent the spread of the AIDS virus. Politicians and public health officials, in cities where I-V drug users congregated, were about evenly divided on this proposition in early 1988, and the Catholic Church was firmly opposed. Some black and hispanic leaders accused those sponsoring the distribution of free clean needles and syringes to lessen the spread of AIDS of being "racists". In addition to the objection that it abetted drug usage, was the belief that the money would be better spent for treatment of addicts. The last objection was probably spurious, since the amount of money involved in a clean-needle-program would be relatively small. That the clean-needle-program would, or would not, be effective in curtailing the AIDS epidemic was the crucial point. Should the distribution of free, clean needles and syringes be proven to limit the spread of the AIDS virus among drug addicts without increasing the use of drugs, and limited data from abroad and Tacoma, Wash. indicated that it did, there could be no adequate reason to oppose it.

Just before the presidential election of 1988, a comprehensive anti-drug bill was enacted by Congress and signed by the outgoing President. It, for the first time balanced the money to be expended ($2.8 billion over two years, in addition to the $3.5 billion previously appropriated) about equally divided between measures to reduce demand and those to limit the supply. However there was only $485 million actually available for added funding at the time of enactment. The previous drug act had appropriated 72% of funding on law enforcement. The new drug act provided that in the years after fiscal 1989, that the 50% of the new funding to go to education programs and the money for making treatment-upon-demand available be raised by 60%.

To help reduce demand, the new legislation for 1989 provided penalties for the possession of any amount of illegal drugs, including marijuana, even if for only personal use. The penalties were a fine of up to $10,000 (depending on income) and permission for courts to suspend federal benefits, such as student or small business loans, federally guaranteed mortgages, etc. However, there were 600 different types of benefits available, and the Act left it to the President to decide by September 1, 1989 which benefits and licenses could be suspended without creating administrative problems, such as a prohibitive amount of increased bookkeeping. Benefits not to be withdrawn were Social Security, Medicare or Medicaid, veteran's or disability benefits or welfare. These penalties and sanctions, to be imposed in a civil hearing which requires only the majority of the evidence to be against the accused, were meant to deter that large population (estimated to be 23 million) not addicted, but who use drugs for "recreational purposes". The Bill did provide the option for the accused to insist on a criminal trial in which a jury could return a guilty verdict only on evidence leaving no reasonable doubt, but the penalty then could include a jail sentence.

The supply side attack was furthered by allowing judges to impose the death penalty on anyone involved in two drug felonies and who committed, or arranged for a murder. If it was a law enforcement officer that was murdered, the murderer need not have a previous record to be condemned to death. Prior to the passage of this bill, federal law provided the death penalty for only two crimes, an act of air piracy or espionage by military personnel. The act further provided for one cabinet-level person, with no other administrative responsibilities, to be the overall coordinator of the federal effort against drugs. Financial institutions would have to strengthen their record-keeping to combat "laundering" of drug money. Chemical makers and distributors were required to file periodic reports on shipment of chemicals that could be used to make illicit drugs.

A proposal to make illegally gathered evidence admissible in court under some conditions (narrowing the exclusionary rule on evidence) was not included in the act, after a serious debate. A Senate proposal that would have mandated random drug testing of transportation and nuclear power plant employees also was eliminated from the final bill. These were concessions to those legislators who feared that these intrusions on the civil rights of individuals would be more harmful than any good that could be accomplished, and whose votes were needed for final passage of the Act. The final measure also required warning labels be placed on alcoholic beverages.

Following upon the above legislation, the Bush Administration, in September 1989, announced its own war on drugs by proposing to increase funding on anti-drug-abuse programs by 118%, to approximately $7.9 billion dollars annually. They recommended that funds for treatment programs were to be increased 53% - from $604 million to $925 million. There was to be an increase of 25% for education and prevention - from $943 million to $1.2 billion; and there was to be increases in prison construction from $734 million to $1.6 billion to provide 95,000 more prison beds. Also, state and local law enforcement matching funds were to be increased from $150 million to $350 million. In addition, schools and colleges were to begin drug-free programs with federal funds; and drug testing was to be required of prisoners, parolees, those who were arrested and workers in sensitive jobs. Also, performance standards for federally funded anti-drug treatment programs were to be established. The entire effort was to be coordinated by, and be under, a federally appointed "drug czar".

The Bush "declaration of war against drugs" received general approbation, both from members of Congress and those outside of government. Some Democratic members of Congress even stated that the funding was still inadequate for the effort required, and that the Bush plan was not bold enough nor sufficiently imaginative, without making it clear what new initiatives they had in mind.

Despite the increased efforts of the U.S. to curtail the supply of illegal drugs, in 1989 the major drug-producing countries sharply increased their production: poppies in Asia, coca in South America, and marijuana in Mexico.

1.5 Summary and Discussion

To reduce the supply of illegal drugs in the U.S. would require that its borders be sealed (200 million cross them annually), mobilization of the military, destruction of foreign sources, zero tolerance enforced, and penalties increased for both dealers and users of drugs. It must be demonstrated that crime does not pay, no matter how deprived that portion of the population from which many dealers and users arise. It is unlikely that these measures could ever be undertaken to an effective degree, either because of domestic or international political considerations[58].

The alternative strategy is to reduce the demand for drugs by increased educational and treatment efforts, and other measures remaining to be tried, as discussed above.

A third strategy is to combine the first two, carried out with as much determination as the entire nation, led by its elected officials, can mobilize. This was the opinion of an influential, usually liberal, newspaper in the summer of 1988[59]. It reversed its previous position by recommending random testing at work or school and abstinence as a condition for bail or parole. These recommendations were added to the call for increase of treatment facilities and broadening of educational endeavors. The enactment of the Drug Act of 1988, to a large measure, pursued this third strategy.

If, as is likely, this combination of measures to curtail the supply and demand for drugs be unsuccessful, it is possible that the option of making addictive drugs legal would be tried. It should be recalled that almost everyone takes some form of mood affecting drug. Alcohol, tea, coffee, tobacco all calm or console or stimulate the mind; tranquilizers and other stimulants are widely used on prescription from doctors. All these legitimate substances also are addictive to a greater or lessor degree. If street drugs were legalized, the billions spent on enforcement could then be used for education and rehabilitation. These billions would be added to by the billions government would collect from the world's largest untaxed business. Also, emphasis could be on spending some of these billions to discover a method that would be certain to break addictions.

In any event, it is probable that the latter course, a crash program in medical research to find a specific medication to treat addiction, should be the focus of governmental efforts.

2. Drugs in Sports

Illicit drugs, especially cocaine, are used by athletes and there have been several well publicized reports of deaths in young athletes from using cocaine alone, or in combination with alcohol. Even more widespread is the use of anabolic-androgenic steroids by young people to increase their bulk, especially their musculature and strength, and increase their capacity to train through speedy recovery from training fatigue. These drugs were developed as synthetic analogues of testosterone in an effort to minimize the androgenic (masculinizing) effect, but maintaining the anabolic (growth-promoting) quality. This has been achieved to a marked degree, but nevertheless they all retain some androgenic power and can cause masculinization of women, in a shorter or longer time depending on dosage and duration of use.

Despite the official opinion that steroids do not help in athletics, there is a general experience among athletes that they do, particularly in sports in which muscle strength is a factor. A survey of the literature gave some credence for the latter opinion[60]. This discrepancy causes a loss of credibility for the medical community as far as the athletes are concerned, and therefore they are unimpressed by physicians' warnings on the bad side-effects of steroids. No deaths from the use of steroids have been reported and the onset of the side-effects are generally delayed, often for years. Moreover, the severity of the side-effects of the anabolic steroids has not been well documented and "there may or may not be serious long-term side effects,"[61].

A study showed that 6.6% of male high school students had used anabolic steroids, and two thirds of these had initiated use when they were 16 years of age or younger[62]. Twenty-one percent of these high school students related that a health professional was their primary source! One report estimates that 1% to 2% of competitors in international sports test positive for steroids; in college competition 5% test positive; and in professional football 7% to 8%[60]. Most informed observers agree that more than 50% of the 9,000 athletes participating in the 1988 Olympics had used anabolic steroids in their training[63].

The anabolic steroids used are synthetic hormones, many available by prescription from physicians, but the greatest number are unapproved by the Federal Drug Administration and brought into the U.S. (principally from Mexico) and distributed illicitly. It was said this market was as much as $100 million annually[60].

The purported ill effects of anabolic steroids are well known, but the desires for fame and fortune are too strong to be resisted, especially by young minority people for whom sports represent their best chance for such successes. Ill effects of anabolic steroids are said to be liver or kidney disease (it was said that jaundice could occur after even short-term use), increased cholesterol production, and reduced resistance to infection. They can lead to aggressive behavior and outbursts of uncontrolled rage (known as "roid rage"). In the long term, there was said to be increased risk of coronary heart disease, stroke, obstructed blood vessels, and liver, kidney and prostate cancer. Other effects, which may never reverse are, in women: masculinization (hirsutism and baldness, deepened voice, breast diminution and clitoral enlargement); and in men: breast enlargement, testicular atrophy and azoospermia, impotence and enlargement of the prostate. When used by pre-teeners and teen-agers they can induce acne and accelerated bone maturation leading to (permanent) short stature. Again, it must be emphasized that the incidence and duration (after discontinuance of steroid) of these adverse effects were not well documented as of 1989[61].

Other drugs used to enhance performance are caffeine and ephedrine which in large doses reduce fatigue. Beta-blockers steady muscular movements and enhance such performance as target shooting. These drugs are taken only sporadically and thus there are no deleterious side-effects. Since they also are used for therapeutic purposes (as treating colds, allergies or, in the case of beta-blockers, hypertension), it could be difficult to ban them. However, since therapeutic or casual use of caffeine or anti-congestants give low urine contents, a case can be made for banning those athletes whose urine content is high at the time of an event.

Are there reasons to object to the use of drugs in sports, other than some have harmful side-effects? Most people have believed in the past, and most still believe, that it is only sporting to "level the playing field" as much as possible. This is demonstrated by classifying many events by weight, especially those requiring strength predominately, and many others by age, and all by gender. In fact, the International Olympic Committee had ruled that the sex of female athletes be verified routinely[64]. Clearly, sporting events are no longer sporting events if some of the contestants use artificial stimuli. Certainly, masculinizing women with anabolic steroids for competition is no different from feminized males competing in female events. "No one would tolerate a racer having coiled springs in his boots! Brass knuckles were ruled out years ago!"

Athletes and their coaches say that *their* use of drugs is "leveling the playing field" because so many of their competitors are using performance-enhancing drugs.

Undoubtedly doctors have prescribed drugs for athletes[62] - and they clearly had been involved in giving transfusions of blood ("blood doping") before races - but illicit drugs also are widely available in gymnasiums and other training facilities where they are distributed by non-professionals[65]. Doctors (those involved in "sports medicine" especially) must resist requests for possibly harmful prescriptions to enhance performance. Indeed it is their *beneficent* duty to campaign against those medications which could have harmful side-effects. The fact that successful athletes become role models adds to the requirement that physicians speak up against drugs and other measures used by some (or now, by many) to gain unfair advantage in competition. It is not apparent what societal good comes from individuals bolstering their performance in sporting events. Doctors have to encourage sports officials to ban drugs in competitive events, and cooperate with them in testing athletes, so as to discourage the use of drugs.

The Bulletin of the Institute of Medical Ethics devoted a whole supplementary issue to drugs in sport[66]. The editor, a frequent contributor to the medical ethics literature, surprisingly used deontological reasoning to reach an opposite conclusion: that there was no logical basis for the International Olympic Committee Medical Commission to ban, or to test for, drugs. He observed that an athlete's use of drugs: "relates to only his own body, so he has not infringed on (his opponents) right to bodily autonomy in any way ....". Also: "The decision of a sports governing body to impose rules that prevent drug taking is therefore inevitably an infringement of the individual's autonomy." This appears to be another example of an ethicist favoring patients' autonomy over doctors' beneficence, and this time with an unbelievable conclusion! This ethicist-editor clearly was confused. Sporting organizations have an obligation to make the competition "even" (i.e. - at one time to prevent professionals from entering competition with amateurs), and to minimize the danger or risk inherent in any sport. Obviously, drugs can increase the risks!

It is interesting that, elsewhere also, efforts to test athletes for drug usage were resisted as an infringement of a competitor's personal rights. The U.S. National Collegiate Athletics Association (NCAA) had outlawed drugs to enhance performance and required random drug tests throughout the year. Two Stanford University students challenged these rules in court, pleading that it was an invasion of their constitutional right to privacy. A California state court agreed with them in 1988, but the NCAA said it would continue its drug testing program, exempting Stanford athletes, while appealing the decision.

Others believed that if an athlete tested positively for the use of drugs, sports organizations should protect the confidentiality of the athlete: "If the athlete or someone else wants to speak up, that is their right."[67] Of course others viewed the situation differently, believing, if drugs are to be eliminated from sports, users have to be exposed.

Anyone with an evolutionary approach to ethics would not likely be distracted by deontological reasoning based on the primacy of individual autonomy. The prescribing of drugs to enhance immediate athletic performance at the expense of probable, or even only possible, future disability should not pose a difficult equation for physicians to solve, even if an evolutionary answer is not always immediately apparent in most other medical ethical dilemmas. Further, there is no perceivable overall advantage to a community that would be derived from an enhancement of individual performance in sporting competition.

CHAPTER SIX. PUBLIC HEALTH POLICY AND INDIVIDUAL RIGHTS (CONTINUED)

1. Rights and Psychiatry

In the evaluation of morality in relationships, both between individuals and between the individual and society, it is assumed that individuals are rational. Individuals who are severely irrational, or whose irrationality is sustained, most often are held not to be morally or legally accountable for their actions. When the irrational behavior consists of the threat of bodily harm to others, there is no dispute as to their right to be protected from such an irrational act. Even the irrational person is believed to have the right to be protected from doing bodily harm to his- or herself. If the irrational act is only one of annoyance to, or interference with, the public and/or harmful to the place in society or career of the perpetrator, the right to protection from the irrational behavior is less freely granted.

With an increasingly liberal approach to individual rights continuing in Western democracies, their legislatures and courts have been more and more loath to interfere with the freedom of individuals, even if the individuals are accused of being irrational. It is difficult to assess degrees of annoyance to society or interference with its activities, and easier to evaluate the consequences of threats of bodily harm, so it is the latter that most often is chosen to be the basis for ordering the restraint of irrational people.

Hesitancy to order restraint of irrational people is added to by the fact that the determination of irrationality is a matter of judgment and all, but especially judges, are familiar with qualified psychiatrists testifying on both sides of the question in the same individual. In truth, even today, psychiatric diagnosis is very much a subjective matter and not anchored on agreed objective criteria[1], and the rate of disagreements for specific diagnostic categories often equals or exceeds rate of agreement[2].

Irrational behavior is most often episodic and its treatment and prognosis can still be a matter of dispute[3], all adding to the dilemma of formulating policy that can properly protect the various rights involved. As in all dilemmas of conflicting rights, zealots further confuse the situation by demanding precedence for their perceived (usually *a priori*) point of view, no matter what that would entail as a consequence.

For instance, libertarians are in favor of protecting the right to freedom of action of even irrational people in all but the most flagrant instances (such as clear threat of bodily harm). They cite slippery slope reasoning as the basis of their position - failure to protect the freedom of the mentally deranged will be followed, step by step, by infringement on the freedom of all. Some go so far as to state that liberty is more valuable than mental health and that no one should be deprived of his freedom for the sake of his mental health[4,5]. Moreover, it is stated if persons become demented, it is because of "the system" in which they live. Foucault in 1965 published his *History of Insanity* expressing the same point of view, and based his opinion on historical facts that he subsequently is accused of treating with "a laxity bordering on disdain"[6] (see below for further discussion of "antipsychiatry").

The association of the success of Western civilization with the increased rights of the individual also gives support to the position of the libertarians. In their righteousness, however, the libertarians fail to recognize the validity of the Aristotelian concept of a mean position on most, if not all, issues. Those who take an extreme position on the solution of any question are too often characterized by an inability to contemplate any modification of it. As a result conflict is deepened, conflict that could have been avoided or shortened if humans were less zealous. Unfortunately, zeal in situations other than moral conflict has been a most important ingredient for human advance and this characteristic probably cannot always be sorted out and made suitable to the occasion.

Thirty years ago civil libertarians, including many lawyers, decided that individuals confined to mental institutions were having their right-to-freedom compromised. They attacked the laws on involuntary commitment as an infringement on the right of an individual to freedom. Strengthening their position were undoubted instances of wrongful commitment, and retention of some patients under commitment for unnecessary lengths of time ("warehousing of patients").

Included in the movement against involuntary commitment were the "antipsychiatrists", a group that included even some psychiatrists. They denied that mental illness even existed, and claimed the diagnosis of mental illness was really a device for exerting social control over annoying or unconventional people. Unfortunately they could use what was taking place in the Soviet Union as an example: political dissidents being diagnosed as mentally ill and confined to mental institutions. These antipsychiatrists, since they did not accept the diagnosis of mental illness, and some libertarian associates who felt nothing should compromise an individual's freedom, took the extreme position of being against involuntary commitment under any circumstance. This extreme position in the 1970's took the passage of only a modest amount of time for its consequences to emerge in the 1980's: the mentally ill being a major, if not the principal, element in the problem of the homeless. The position of the antipsychiatrists was contested on philosophical as well as clinical grounds, with great cogency, by an experienced clinical psychiatrist[7,8].

The more liberal portions of the community supported the attack against the involuntary institutionalization of mental patients, their position being that patients' rights would be better observed, and it would be more humane, if patients could be provided for "in their communities". This objective was pursued prior to increased provision having been made for the care of these patients in the community and without scientific evidence that, in fact, community care could be efficacious[9].

It should be noted that new anti-psychotic drugs had been created that added to the optimism that mental patients could be cared for in the community. This, nevertheless, proved to be, to some extent, illusory - both because the drugs did not perform to the degree expected of them, and because of the frequent failure of patients to take medications as directed, or failing to take them at all.

Another claim that proved to be illusory was that increased environmental stimulation would be beneficial, especially to those with negative symptoms. Negative symptoms are poverty of volitional acts or of emotions due to schizophrenia and/or depression. While improvement occasionally occurred, on the whole, negative symptoms were handicaps to patients for adjusting "in the community", and the added stress of the demands of community living more often added to their problems.

In summary, the "return to the community" dictum for mental patients can best be viewed as an ideologic rather than a therapeutic movement.

Another important fact supporting the libertarian and liberal approaches was the feelings of guilt so natural to families of mental or severely handicapped patients. The guilt feelings prevailed until the release of their relatives from institutions disrupted their lives. Now that most institutions for the mentally handicapped are emptied out, the parents of mentally handicapped people are overwhelming in favor of retaining such hospitals[11].

Other circumstances conducive to the civil libertarian purpose of reversing the previous approach to involuntary commitment were: first, the trend to liberalism so characteristic of Western democracies (Italy passed a law in 1978 to gradually phase out all of its psychiatric hospital); and secondly, the cooperation of state authorities who collaborated because they saw a partial solution to their chronic budgetary problems by deactivating mental institutions, perceived as inordinately expensive anyway. The change in atmosphere created by increasing medical malpractice suits in the U.S. (fueled in part by the rising emphasis on patients' rights) undoubtedly further reduced any remaining ardor of psychiatrists for involuntary commitment procedures. In the U.S. the number of institutionalized mental patients fell from 500,000 in 1950 to 100,000 in 1982, despite a 1/3 increase in the total population of the country in the same period of time. The figures for the U.K. were roughly similar, in proportion: in England, the number of psychiatric beds peaked at 148,000 in 1954 and in 1990 there were about 64,000 remaining.

Michels and Eth[10] pointed out how premature was the shift from institutional to purported community psychiatric care, and the lack of research evidence to support such a move. Indeed, the net result was a reduction in available facilities of any kind for psychiatric care. They stressed that the impact on patients' families was deleterious and that the negative impact on the neighborhoods was often striking. Nevertheless they offered, what they believe to be,

philosophical support for community care rather than institutional
care of psychiatric patients[10]:

> "Behind any discussion of the choice of
> a specific mental health policy looms an
> unarticulated question of competing models
> of ethical theory. For example, some would
> argue that institutionalization of the mentally
> ill is preferable because it protects the family
> and neighborhood from the burdens and risks
> of community care. The proponents of this
> policy might not realize that the foundation
> of their belief is the contemporary ethical
> theory of rule utilitarianism. The utilitarian
> approach to social justice tends to favor the
> greatest good for the largest number. With
> society as a reference point, utilitarians would
> argue that the largest number of people are
> served by the distant incarceration of the
> mentally ill. Since no one can accurately
> predict whether a given citizen will become a
> psychiatric patient or remain well, there is no
> *a priori* discrimination in a hospital-based
> system. Further, since there are far more
> healthy community residents who benefit from
> the hospitalization of the few who are ill, the
> moral calculus points toward hospitalization.
>
> "The position favoring a community
> mental health center policy might be
> supported by a different ethical theory - one
> that emphasizes concern for the distribution
> of sacrifices imposed by a mental hospital
> based system. It would argue that the major
> burdens of an institutional system of care falls
> on the patients who are already the
> unfortunate victims of mental illness. Justice
> would be better served by a policy that allows
> patients already afflicted by mental illness to
> be compensatorily rewarded by a system that
> favors their care. in this way the interests of

the well majority are overridden in order to provide advantages for the ill minority. The philosopher Rawls (1971) convincingly advocated a procedure for producing this outcome.

"In Rawls' procedure, a community member is asked to imagine the following hypothetical situation. He is to act reasonably but is to decide on a plan while cloaked in a 'veil of ignorance'. That means he is completely unaware of his own age, social status, natural assets and liabilities, interests, etc. He does, of course, have a general idea of human nature, including the values of personal well-being, functional capacity, and the happiness of fulfilling life's goals. For example, the goal of this thought experiment would be for the community member to choose a plan for psychiatric care for the mentally ill - either community or hospital based. He is assumed to have a natural and typical self-interest but will choose fairly and without exploitation since he must make the decision without knowing whether he himself is, in fact, mentally ill or not. Our anonymous community member, unaware of whether he is a patient, a relative, or a neighbor must choose a plan for psychiatric care. He will certainly wish to maximize the general welfare but will be careful not to ignore the few who are most impaired since he himself might well be one of them. The greater risks of deterioration in a state hospital must weigh more heavily than the lesser risks of the smaller harms to family and neighbors in the community care of the mentally ill. Further, the certain deprivation of a patient's personal freedom within an institution is unmatched by the potential loss of liberty a relative or neighbor might suffer. Although the deleterious effects of community care are well documented, they would fall predominantly on the well relatives and more advantaged community members. Consequently, anyone blind to his status as patient, family, or neighbor would seek to avoid the devastating loss of liberty and danger of deterioration involved in institutional care. However, from the family and community perspective one would demand local mental health resources to minimize the largely avoidable social sequelae of insufficient aftercare and support. In a well-funded community mental health system everyone is entitled to the same degree of personal freedom of movement. The burdens and harms of community care that do exist would tend to spare the already disadvantaged mentally ill, who would also be the recipients of the principal benefits. The intrinsic fairness of this pattern of distribution is based on the premise that the inequalities of mental illness are open to all and are of such magnitude as to demand special consideration."

It was felt necessary to give this extensive quotation to illustrate the theoretical confusion that besets the problem of rights in the psychiatric field. The rationality of Michels and Eth in favoring their formulation of the Rawlsian approach for the care of mental patients, especially after so clearly having reported on the failure of community care of mental patients, escapes me. The need is only, by preliminary investigation, to be certain of consequences and then make adequate preparations before there is application of any abstract principle.

The success in closing or reducing the size of mental hospitals in the 1960's and 70's spawned, or made more obvious, another problem in the 1980's: the homeless, particularly in the rigorous climate of the northern cities. There were no accurate figures (as of early 1990) on the number of people who were homeless in the U.S.: some estimated 2 million, while the Department of Housing and Urban Development estimated 350,000, a figure supported by a study in 1986 by the National Bureau for Economic Research[12]. The Bureau of the Census is committed in 1990 to determine the number of homeless as accurately as possible.

Though the data were not clear it was agreed that a large, if not the largest, percentage of homeless people was the mentally disturbed who previously would have been institutionalized when they became too disruptive to be tolerated at home[13]. A sampling of New York's homeless in 1987 revealed that 96% had at one time been in a psychiatric hospital[14]. In Washington D.C. St. Elizabeths Hospital, the capital city's mental institution, had been reduced from 8,000 inpatients in 1950 to about 1700 in 1988, with "the problem of the mentally ill...literally spilled into the streets"[15]. A panel of the National Academy of Science reported late in 1988 that lack of affordable housing was only part of the problem and that the vast majority of urban homeless suffer from major dysfunctions, many of which preceded homelessness[16]. A study, done in Philadelphia, found that 78% suffered either from mental illness, substance abuse, or severe personality disorders; a comparable figure from a Boston survey of adults in shelters was 90%; a 1989 report on the homeless in Baltimore stated 80% of women and 91% of men had serious mental problems, including 41% of women and 31% of men with either schizophrenia or manic-depressive disease[17]. In Great Britain, too, a study reported in 1989 revealed that the largest component of long stay residents in hostels for the homeless were severely affected psychiatric patients discharged into the community[18].

Another consequence of the policy of deinstitutionalization was an increase of criminal acts, including purposeless murders, by individuals obviously demented and whose families failed in their efforts to commit them involuntarily; or else such people had been discharged from mental institutions, obviously prematurely. Also, the closing of public psychiatric institutions caused a tripling of the private care sector for hospitalization of psychiatric patients (to 35% of the total number of such beds in the period from 1975 to 1990) [19]. This may be viewed as a further tiering, according to wealth, in the care of psychiatric patients. Also, It became apparent that releasing long term mental patients into the community raised the issue of the need for new long term social care as well as new psychiatric services. Nonetheless, in the U.S., community mental health centers tended to concentrate on psychological treatments for people with minor disorders[20].

Of course the most zealous on behalf of the homeless and in decrying the lack of public support for the homeless are the ones whose previous zeal had been so instrumental in creating the problem. The situation of the homeless was critical and required attention but what causes wonder is that prime creators of the problem continued to take center stage, unabashedly, and with continued great righteousness. As late as 1988 a panel of the National Academy of Science (NAS) charged with examining the health problems of the homeless and made up of health care professionals (not practicing physicians) expressed outrage at the plight of the homeless and recommended more housing and extension of health insurance to them[16]. The president of NAS thereafter commented: "the language was charged and polemical and emotional" and that the recommendations went beyond the expertise of the panel. In early 1989, a feature article in a leading United States newspaper, reviewing the homeless problem and its causes, did not even mention the closing of psychiatric facilities or the mental status of those homeless[21]. Also, an editorial in the Journal of the American Medical Association, by a presumed expert on the problem, commenting on the dimensions of the mental disease in the homeless, nevertheless said: "We must complete the deinstitutionalization of the mentally ill we began 30 years ago by providing adequate housing, halfway houses, outpatient mental health care, crisis intervention, brief inpatient treatment programs, and longer inpatient treatment for those that need it."![22]

By 1987 legislatures were reversing their stand on involuntary commitment. The newest changes reversed the previous trend that made bodily danger to themselves or others the only legal grounds for involuntary commitment. Six states already had adopted, by 1987, a new standard that made it possible to involuntarily commit mentally disturbed people who were unable to provide for their own basic needs, such as shelter, or who would "suffer an abnormal mental, emotional, or physical distress" if they were not hospitalized. In two thirds of the remaining states legislation for similar changes had been proposed. All such changes were in keeping with a model law devised by the American Psychiatric Association in 1983. While these changes were strongly supported by psychiatric associations and organizations of patients' families, they were vigorously opposed by some mental health administrators and still by some civil libertarians and lawyers. The administrators were fearful of the overcrowding and actual lack of facilities in institutions which had been curtailed, and not yet restored. This in fact became the situation in those states which had already made involuntary commitment easier.

Another facet of the law, at least up to 1989, that made treatment more difficult, and possibly had prolonged the stay of some patients in institutions, was that many courts had ruled that patients, no matter how irrational, had the right to refuse treatment. Many ethicists supported these judicial decisions (and may have contributed to them). Lawyers not only pleaded that it was a patient's right to refuse medication but also that drugs used for mental illness commonly had side-effects, such as tardive dyskinesia. Courts had sustained the right of even involuntarily committed patients to determine their own treatment or at least have their objections to treatment reviewed by a court[23].

In February 1990, the Supreme Court decided that prisoners could be forced to take anti-psychotic drugs against their will and without a court order, as long as the medical decision is subject to a fair review by prison doctors and officials. The majority (6 to 3) opinion stated "an inmate's interests are adequately protected, and perhaps better served, by allowing the decision to medicate to be made by medical professionals rather than a judge." Experts were reported to have said the same principle conceivably could be applied to thousands of mentally ill persons involuntarily confined to mental institutions, but not unless greater protection would be given to doctors and hospitals under state constitutions or laws[24].

A review of confinement for mental disease around the world, published in 1988, stated that hospitals in the West were continuing to release patients. But in the East (Japan, China, India, Bangladesh) the number of psychiatric inpatients was growing all the time, with blatant denial of the civil rights of many, particularly in Japan[25]. The author of this review ruefully concluded that neither trend appeared to benefit the patient and "after 30 years, the temptation for many seems to be to pillory community care as yet another solution that has failed...". Actually, he observed, discharges from mental institutions in the West were too precipitous and too broadly carried out, before community facilities were prepared.

There was yet another deleterious aspect of the diminution of public hospital facilities for the care of severely ill mental patients. Psychiatrists complained in 1988 that many such patients had nowhere to obtain the modern, psychopharmacological treatment then available for their illnesses, but which can only be administered in an inpatient setting[26].

The solution of the dilemma arising between the rights of mentally disturbed individuals and the rights of their families and the public, according to the evolutionary theory of rights proposed in this book, lies in the evaluation of the consequences of giving priority to one side or the other. This essentially utilitarian approach requires that data be accumulated before change is made on the importuning of zealots who had drawn their conclusion from what appears to them as obvious (*prima facie*) logic.

Wyatt and DeRenzo[27] had pointed out, in an editorial in Science, that America's homeless crisis began in 1963 when de-institutionalization became law and hundreds of thousands of mentally disabled patients were released from large institutions to the streets. "This situation occurred because a social welfare movement, based on virtually no scientifically gathered data, became public policy". They found no reason to believe that current concern for the homeless and the inadequate solutions offered would not create new, possibly more serious problems. They pleaded for well-controlled studies to be designed and carried out, no matter how difficult, before new mistakes were made as the result of the inordinate drive for action in our "feeling" community.

The rational approach, as recommended above, in 1989 appeared to be a distinctly utopian one. The wonder is that rational solutions are ever attained at all. However, in truly democratic societies they eventually are achieved in important issues because they touch enough of the electorate for the majority to enforce the view that best serves them. It may well take an inordinately long time for this to occur, but all that is required is that democracy be preserved, and that it not be permitted to be destroyed, or abridged by zealots or fundamentalists - no matter how well motivated or moral they appear.

For instance, the Soviet Union, which had not had a democratic system, appeared in 1987 to becoming a more "open" society. This can be said to be the result of the compulsion of economic competition, now that war is not an option - because of the impossibility of contemplating an atomic one. It might be said that an evolutionary change is occurring in their culture with the civil rights of the individual, so necessary for economic efficiency, receiving more emphasis. Thus, under the glasnost and peristroika of Gorbachaev, a party publication condemned arbitrary diagnosis and abuse of power in Soviet psychiatry[28]. While the article did not refer to the previous labeling of political dissidents as mentally disturbed, it specified similar abuses in other situations - which certainly was a large step in that direction. This was followed, in January 1988, by the Soviet authorities promulgating new laws giving patients, or their families, the right to appeal psychiatric diagnoses in court. The authority over "special" psychiatric units, which were used to confine dissidents, also was transferred from the Interior Ministry to the Health Ministry.

2. Rights of the Handicapped and Disabled

The individuals in this category are numerous and varied. Included are children born with physical and/or mental disability, adults with physical and/or mental disability, adults with chronic diseases or who have lost a limb, sight or hearing. Adults often are included whose mental disturbances can be classified as only aberrations. It is generally agreed for purposes of legislating access to, and construction of, buildings and public facilities that 5% of the population is physically disabled. The library of Congress estimated that there were 43,000,000 Americans in 1989 with some form of mental and/or physical disability or handicap.

The liberalization in the attitudes of Western societies, already abundantly referred to, has been extended to these groups, and some would say overextended. Contributing to the public sympathy for the disabled is the special responsibility felt for the relatively small number resulting from wars. The activity and visibility of the disabled veterans of the Vietnam War, in particular, has contributed to the recent political clout of the disabled. The disability rights movement has been encouraged by the relatively recent scientific advances of our culture. Innovations in medical care has kept many of them alive and in relatively good health, as for instance paraplegics and even quadriplegics; the development of computers has allowed the hearing and speech impaired to use telephones; the advancements in motorized wheel chairs has given many more mobility and permits them to do more for themselves with the potential for enjoying fuller lives.

An elaborate bill of rights already had been set for them by law: to be educated to the limit of their capacity "in the least restrictive environment" and at public expense; to join the regular work force and not to be discriminated against in this endeavor; the right to be supported if unable to work. Despite only 5% of the population being physically disabled, a 1988 amendment to the Fair Housing Act in the U.S. requires 100% of new residential buildings and its units be made accessible to the handicapped, at severe increases in costs for all. Some localities (as New York and New Jersey) already had even more restrictive building regulations, such as including all residential units being renovated as well as new ones, and requiring all units be included, not just those built with public funds. The building codes of most localities require only 4% or 5% of all units constructed be provided with facilities for the physically handicapped.

The two ethical questions involved are to what extent the community at large should be taxed to support the rights of the disabled, and how far to extend the classification of handicapped and disabled? The latter problem arises, in particular, as to whether the mental and emotional aberrations arising from the complexities of living qualify one to the rights of the disabled? The same problem is encountered in classifying the victims of certain disease processes such as AIDS. An added aspect of these problems is: how much disability need be present for an individual to acquire the rights of the handicapped?

In 1973, Congress passed the Rehabilitation Act forcing those facilities which were built with federal assistance to modify any physical features that could be an obstacle to the handicapped. This has caused the expenditure of billions of dollars on school buildings, mass transit systems and sidewalks of towns and cities. There are no studies on the cost effectiveness of these expenditures in alleviating the plight of the handicapped. Isolated reports question the effectiveness of this law. For instance, in New York 1,362 buses had wheel chair elevators and only 10 to 20 people per day used them. Subway station elevators cost $1 million each and there were 88 decaying stations in New York City. The City could not find the money to both rehabilitate the stations and add the elevators too[29]. The elevators in systems so equipped are seldom used - in Washington, D.C. 29 disabled per day use the elevators and in Atlanta only 5. Because of the law millions of non-handicapped passengers are inconvenienced, or even endangered, because this restriction on the use of limited funds prevents their application for normal maintenance of public facilities.

As of the summer of 1989 the likelihood of requiring empirical evidence of the net benefit of modifying structures for the handicapped was small or non-existent. Indeed, legislation was pending in the U.S. congress (Americans with Disabilities Act) to extend to private industry the existing laws prohibiting federal agencies and federal contractors from discriminating against the handicapped in hiring and promotions. The pending bill even would broaden the provisions of the 1973 act to require employers to provide special services and devices for those with impaired hearing or vision. Also, the new measure would mandate elevators in new commercial and public buildings of more than two stories and provide the disabled with the means to enter and exit (including restaurants, lodgings, places of entertainment, doctors' offices, etc.). The telecommunications industry calculated it would cost $250 to $300 million per year to provide service to people with hearing or speech impairments. The Greyhound Bus Company asserted it would have to spend $40 to $80 million annually to equip their new buses with wheelchair lifts, and that any such increase in costs would necessarily decrease their services to small towns.

A separate measure, the Civil Rights Act of 1990, also was introduced in Congress which amended the 1964 law to permit compensatory and punitive damages for victims of job discrimination, including the handicapped and disabled. This bill was supported by a coalition of civil rights organizations that included groups representing people with disabilities. They argued that the threat of large jury awards was the only effective way to insure fair treatment of blacks, women and the handicapped or disabled in hiring and promotion. Business groups, on the other hand, feared a rush of litigation and of huge awards from juries. The threat of unlimited damages for plaintiffs in job-bias suits would have a chilling effect on personnel decisions and force companies to hire and promote unqualified people to keep themselves out of court. The National Association of Manufacturers feared, especially now that 43,000,000 disabled or handicapped people would be added to those covered by civil rights legislation, that the nation would go down the same road taken in the product liability problem[30].

The Federal Government itself already was spending between $70 and $75 billion per year on the handicapped by 1989 (via more than 50 programs) and it was admitted that the added costs of the pending new act, or its net benefit and inherent justice for the whole of society, were unknown. Another doubtful aspect of the bill was its definition of disabled - a physical or mental impairment that "substantially limits" an everyday activity like walking talking or working - is so broad that it includes about 43 million people or one in five Americans. Conditions included were: arthritis, AIDS, reformed alcoholics, and drug abusers; excluded were people with emotional disorders like kleptomania and compulsive gambling. The Americans with Disabilities Act was receiving broad support in both Houses of Congress and a lobbyist for the U.S. Chamber of Commerce was quoted as saying: "No politician can vote against this bill and survive."[31]

In addition to sympathy for the disabled and the recognition of their "rights", a more pragmatic motivation for helping them perform and/or become more mobile should be noted. It is that in many of the developed industrial nations there was, or still is, a labor shortage. Insofar as the measures that train or make the disabled more mobile help answer labor shortages, that should be entered into the equation determining their economic utility. Precise data on this point would be helpful, and the recital of anecdotes is only distracting.

In 1975, the Education for All Handicapped Children Act was passed in the U.S. and in the next decade it resulted in expenditure of over $8 billion. By 1987 one in each 10 public school children was covered by this act, about 4.3 million children in all. Proponents said this law, by compelling schools to place handicapped students in regular classes, had shown that separate, isolated education was not necessarily in the best interests of the disabled. It was also said to be a model inspiring advocacy for the handicapped in other spheres of life and increased the likelihood that handicapped children could be brought closer to being self-sufficient adults.

Critics said that the law had proved to be too expensive and that it had led to tens of thousands of normal students being classified as disabled. It had led, for example, to compulsion of a school to provide periodic catheterization for a spina bifida child and thus a school board expenditure for one mentally defective and physically handicapped child of more than $25,000 per year. It was said the law has led to more classroom disruption by emotionally handicapped children who were required to be placed in the "mainstream".

The Supreme Court, in January 1988, upheld decisions by lower courts which interpreted the 1975 law to mean that disruptive, emotionally disturbed children cannot be expelled or removed from public schools for more than 10 days, even to protect others from physical assault, without the permission of parents or a judge. The Court, in their 6 to 2 decision, said that Congress did not trust school officials to protect the rights of disabled students they consider disruptive. The Department of Education reported that there were 385,000 children, or 8.7% of those enrolled in the special education program in the 1986-87 school year, described as "emotionally disturbed"[32].

Of course many anecdotes were available of remarkable success with isolated instances of handicapped children because of this law. The real problem was that there were no comprehensive data available, with suitable control studies, upon which valid conclusions could be reached as to the true effectiveness of the law; or even as to whether the good results achieved outweighed the harm done to the community as a whole.

Another aspect of the rights of the handicapped was addressed by the authorization by The House of Lords in England for the sterilization of a mentally handicapped girl[33]. This epileptic 17 year old with the mental understanding of a six year old child was noted to have an uncontrollable sexual drive. It was judged she could not handle ordinary contraceptive techniques. Should she become pregnant, it could not be diagnosed in time to abort her because of her obesity and usual menstrual irregularities. Further, since she would panic with the usual pains of delivery she would need to be heavily sedated making vaginal delivery dangerous. Therefore Caesarean section would be necessary. Should she have a section done, it was judged she probably would open up her abdominal wound repeatedly. For these reasons and for her own best interests, sterilization was authorized. This reversed a lower court decision that stated a non-therapeutic sterilization was an intrusion into the rights of a mentally handicapped individual. Even if the women had reached the age of majority, the Law Lords argued, the common law principle of *parens patriae* - that the state can look after those who cannot look after themselves - would apply. The lower court had denied the application of this principle.

Despite their authorization in the above case, the Law Lords made clear that a doctor would still need a court order for sterilization in other similar cases; the consent of the parents would not be sufficient authorization. It was also emphasized that authorization was on the basis of the handicap's welfare and not for the good of society. In February 1988 the Iowa Supreme Court in a 7 to 1 decision said lower courts could authorize the sterilization of mentally retarded people but refused to say when such a procedure was appropriate.

In late 1989 it was reported that laws for the sterilization of the mentally retarded were being enacted, and the procedure widely applied, in China[34]. The purpose of the law was to raise the quality of the population and of the Chinese nation. Geneticists criticized the policy on the basis that it would not significantly decrease the number of retarded children born. It was likely that less than half of mentally retarded persons acquire their disease genetically. Also, about 1% of the world population suffer from mental retardation and it would take about 20 generations to reduce the frequency of a gene from 1% of the population to 0.1%. It should be recalled in this connection that there have been less than 300 generations in all of recorded history. These last facts are the best arguments against eugenic movements.

The same concerns as expressed for the institutionalization of the mentally ill several decades ago were voiced on behalf of the mentally deficient and handicapped. The result was the closing of many state institutions in the early 1970's with the call for the providing of group homes for the handicapped and mentally retarded. Such group homes were never set up in sufficient numbers or with adequate facilities to compensate for the loss of state institutions. The population of the retarded and handicapped in state institutions dropped from 141,000 in 1977 to 91,000 in 1988, despite the far greater overall population in the latter year. Many mentally retarded had now to be cared for at home, to the anguish of their parents and relatives. The pressure was kept up on the remaining state facilities with demands that the severe mentally retarded be given more instruction and recreation, and indulged in more adequate "verbal exchange"[35]. Even though these remaining institutions were greatly improved, "the staff members at most, rather than teaching basic eating and bathing skills, simply toileted, bathed, groomed and fed the clients, sometime with no verbal interchange at all."

In desperation many families took advantage of that provision of the Medicaid Law which paid for care in nursing homes and placed many retarded and mentally ill relatives in them. The average annual cost of caring for a patient in a nursing home was $25,000, and in 1986 the outlay by Medicaid on nursing homes was $15.8 billion (42% of the $38 billion spent by Medicaid). Nursing homes were required to provide only custodial and very limited nursing care. The number of patients who were confined to nursing homes solely because of mental illness or retardation was not precisely known: estimates ranged from 33%, of the 1.6 million nursing home residents by the National Institute of Mental Health, to 4% by the nursing home association.

Congress, led by a liberal House committee chairman, stating their purpose was to assure that the mentally ill and retarded would receive the psychiatric and specialized treatment they deemed was needed (but also in an effort to reduce the costs of Medicaid), amended the federal budget legislation of 1987. This new law required that, after January 1, 1989, nursing homes refuse admission to people seeking care solely for retardation or mental illness. Also by April 1, 1990, all such residents who had been confined in them for less than 30 months must be placed elsewhere. The Government was to issue regulations defining retardation and mental illness for purposes of the law, but the law did specify that those with Alzheimer's disease and those requiring round-the-clock non-psychiatric nursing care were to be exempted from its provisions.

Congress felt that the states would be forced to widen the activities of their community centers, like half-way houses and group homes, that could provide intensive psychiatric care. Of course such capabilities were nowhere near to being sufficient for the demand for them, even before the burden to be added by the new amendment to the Medicaid Law. The only certain effect of the new Law would be to increase burdens on families and the numbers of the homeless.

In 1956 the Social Security Law was extended to provide support for totally and permanently disabled adults, even if less than 65 years old, and by 1986 the expenditures for this disability program amounted to $18 billion dollars per year, supporting 2.6 million individuals. When the conservative Reagan Administration took over, in an effort to preserve the Social Security System and reduce the need for government expenditures for this purpose, it removed 100,000 (<4%) from the disabled rolls of the system. This was done under the regulation of the Act which denied disability benefits to people who suffer only "slight abnormalities" without consideration to age, work experience or education, rather than medically severe impairments. Many of those whose benefits were discontinued appealed, eventually to the courts. Generally the lower courts were sympathetic to the claimants and this was supported by the reaction in Congress (mostly Democratic legislators) and by the press.

However, in June 1987 the Supreme Court in a six to three decision upheld the Social Security regulation under which the disability claims had been disallowed. The specific case the Supreme Court decided involved a female former travel agent and real estate broker who sought disability benefits on the basis that she could not work because of flat feet, an inner ear dysfunction, dizzy spells, headaches and an inability to focus her eyes. The Supreme Court, upholding the Social Security regulation, remanded the case back to the lower court for determination as to whether the medical evidence justified the conclusion that her impairment was not severe.

As a former practicing neurosurgeon, I can attest to the fact that the unconvincing symptoms recounted above were typical of the majority of patients I reviewed for purposes of determining their disability status after they had been dropped from the Social Security rolls. The problem, from this experience, was that there were a very large number of individuals on Social Security disability who were not totally and permanently disabled (certainly 4%, the percentage of recipients dropped early in the Reagan Administration, would seem to have been a minimal number). These decisions were nevertheless difficult to make owing to the inability of physicians to be precise in the evaluation of the actual severity of subjective symptoms, even when they are the result of obvious organic disease. Subjective symptoms are heavily influenced by the motivation of the patient, or lack of it (as everyone is aware). The problem was compounded by a 1986 Supreme Court decision that "mentally disabled people" had the right to sue for Social Security disability benefits. In this decision the opinion was expressed that Social Security officials had a "fixed clandestine policy" to deny disability benefits to people with mental illness. The problem, of course, is that psychiatric diagnoses and prognoses are even more difficult to evaluate than physical complaints. Indeed, it has been suggested that the opinions of psychiatrists and psychologists on diagnoses and prognoses are so variable (and unempirical) that they ought not be considered in any legal proceedings[36].

The ethical problem faced by physicians is where to set their "thermostats" to balance their judgment as to the relationship of their patients' complaints to the actual amount of disability present. In addition to all the personal factors of the doctor-patient relationship affecting this balance are physicians' moral sense as to how they should balance the right of their patients to support for disability and the need to control expenditures for the good of society as a whole. Physicians conditioned to beneficence by their Hippocratic tradition find it far easier to favor individual patients in front of them than the remote needs of the whole of society. Even our whole society favors leaning to the side of the individual! This is the problem faced by physicians in all forms of disability evaluations - personal injury litigations and workmen's compensation cases included.

Several solutions were suggested by non-practicing physicians, limiting themselves to the problem of evaluating patients for short-term work or school releases[37]. The first was for physicians to refuse to do such evaluations, thereby forcing society to adopt another approach to the problem. Such other approaches include "no-fault absenteeism" in which all excuses, medical and otherwise, were treated alike with a reduction of benefits and/or restructuring of payment systems to create work incentives (and discourage non-work). Since this was unlikely to be adopted, at least in the near future, they suggested that the doctor warn the patient when they come for evaluation that the usual doctor-patient relationship does not apply, and in fact the doctor represents the school or employer. The authors themselves recognized the impracticability of this suggestion and finally suggested physicians continue to do these evaluations, but only in the context of treating patients. For example, if there was nothing physically wrong with a patient requesting time off, then, automatically, he or she was suffering from an emotional stress and if granted time off because of it, then they had to comply with treatment for their emotional stress.

The above obviously inadequate suggestions, at least from the practicing physician's point of view, leave the solution of these problems to the political arena. There, it will have to be determined how to frame the various legislations that regulate workmen's compensation and negligence remuneration that would be just to the individual, as well as to the whole of society. In the long run, and it may be an intolerably long run, the proper solution will be achieved depending upon what is best for society. My guess is that society will become less tolerant of the increasing number of extravagant and false disability claims and, perhaps, legislate controlled "no-fault systems" (presently most widely in effect in New Zealand) that might prove to be the eventual best answer to these problems.

3. Testing for Genetic Disease

Advances in molecular chemistry are making possible the identification of carriers of genetic disease and the testing of fetuses *in utero* for the presence of genetic malformations. Presently, the carriers of inheritable diseases that result from a single gene abnormality are the only ones being identified directly. Most diseases due to single genetic defect are being diagnosed by identifying a genetic marker and not the gene defect directly. A marker is a length of genetic material lying close to the defective gene on a chromosome. However, in order to make the diagnosis it is necessary to correlate the marker with the same marker in a family member (and preferably two) known to have the disease. The fact that the marker and the genetic defect are so close together on the same chromosome makes it almost certain that they will be inherited together.

Examples of inherited diseases identified by markers were, as of 1988, cystic fibrosis (30,000 cases in U.S.), Duchenne's muscular dystrophy (50,000 cases in U.S.), Huntington's dementia (or chorea, 25,000 cases in U.S.), adult polycystic disease (400,000 cases in U.S.), neuro-fibromatosis (100,000 cases in U.S.), hereditary emphysema (40,000 cases in U.S.), adenomatous polyposis of the colon and retinoblastoma.

There have been conflicting reports of chromosomal locations associated with manic-depressive psychosis, schizophrenia and Alzheimer's disease, each of which affects millions of Americans. Although these mental diseases often tend to run in families, by early 1989, there was no certain evidence that necessarily meant they were genetically caused. Therefore the principal search, at that time, was for genes that may predispose an individual to a particular mental disorder rather than cause it directly.

Identifying a carrier of a genetic defect (suspected because of a family history) will not benefit the individual by preventing the disease. It does furnish information as to which family members would develop the disease and thus provide the ability to make rational plans for the future. Also testing would inform adults on the risks of propagating or, if the test were negative, relieve their fear for the future. Most importantly, testing of fetuses can be done *in utero* and genetically defective ones identified early in pregnancy.

By 1988, some 200 metabolic and chromosomal disorders could be diagnosed in a fetus, and it was believed it would be possible at some time to so detect all of the 3000 known single-gene defects in humans. Identifying the gene causing a disease could enable the identification of the abnormal protein it creates and thus eventually, perhaps, lead to an effective treatment. By early 1989 the gene responsible for sickle cell anemia and Duchenne's muscular dystrophy had been identified and there was promise that the genes, or their mutations, causing cystic fibrosis (actually accomplished by late 1989), neurofibromatosis (Elephant Man's disease) and Huntington's disease would soon be known. Also, bio-engineering (see Chapter Seven) gave promise of altering the genetic structure of cells and thereby cure some inherited diseases.

A remarkable improvement towards diagnostic certainty was the application of DNA amplification by the polymerase chain reaction (see Chapter Four for its use in diagnosis of the AIDS virus) to the diagnosis of genetic defects from blood, chorionic villus (see below), or other tissue samplings[38]. It permits the direct identification of the DNA fragment of interest (for instance in cystic fibrosis as of 1989) instead of using a radioactive probe as a marker. This technique, which requires only a few cells or even only a single cell from the sample being tested, is also applicable to determining possible genetic defects in embryos created *in vitro* that are being considered for artificial implantation (see Chapter Nine).

Other congenital malformations, such as heart deformities or neural tube defects (open spinal cords) are called multi-factorial. That is they are partly genetic in origin, and partly due to infection or malnutrition or other "environmental" factors. Some of these, too, were being identified in utero, mostly as a result of improved ultrasonographic techniques which in addition to producing clearer images of the fetus, also permitted the obtaining of samples of umbilical blood.

As of 1988 there was little data on the false-positive rate for genetic testing, nor was there a forecast for such a percentage at that time. There were data on the percentages of failure to identify correctly those who would develop genetic diseases. For instance, in families with the genetic fault for Huntington's disease, 95% of individuals who were going to manifest symptoms of the disease (a dominantly inherited disease with involuntary abnormal movements and dementia, onset usually between ages 30 and 50) could be identified[39]. On the other hand, such at-risk individuals could be given only a 70% assurance that they would *not* develop Huntington's disease[40]. Individuals (and fetuses) at-risk to inherit Duchenne's muscular dystrophy (occurring once in 3000 male births and fatal in the early teens) were identifiable only 75% of the time; although, a late report stated that the failure-of-identification rate had been reduced to less than 5% in male fetuses, by using chorionic villus sampling (q.v.)[41].

The failure to identify a higher percentage of individuals who would develop genetic disease was most often due to difficulty in locating family members who were cooperative and whose diagnoses were correct. (This was so because the diagnoses of most genetic defects by 1988 still was being accomplished by associating markers in at-risk individuals with the same marker in a kin, known to have the disease.) For instance, the diagnosis of polycystic kidney disease in the adult, with a 17% to 34% false negative rate (by ultrasound), continued to be difficult. Also, some mentally disturbed patients were found to be incorrectly labeled as Huntington's disease when in fact their dementia was ultimately proven to be from other causes.

On occasion, the procedure for diagnosis of potential genetic disease in a child had been complicated by clear evidence of false paternity; a circumstance posing its own ethical dilemma. Withholding such information and protecting a marriage and/or a child from possible harm by an emotionally disturbed disproven father seems to be the beneficent duty of a physician. However, some ethicists probably would believe this to be paternalism as well as a deviation from the moral duty to tell the truth. Consequentialist reasoning, on the other hand, does support the paternalistic approach and would be preferred by most doctors, if the fear of a possible future malpractice action by the deceived father would not be a factor.

Tay-Sachs disease, Sickle cell anemia, thalassemia and cystic fibrosis are recessive autosomal diseases. This means that both parents need to be carriers to produce a child with such a disease, and that there is no sex linkage. Huntington's chorea, on the other hand, is a dominant autosomal (not sex-linked) disease, meaning that only one parent need be a carrier for a child to be afflicted. Another feature of Huntington's disease is that it most frequently comes on in maturity with its victims having the opportunity to procreate, so there is not a good chance for natural selection to work.

Genetic screening means testing individuals in known afflicted families, or in population groups at-risk, to determine whether they are carriers of genetic diseases, and/or testing fetuses while still in the uterus to determine if they have genetic disease. In the former situation undesirable mating could be avoided, or the bearing of children decided against, or, at the least, the odds of having an afflicted child forecast. In the latter situation, if an afflicted fetus is disclosed, termination of the pregnancy would be an option. It is emphasized that screening for carriers of genetic diseases must be preceded by an educational program to avoid anxiety by making sure that persons testing positive does not mean they have the disease. It also must be accompanied by a program for counseling those who test positively so that it is certain that they know their options on reproducing and to be certain the educational program had been effective. It is important that provision be made for absolute confidentiality of the results of testing so that those who test positive suffer no stigma or penalty, as being denied health insurance.

There are genetic diseases that are detectable prenatally and are treatable, such as congenital adrenal hyperplasia. Such a circumstance (treatability of a defect) adds to the difficulty of parents and the doctor in deciding to abort or not. It even poses the question whether it is right, or not, to screen for congenital adrenal hyperplasia, especially in view of the unnecessary anxiety that is produced by the particular high false-positive rate associated with its test[42]. An obvious compromise is to screen only in areas with high incidence for this genetic defect, as apparently exists in Alaska.

Some, probably a majority, object to any legislation mandating genetic testing of individuals of families known to have genetic disease, or who are of a population that is at special risk. Examples of the latter are blacks at-risk to sickle cell anemia (8% in the U.S. are carriers), ashkenazi jews liable to Tay-Sachs disease (1 in 3600 births as compared with 1 in 360,000 in the general population) and thalassemia rampant on Cyprus and Sardinia. Mass testing had been remarkably successful in reducing the incidence of Tay-Sachs disease and thalassemia[43]. There had been resistance to screening for sickle cell anemia (on the basis that it represents racial discrimination) and there has been no reduction in its incidence. Opposition to mass testing for the sickle cell trait recently had diminished; perhaps because testing of fetuses prenatally became possible. There was even hope that it would be possible to tell the severity of the disease in the fetus and help parents' make a decision whether to abort or not[40].

Another reason for the failure of the screening program for sickle cell disease was the lack of preparation for fully adequate campaign for education and counseling[44]. This resulted in considerable confusion and anxiety. Many of those identified as carriers mistakenly thought they were afflicted with the disease. And all too often confidentiality was breached, and in some cases, carriers were stigmatized and denied health insurance. By contrast, in the Tay-Sachs program the educational process went on long before any testing was done, and the entire program was carefully targeted to the only 1 to 2 million ashkenazi jews of reproductive age.

There also was resistance to testing for Huntington's disease: only 65 of 349 people with a family history agreed to be tested to determine whether or not they would develop the disease[45]. The reason offered was the awareness that nothing could be done to prevent the affliction or cure it, if symptoms did develop. (The suicide rate of 5% in families with the potential of developing Huntington's disease is high.) In the U.S. there are about 25,000 patients with Huntington's disease and 125,000 people at risk for developing it. Canada, with 3000 patients and perhaps 20,000 at risk for developing Huntington's disease, in 1988 instituted a program that offered a nationwide ability to test anyone 18 years old or older who had a relative suffering from the disease or had died of it, and voluntarily requested the genetic test[46]. It was to be available through genetic counseling centers who must provide psychological support for those whose tests were positive. Fourteen medical centers in Canada were to participate in the testing, and the program was estimated to cost from $800,000 to $1,200,000 over a three year period, and would include research on the disease as well as testing for it. The funds were being supplied by the government and private sources. In the U.S. there were only four centers with the capability to do the test, and 3 of the 4 were on the east coast. A commercial firm announced its capability to perform the test and their charge was to be $2,750 per test.

By 1989, demand for testing for Huntington's disease had fallen off, because both of its untreatability and cost, and the Columbia-Presbyterian Medical Center had begun to phase out its screening program. Some individuals expressed concern that if their test were to be positive that they would suffer discrimination in insurability and employment. This was especially true for those who had to rely on their insurance to pay for testing, with the consequent necessary break in "confidentiality". A further discussion was whether more harm was being done than good accomplished, especially considering the psychological damage done to asymptomatic persons testing positive with a 5% chance their result was a false-positive. A severe added expense was the counseling believed to be necessary prior to testing[47]. A recommended counseling program would consist of five 90-minute sessions prior to testing individuals with a 50% chance of being carriers of the defective gene.

While testing for Huntington's disease carries no therapeutic implications, there are other familial genetic disorders that also come on in adulthood, but if the individuals could be diagnosed early as to whether or not they are carriers, their care could be altered[48]. For example, if young individuals in families afflicted with adult polycystic kidney disease or familial adenomatous polyposis coli were found by genetic testing not to be affected, they would be spared repeated, often onerous, anxiety provoking investigations: renal and blood pressure studies in the former and colonoscopies in the latter. These observers[29B] suggest even in instances of individuals in families with untreatable genetic diseases that come on in adulthood (as retinitis pigmentosa or muscular dystrophies), knowledge as to whether or not they have the genetic defect could be helpful in planning their lives, such as picking a career. They did recommend there be empirical studies on the physical and emotional effects of genetic testing on the children of such families (diagnosed as having serious genetic disorders) to help answer questions raised in making decisions to test or not to test.

An objection to testing for fetal genetic disease by amniocentesis, or any other invasive test, is the possibility of inducing an abortion or miscarriage. Another objection to prenatal screening is the fact that the only way to avoid a defective child, if the test is positive, is by abortion. As is well-known, many in society take a fundamental position on abortion, denying that there can be any reason for it being carried out. On the other hand, failure to recommend testing in the above situations had been used as grounds for malpractice suits against doctors.

Amniocentesis, the most common method of prenatal screening is usually done at or after 16 weeks of gestation, though some doctors are beginning to perform it as early as the ninth week[49]. It is almost totally accurate and about one in 240 of amniocentesis procedures results in miscarriage[50]. The newer procedure for prenatal testing is chorionic villus sampling which can be done after only 8 to 12 weeks of pregnancy. This permits earlier diagnosis and safer abortion, should it be indicated. However, chorionic villus sampling is said to carry a slightly higher risk of inducing miscarriage than does amniocentesis. Another drawback of chorionic villus sampling is that there may be a significant rate of false-positive results: that is when a normal fetus is reported to be abnormal. The procedure is relatively new and improving results were being reported. Transabdominal chorionic villus biopsy recently has been reported to have been done safely in a series of patients (127 cases) in the second and third trimesters[51]. The purpose was to diagnose the presence of chromosomal abnormality in fetuses at high risk for such a defect. Chorionic villus sampling can provide results more rapidly than amniotic cells obtained by amniocentesis - in 36 hours as opposed to two or three weeks - a difference of time that is of critical importance for management decisions in late pregnancy.

Amniocentesis and chorionic villus sampling are costly procedures: about $500 each (as of 1988). Yet when their total cost is balanced against the cost entailed in the support of defective and handicapped people whose births could have been avoided, there is no question prenatal screening is cost effective. Another important consideration in favor of these procedures is the vast amount of suffering they can make avoidable, both for the parents of defective children and for such children themselves.

Prenatal testing for the presence of genetic disease in the fetus had become more and more extensive. It is sure to be used even more when tests for the common genetic disorders are perfected. Presently, pregnant women over 35 years of age (7.5% of all pregnancies) should be tested for the possibility of their fetuses having Down's syndrome (Mongolism) or other trisomy disorder (an additional, third, chromosome in an otherwise normal diploid cell). A pregnant women over 35 has about one chance in 270 of delivering a mongoloid, and 35% of all mongoloids occur in pregnancies of women over 35 years of age. Other indications for testing for genetic defect in a fetus are: if a mother is under 35 and has a history of delivering a genetically defective child previously; if one of the parents is a known carrier of a genetic defective disease; if there is a family history of neural tube defect (spina bifida and/or anencephaly).

Neural tube defects (NTD) do occur frequently in families but about 90% of children with a NTD are born into families without any previous history for NTD. They arise from a number of factors, that is they are multi-factorial - genetic and otherwise. As a group they are a leading cause of stillbirth, death in early infancy, and handicap in children. It is estimated that between 5000 and 8000 infants are born with NTD every year, that is one in every 500 to 1000 births.

A high level of the chemical alpha-fetoprotein in the amniotic fluid at the 16th week of pregnancy will identify all anencephalic fetuses and 90% of those with spina bifida, the undetected cases being the mild ones. Ultrasound scanning (a non-invasive test) is also an efficient means of identifying a fetus with NTD in utero. Recently radio-immune assay of alpha-fetoprotein in the maternal serum has become available. It is much less sensitive than testing the amniotic fluid but it can be used to screen pregnant women without risk to mother or fetus, and it is less expensive than amniocentesis. If the mother's blood has a high level, it indicates a problem and the need for further testing (ultra-sound and/or amniocentesis). About 5% of elevated levels of alpha-fetoprotein reported in maternal blood are falsely positive for NTD in the fetus. The anxiety this might occasion is offered as an objection to mass screening, principally by anti-abortionists.

A low level of alpha-fetoprotein in the maternal blood may indicate a chromosomal defect in the fetus, the most common of which is Down's syndrome (Mongolism). Five thousand such children are born annually in the U.S., and about 900 in Britain. While Mongolism does occur more frequently to mothers over 35, actually 65 to 80% of all such children are reported to be born to women under 35. Therefore this disclosure of the possible significance of a low alpha-fetoprotein level in the maternal blood was an added reason that this harmless test be used as a screen at 16 weeks in all pregnancies, in the opinion of some experts[52].

Another opinion was that the sensitivity, specificity, and predictive value of a low alpha-fetoprotein level left much to be desired[53]. In 1988, it was said the increase in amniocentesis to verify that a low alpha-fetoprotein level was the result of a fetus with Down's syndrome well could result in greater loss of normal fetuses than the number detected with Down's syndrome. Most investigators seemed confident that future progress will make screening for trisomy defects in fetuses early in the second trimester a sufficiently accurate procedure to satisfy everyone, and perhaps also eliminate the need for recommending routine amniocentesis for pregnant women over 35 years of age. One report in October 1988 did just that[54]. It stated an improved detection rate of pregnancies with fetuses having Down's syndrome (>60%) with a lower false positive rate (<0.5%) was achieved by matching the results of testing for the blood concentrations of alpha-fetoprotein (slight decrease), unconjugated oestriol (slight decrease), and human chorionic gonadotrophin (slight increase) with the age of the women. All women with positive results had amniocentesis before being aborted. Routine use of this combination of tests could eliminate the need for routine amniocentesis in pregnant women over 35 and reduce the number of Mongoloids born in the U.K. from 900 to 350 per year with an actual decrease in the 5% rate of amniocenteses being done for this purpose.

The fourth King's Fund Forum on screening for fetal and genetic abnormality was held in London from 30 November to 2 December 1987. A panel of 12 took evidence from experts in many disciplines and then issued a consensus statement[55]. They found that there were three factors contributing to the growth in the testing for genetic and congenital impairments: 1) a continued decline in mortality and morbidity due to other causes had increased the proportion due to genetic and congenital abnormalities; 2) advances in molecular biology had improved the means to identify carriers of deleterious genes; 3) recent initiatives were focused on disabled people.

Concern was expressed to the panel about developing screening programs, particularly those in which termination of pregnancy was an option. It was also feared screening would, in fact, be a form of eugenics; it would divert funds from areas more sorely in need, the disabled for example; it would favor the mother's freedom of choice over the claims of the fetus and the sanctity of life; screening high risk ethnic groups would promote racist attitudes; screening would stigmatize the disabled and their families; and finally it would overmedicalize the reproductive process.

On the other hand screening could provide a means to improve the well-being of women and their families; it could lead to a reduction of the amount of disability with which society has to contend; it could assist in making an informed decision before pregnancy, permitting the avoidance of a high-risk pregnancy; provide the option to abort or else to take steps to prepare for the care of a disabled child; it would allow optimal management of delivery and post-natal treatment when fetal abnormality has been identified.

It was pointed out that at least 6000 (one per hundred) babies born alive each year in the United Kingdom were seriously disabled despite nearly 2000 planned terminations for fetal and genetic abnormalities. The evidence was that the screening programs paid for themselves, but many believed that even if not, the social and clinical outcome justified the programs.

There was evidence that a conscientious objection to abortion on the grounds of fetal abnormality was the view of only a minority in the U. K. The forum came to no consensus on the meaningfulness or extent of the "rights" of the fetus. There was a consensus that a woman's informed and considered decision not to participate in a screening program should be respected; if there be a conflict between the parents, it was the woman's decision that should prevail; the decision as to whether abortion will or will not ensue should not affect access to screening; the sex of the fetus must never be a reason for abortion; the confidentiality of persons screened must be observed at all times; governments should make certain that screening is available to all on an equitable basis.

It can be inferred, from the reading of the report, that there was a panel opinion that genetic screening should be encouraged, programs broadened to keep pace with scientific advances, and that the government support these efforts with more funds.

Lawyers said that doctors need informed consent to do genetic testing and were liable to suit if they informed spouses or family members of the result without the explicit permission of their patient. An ethicist[45] urged legislation to limit any right of third parties (insurance companies, employers, etc.) to obtain the results of genetic testing. The analogy to AIDS was referred to: its incurability, the prolonged incubation period, and the need for confidentiality on test results so as to protect the rights of the victims. The right to privacy was given as the basis for objecting to mandatory genetic testing of adults, mothers prenatally or newborns, and the opinions of other ethicists on this point were cited. That eventually it would save money for third parties was not thought to be a valid reason to do such testing. It was said that the threat to society by genetic disease did not seem to be of sufficient magnitude to offset moral objections to the mandating of testing for it. How much voluntary testing of adults and fetuses prenatally will be done depends upon how much suffering the afflicted families are willing to endure.

There are precedents for requiring routine testing for genetic diseases in the newborn. It has long been the law to instill antiseptic into the eyes of newborns to prevent ophthalmic gonorrhea. Presently, all states require testing for phenylketonuria (PKU), because the 300 infants born each year in the U.S. with this autosomal recessive genetic disease can be treated by diet to reduce its ravages (mental retardation). The same blood sample from newborns used for testing for PKU (the Guthrie test) also has been used in recent years to screen for low (but treatable) levels of thyroid hormones. It was argued by pediatricians that more such routine screening of newborns should be done (for sickle cell anemia and metabolic diseases etc.) to prevent future suffering.

While there was no consensus for mandatory genetic testing up to 1988, the legal exposure of physicians for failure to test had already been demonstrated. This was expressed in two new legal concepts: wrongful birth and wrongful life[56]. "Wrongful birth" is a term to describe the basis for malpractice actions in which the parents sue the doctor for negligent conduct that results in the birth of an impaired child. These actions have generally arisen when physicians had failed to offer amniocentesis or had failed to give accurate counseling on the risks of congenital abnormalities. Wrongful birth has been accepted as valid in many jurisdictions. The concept of "wrongful life" is very similar to that of "wrongful birth", but the legal action is brought on behalf of the infant. It is not claimed in either concept that the doctor caused the impairment, but that the physician's negligent conduct permitted an infant to be brought into existence in an impaired state. As of 1988, three state supreme courts had recognized wrongful life actions and seven had rejected the concept.

A physician commenting on these concepts (wrongful birth and wrongful life) believed that it is the principle of beneficence that dictates physicians provide adequate prenatal counseling to parents[56]. It was his opinion also, that any child had a right to have informed parents and to have them make decisions in his or her best interests.

He rejected the principle of patient-autonomy as the basis for physicians' conduct in these cases. Parents' autonomy would dictate that they had the right to any and all information that they deem appropriate for control over their reproductive lives. He suggested that such grounding was undesirable and inconsistent with present practice. Prenatal counseling, correctly in his judgment, was being offered only to those in high risk groups. He went on to explain this practice *in extenso* and convincingly. A telling argument was that a normal young couple could have a child with Down's syndrome, despite the length of the odds for this to happen. In the view of this observer, the principle of autonomy would permit them to recover from the physician for their bad luck on the ground they were not informed of this possibility. The odds of a Mongoloid child being born to healthy young parents (and having no previous abnormal children) were far lower than those for miscarriage from amniocentesis, small as were the latter. Nevertheless, it was conceivable that someone, even a bioethicist, would testify that the young couple should have been informed of the possibility of a Mongoloid child, even if the doctor would have refused to do the amniocentesis, if demanded of him. This is a poignant example of what is expected of physicians by ethicists using the principles of patients' autonomy and right-to-know (see Chapter Three).

How these conflicts on genetic screening will be solved is not predictable for certain at the time of this writing, but one can be confident they will be solved in favor of what is best for the community as a whole. Since the intelligence of *Homo sapiens* is the result of evolutionary development, it seems reasonable to assume that the products of intelligence are used for the advantage of that species. This has been amply proven in the past. Therefore techniques for avoiding genetic misfits, developed by this intelligence, will be similarly utilized to the advantage of the species. Indeed, the ability to assure that offsprings are not diseased or deformed seems an even more direct evolutionary purpose than are many other products of man's intelligence.

An important item in arguing for the use of genetic testing of fetuses early in pregnancy and to eliminate those that are defective is that it is only strengthening a natural process. The commonest cause for spontaneous abortion, often occurring so early in pregnancy that the event is unnoticed by the woman, is a genetic defect in the fetus. Spontaneous abortion is nature's method to spare the species of useless, or even deleterious, individuals.

It should be carefully noted that assuring that offsprings are not diseased or deformed is different from improving the quality of human progeny. The latter phrase implies an eugenic purpose, or even the creation of a master race - which had been rightly labeled an anathema in the past[57]. The reasoning used in Chapter Two, that equal opportunity for the masses is necessary for the creation of the maximum number of elite minds, supports the opposition to eugenic programs as conceived in the past. However, and to repeat, the alleviation of individual genetic defects should not be confused with any objective to redefine mankind by genetic engineering. This will be discussed further, in Chapter Seven, in relation to the definition of the human genome.

CHAPTER SEVEN. EXPERIMENTATION and RESEARCH

Experimentation on living creatures is one of the ways the science of medicine is advanced. Some people believe experimentation on lower species requires more circumspection than when done on humans, because of the inability to obtain informed consent. A few enthusiasts for animal rights feel it is wrong to do any research using animals, and label those that conduct and condone such activities as prejudiced speciests. Nevertheless, the vast majority of people believe that human experimentation raises far more pressing moral issues than does experimentation on animals.

1. Research on Humans

The very thought of using human subjects for research arouses fear that some individuals will be misused for the benefit of others. To allay this fear, both deontologic and utilitarian reasoning have been utilized to set rules for human investigation. At first, the utilitarian concept, doing what was in the best interest for the greatest number of individuals, was offered as justification, and subjects were to be protected by physicians' beneficence: to do no harm, to maximize benefits, and to minimize injuries.

More recently, the deontologic principle that physicians have the duty to respect the autonomy of the person has been advanced as better protection for those humans used for research.

Indeed, that this latter principle is an absolute necessity was emphasized by the reporting of research in the U.S. causing irreparable harm to, and without the consent of, its human subjects[1]. Also contributing to this sentiment are the memories of the horrors of Nazi experimentation on prisoners considered to be of inferior races. It is of passing interest that the written comments condemning the Nazi doctors for their experimentation on human subjects were based on their lack of beneficence and violation of the Hippocratic oath much more than on their transgression of the autonomy of their subjects. Perhaps the latter was so obvious that the ethicists concentrated only on the former.

Because of the appalling experiments mentioned above, Federal Regulations were issued in 1966 to protect human subjects of research. The first two requirements were informed consent and that the risks were to be minimal and reasonable in relation to the expected benefits. In addition, the regulations mandated that there be peer review approval of projects prior to their being started. This meant that ethics committees for research be set up in institutions in which, or under whose aegis, research was intended. These committees were charged with not only having to approve protocols for obtaining informed consent, but also to agree with the investigators' assessment of relative risks to, and benefits for, the intended subjects, and also the feasibility of the projects achieving their goals.

The completely informed consent of an intended subject now is agreed to be the *sine qua non* for the two categories of human research: clinical research - concerned with treatment or diagnosis of disease, and non-therapeutic bio-medical research. The latter, presumably, is for the better understanding of the human body and, ultimately, for the benefit of the species.

Informed consent comprehends that it be voluntary and that the intended subject be adequately informed of the aims, anticipated benefits and potential hazards of the study. An exception to this rule, as perceived by practicing physicians, is when a patient is included in a clinical study of a form of treatment in which there is no alteration in the care of the patient between groups; that is when the patients are to receive a standard form of care from their usual medical attenders. The only difference is to be in record-keeping and, of course, the confidentiality of the patients was to be vigorously maintained. The objection to informing the patients of their participation in the latter type of clinical research was that it could only raise doubts in their minds as to their care. Most importantly, research had shown that the subjects' understanding of technical aspects of research design was so inadequate that, in fact, informed consent can never be achieved[2].

In instances where the condition of the patient involved in clinical research is such that it be a barrier to communication or places the patient in a position that rational judgment cannot be made, it is recommended that a lay surrogate be used to give informed consent. A responsible family member usually is considered the best surrogate. This raises the question, which is also an issue when patients themselves give consent: how educated must one be to give consent truly? The complexities of describing the natural history of disease, the treatment being offered, and the possible advantages and disadvantages of the suggested therapy are so great that they well could try even expert surrogates. A study in Canada is reported[3] in which 118 physicians who treated pulmonary tumors were asked: "how they would wish to be treated if they had non-small-cell lung cancer?". They were given four different treatment regimes and asked if they would consent to take part as subjects in a clinical trial. The percentage of respondents who would consent to each study varied from 11% to 64%. Many of the reasons for refusal were that the physicians felt that the trials offered were unacceptable options for treatment. This study pointed up the difficulties in carrying out clinical trials on the basis of completely educated, informed consent that is demanded on behalf of patients' autonomy.

If further research confirms that in many instances absolute, educated informed consent is not possible - then such a scientifically powerful tool as randomized, controlled trials often will have to be placed in ethical balance with informed consent that is necessarily limited in scope. These commentators[3] were saying, in other words, that if some therapeutic trials were to be done, an utilitarian justification that experimentation on some humans for the benefit of all would have to suffice (really an evolutionary point of view). It was to be presumed that such clinical trials thereafter would be closely monitored by ethics committees and, hopefully, by a re-inspired physician-investigator beneficence.

Although the procedure set by the U.S. Federal Regulation of 1966 received general endorsement, it has by no means achieved the goals set. Ingelfinger [4] in 1972 suggested that often it is impossible to obtain an educated informed consent; he was the first to point out the complexities of this problem so recently confirmed experimentally[2]. Even peer review has its flaws. The term "peer" is too often construed to limit the committee to just investigators who themselves, in the future, could come before the committee. At that time It would be possible that the committee included the scientist whom they were then trying to judge. Therefore, peer investigators often cannot review the stakes in question as would non-investigator clinicians or laymen.

Few, if any, committees monitor the course of projects as closely as recommended. For instance, in the course of projects there can be changes in the benefit/possible-harm ratio that would indicate prompter terminations than had been anticipated[5]. Moreover, testing of 32 research committees by offering them projects known to be flawed, revealed a shocking failure to detect the flaws, failure to apply their own criteria, the raising of "red herrings" by some, and generally a lack of effectiveness[6].

Some ethicists feel it is proper to prohibit the use of healthy volunteers in any research that exposes them to any possible harm. This presents severe problems in many investigations considered of vital importance. For instance, in the search for a vaccine for AIDS it is necessary to use healthy volunteers to prove its efficacy and a sufficient degree of freedom from undesirable side-effects[7]. To help overcome this problem some researchers proposed to first vaccinate themselves before using other volunteers. Another procedure suggested to help overcome or diminish the ethical issue of using healthy volunteers was to use as subjects, for testing vaccines against AIDS, only spouses of infected hemophiliacs or intravenous drug users who had not yet acquired HIV. This approach raises the question of the propriety of exposing such individuals to infection, when they might have been using protective measures or could be informed of them. Another example of vital research requiring the use of healthy humans is in the development of a vaccine against malaria. It requires not only vaccinating healthy volunteers, but also eventually injecting them with live parasites[8].

The history of using healthy volunteers even since World War II is shocking. Exposure to dangerous amounts of radiation between 1945 and 1971, with and without consent, has been well documented[9]. It has been stated that the use of prisoners, inmates of mental institutions, and employees of the firm or institution doing the experiments are unsuitable subjects, even if "informed consent" had been obtained. A working party of the English Royal College of Physicians reported that healthy medical students in close contact with investigators are undesirable subjects, since they might be persuaded to participate against their better judgment; and no financial inducement should be offered for the same reason[10]. The Committee of Ministers under the terms of the Statute of the Council of Europe in early 1990, after detailing the necessity for informed consent in carrying out research on human beings, for the research to be ethical added that: the interests and well-being of the person undergoing medical research must always prevail over the interests of science and society; no one should be forced to participate; persons deprived of liberty may not undergo medical research unless it is expected to produce a direct and significant benefit to their health; potential subjects of medical research should not be offered any inducement which compromises free consent, and persons undergoing medical research should not gain any financial benefit[11].

Clinical trials often require that there be randomization of patients involved. That is patients, either by drawing of lots or alternation, are subjected to one of two or more treatment variations, or receive a placebo. *A priori*, it is unethical to compare a new treatment with no treatment when an old treatment is known to be effective. When two treatments are to be compared, they must be considered the two best treatments available and there must be no known difference between them in effectiveness or accompanying hazards. In this regard, an ethicist would place an impossible burden on investigators[5]. He suggested that a clinical researcher, to be ethical, must terminate a clinical trial as soon as it is begun "to be felt" that one arm of a trial was better for the patient than the other. Many solutions were offered on how the investigation could be continued and ethics preserved. But in the view of another ethicist, investigators would be required "to seek all information relevant to a patient's treatment", and "this can never be absolute, since the clinician would have to spend all his time reading the literature."[12]

Still another medical ethicist asked (without offering answers): "How do you ethically do a randomized trial on physicians' services? Suppose you want to find out, for the purposes of cost containment, whether certain tests are unnecessary. Do you get consent from the physicians as well as from patients? What if the patients refuse to participate?"[13] He went on to be concerned about the question of discrimination in the exclusion of some individuals from trials because of the fear of AIDS or because they were drug abusers and,therefore, judged to be unreliable.

An obviously thoughtful English clinical investigator raised issues that are likely to result from present trends that hamper medical research[14]. He observed that the animal welfare lobby made it difficult, if not impossible, to pursue certain types of animal experimentation and hostile, ill-informed criticism of clinical research was bludgeoning governments into legislation that frighten both doctors and patients away from participation in clinical trials.". ...how haphazard much of what passes for medical knowledge really is, and how much more awful medical practice would be were it not for trials". He pointed out that it was considered ethical for a surgeon to do a mastectomy for early breast cancer for 10 years and then suddenly switch to a lumpectomy and irradiation for the next 10 years, and compare the two approaches. For a surgeon to randomize his patients, without their knowledge, between the two treatments in order, eventually, to determine the answer to a question that has been present for 50 years would generally be considered unethical. Yet for a specific patient, either approach would represent a not dissimilar haphazard method. The first approach more informal and retrospective and thus more unreliable, nevertheless looked upon as ethical; the second, a reliable comparison of alternative therapies, is not considered ethical.

This surgeon well recognized the need for a protocol to be scrutinized by committees, mostly to protect patients against investigators more concerned with their careers than their patients. He went on to point out the arguments for and against informed consent: a most telling one being the discomfiting of patients by honest clinicians presenting their own doubts and being answered "Well if you don't know how to treat me, I will go to someone who does". This scenario was compared with the apparent triumph of those doctors with excellent bedside manners and an immunity to disturbing uncertainties. "If more and more patients are lost from the honest clinician who admits his ignorance to the dogmatist who already 'knows' the answers, it will become more and more difficult to produce good evidence as to the real facts." He suggested that the reality of informed consent may well defeat the ability to sort out the differences in clinical outcomes of variations in treatment.

Later, he and his colleagues went so far as to argue that in certain circumstances patients need not be informed that their treatment will be decided by entry to a randomized control trial, to prevent the distress that may be caused by having to make such a decision themselves[15]. They recommended that such decisions be made by a national ethics committee, arguing that patients' autonomy needs to be over-ridden at times by the principle of justice on the utilitarian basis that the resulting increase in scientific knowledge will benefit the greatest number of patients. They further observed that "the principle of non-maleficence should overcome that of autonomy". In other words, one should not have to risk upsetting patients for the sake of getting their consent to being used as a research subject.

The gloomy prognosis for the future of clinical trials, because of continued insistence on informed consent from participants, was reiterated in a meeting on breast cancer trials held in Oxford, England during October 1988[16]. Apparently investigators on one side and lawyers and ethicists on the other were unable to reconcile their differences. The latter insisted: "If trials fail through lack of recruitment, initiatives will have to be taken to ensure that the choices are truly equal and that the public and the profession are better educated and better able to communicate with each other."

British doctors continued to object to any requirement in conducting clinical trials that required absolute informed consent[17]. They pointed out that the detailing of every remotely possible bad effect of any treatment would frighten off patients and "make large-scale randomized trials impossible". It was suggested that such a policy on informed consent in the U.S. "is first and foremost to protect doctors from litigious patients and rapacious lawyers. Consent forms itemizing every remotely possible side-effect scare off even the most intelligent patients so that in the USA 98% of cancer patients vote with their feet and patients in Canada and Europe have to be exploited to gain the knowledge that may improve their treatment."

In Chapter Three we, too, inveighed against informed consent, and expressed resentment of suggestions from medical para-professionals (medical ethicists, medical sociologists etc.) "to learn to communicate better". However, it was in the context of clinical practice that this was done. When it comes to research, and certainly random-clinical-trials are research, remonstrances against informed consent seem more out of place. Research on human subjects has dimensions beyond clinical practice, therefore participation should be entirely voluntary and the protection of reasonably informed consent is a necessary requirement. Reasonable informed consent in research must be regarded as just another problem to tax the ingenuity of dedicated investigators.

The requirement of informed consent becomes a special issue in clinical research involving children and the aged. Many of the latter, having lost much of their intellectual capacity, have no more ability to give informed consent than young children. A group of investigators reported on unexpected results of using proxies to obtain informed consent[18]. One hundred-sixty-eight elderly patients in nursing homes were involved. They were unable to decide for themselves whether to participate in a prospective study on the morbidity from long term use of catheters, presumably for the control of urinary incontinence. The proxies were overwhelmingly family members - daughters, sons or spouses - and the research was presented to them as posing minimal risk. Seventy-eight proxies of the 168 patients (46%) refused treatment. The reasons given were that research should not be done in nursing homes, that the study would disturb the patient, or that a patient if able would have refused consent, or the proxy, if himself were asked, would refuse to participate in the study. A result, ethically upsetting to the proxy procedure, was that of the 55 proxies who believed the patient would have refused consent, 17 (31%) nevertheless gave consent in apparent opposition to the patients' wishes. Moreover, of 28 proxies who said they would not have participated in the study themselves, 6 gave consent. If the researchers had known the proxies were acting contrary to the wishes of the patient, they would not have used those patients. It was felt the results of this study may be an important obstacle to research among the elderly.

Lawyers, including a leading medical ethicist, commenting on this study of incompetent patients in nursing homes had several suggestions[19]. One was a nursing home council, composed primarily of residents, to review and approve any protocol before research could be conducted at their facility. They stressed that too often patients in nursing homes are viewed as incompetent and inferred that legal determination of a patient's incompetence was necessary. When consent by proxy was appropriate, then legal guardians and those with powers of attorney in hand should be the proxies. In the absence of specific instructions from the patient, no proxy should volunteer another for non-therapeutic research experimentation that carries any risk of harm with it. In essence they did not believe incompetent elderly patients who had not given prior power of attorney designating someone to make decisions about participation in research should be used in such an enterprise. It may also be concluded that researchers should avoid using mentally incompetent people in their studies[20].

A respected newspaper[21], in an editorial, questioned the Food and Drug Administration's restricting of a new drug possibly helpful in the treatment of Alzheimer's disease, until its safety had been established. Their point was that if irrational, risk-conscious decisions were made by families and doctors to administer the drug to patients with such a devastating disease, it is contrary to the Hippocratic tradition to withhold the drug. Seriously ill patients are already being harmed beyond bearing and no help should be denied them, even if unproven. This is still another view on autonomy versus beneficence.

Children as subjects of research obviously pose special questions, principally in relation to informed consent. Reacting to this special problem the (British) Institute of Medical Ethics formed an *ad hoc* committee to survey the problem[22]. They suggested that research review committees should be 5 to 12 in size and include a general practitioner, a nurse, and a genuine lay member. Any enlargement of committees beyond these numbers generally reduced their effectiveness. The most important issue is the scientific validity of the proposal, since it is pointless to discuss ethical issues if the project be scientifically unsound. When the investigation proposed to be done is on children, the committees should satisfy themselves the project can only be done on children and holds the prospect of considerable benefit to children. The benefits should substantially outweigh the risks. Non-therapeutic research on children is justified only if the risks are minimal - that is, a risk of death of less than one in a million, a risk of a major complication of less than 10 in a million or a risk of a minor complication of less than one in a thousand. Investigators should themselves explain projects to parents, and if the risks are more than minimal they should give written explanation and time for the parents to consider. Children age seven or over should give their own assent to a procedure, in addition to the consent of the parents. "If the child is between 7 and 14, his unwillingness to take part in a non-therapeutic investigation should be binding, but his parents could override his unwillingness to take part in therapeutic research. Over 14 the young person's view should be paramount, though parental consent is still required legally until 16 for therapeutic, and until 18 for non-therapeutic research."

American medical ethicists expressed the opinion that the requirement for informed consent from older children themselves (6 to 7 years or older) be extended to even a therapeutic procedure that was no longer experimental[23]!

A committee of the British Royal College of Physicians believed no remuneration should be offered parents of children solicited as subjects of research[10]. They feared a financial consideration could persuade parents to consent against their better judgment. In the view of the Institute of Medical Ethics the responsibility of the investigators for the ethics of their research cannot be emphasized too strongly. They saw a possible drawback to research ethics committees insofar as they may appear to relieve investigators of some of these responsibilities.

One of the most difficult subjects, to the Institute, was informed consent in controlled trials, particularly in the newborn. The Institute's policy, which is strict in its requirement for informed consent, was seen as imposing a double standard, since ethics committees cannot stop new treatment being tried in an uncontrolled way. The Institute thought, however, that the number of times that innovative treatments would be tried without being submitted to ethics committees would be limited.

A court decision in Canada, in 1988, may make it illegal to carry out any non-therapeutic research on children in that country[24]. The decision was that no one was legally able to consent to a sterilization operation on a mentally retarded woman. It was held that consent to procedures on legally incompetent people (such as children) was only valid if the procedures were intended to be of direct medical benefit.

Medical research was a very limited enterprise until this century, as was communication. Consequently, abuse of the subjects of research received but limited notice. Moreover, in the use of human subjects it was very often the investigator himself, or his relatives and/or acquaintances that were utilized[25]. Very slowly clinical investigation expanded, but it was not until after World War II that scientific advances and economic support permitted it to reach the dimensions of the present era. This vast expansion coincides with that of the present day communications media. Therefore transgressions of obvious ethical principles in clinical research often are brought quickly to the attention of everyone. The reasons for these transgressions were touched upon above. Also in this recent era the new field of medical ethics, populated largely by non-physicians, came into being and undoubtedly has contributed greatly to the attention given to ethical derelictions in clinical investigations. Even though medical ethicists are recognized to serve a useful role in research on humans, on occasion many investigators would compare their role to that of the animal rightists in research done on animals (see below).

It is self-evident that advances in medical care have contributed very significantly to the success of the species *Homo sapiens*. Since this requires research be done on human subjects, the utilitarian concept of the greatest good for the greatest number is offered as its justification. An evolutionary theory for the origin of ethics justifies clinical research on precisely the same ground. This reasoning, however, in the past was used also to violate unjustly the rights of subjects and commit experimental horrors. This made clear to society, now *evolved* to one that recognizes the values of individual rights, that adjustments were sorely needed. These were provided by governmental action and the ready cooperation of a medical profession that was chagrined by the violations of its beneficent responsibilities by a few of its members. Today, when it is thought to be imprudent or impossible to seek totally informed consent in projects believed to be vital, individual patients are protected by the requirement that committees of physicians make sure investigators observe their pledge to the principle of beneficence.

While it is unmistakable that safeguards are necessary to prevent the exploitation of individuals in medical research, and that in contemporary society these are in place, constant vigilance is necessary as well on the other side of the issue. This means not only must firm observance be given to protection of patient subjects, but that necessary projects not be halted by religious, ethical or civil-libertarian fundamentalists. A good example of fundamentalist objection to medical science is their resistance to vaccination against whooping cough. They believe that the relatively many deaths from the disease are to be accepted rather than the very rare one occasioned by the vaccine itself (one per million children vaccinated). They believe society is not responsible for deaths caused by nature's scourges, but only for those it provokes. On the other hand doctors are motivated by the principle of "statistical morality" that insures the least harm to the most people (v.s.).

Research ethics committees must protect society from zealots on either side, by ruling out studies whose transgressions of rights are too flagrant, and yet sponsor studies of great value despite the inability to completely satisfy patients' autonomy. They must not allow the detailing of anecdotes of the blatant transgressions of few investigators to interfere with progress. Thus, in the final analysis the protection of the subjects of research and of society rests most heavily on the moral integrity of physicians, which should be at apogee in the academic milieu of investigators and peer reviewers. Physician-investigators are expected to assert their beneficence to the utmost to protect their human subjects from harm. This means they must use their best professional judgment in being certain that the potential harm to the subject is remarkably outweighed by the potential for their ultimate good (another way of stating the principle of statistical morality). Patients must not be exposed to any risk that is not inherent in their disease and the treatment concerned must be one that gives patients the chance of improvement.

2. Animal Experimentation

Preparation for this book, in part, relied upon a survey of the daily and weekly press. Surprisingly, the number of articles concerned with animal rights, animal experimentation and preservation of various species equaled or surpassed those on the many other current bioethical issues. It is obvious that animal welfare groups, of which there are over 400 in the U.S. and Britain alone, are increasingly influential. In recent years a referendum to ban all animal experimentation appeared on a ballot even in Switzerland. Although it was defeated, the number of votes in favor was impressive. The City Council of Cambridge, Massachusetts in May 1987 banned the classical LD-50 toxicity test for chemicals and drugs (that dose that results in the death of 50% of animal, usually rats) and the Draize eye-irritancy test (drugs or chemicals dropped into the eyes of rabbits). Only one company in that city had been using either test, but area researchers noted other ordinances on the use of animals in research were pending, and they feared a total ban on the use of animals in research.

The English Parliament passed an Animals Act in 1986, the first one since 1876, that had many restrictive regulations sure to add to the complexity and cost of research. One requirement is that investigators must consider the use of alternatives before using animals for experimentation, and sign a declaration to that effect. The Home Secretary must be satisfied that not more animals are being used than necessary and that thorough consideration had been given to minimize the suffering of animals. The U.S. Congress had approved an Animal Welfare Act in 1966, strengthened it in 1970 and 1976 and most recently amended it (December 1985) to require laboratories to exercise dogs and to provide improved facilities to promote the psychological health of primates. On the whole, the English Animals Act places more restrictions on investigators than does Government regulations in the U.S.

The U.S. Public Health Service requires every research institution to have an animal-care-and-use committee with a veterinarian and an outside member on it. These committees must review all research protocols involving animals and they must inspect the facilities twice a year. Institutions must submit exhaustive information on their animal care program and, if not already approved by the American Association for Accreditation of Laboratory Animal Care, give assurance their facilities meet that association's standards. The National Institutes of Health issued a "Guide for the Care and Use of Laboratory Animals" that gives directives in excruciating detail. Investigators are choosing to go along with these regulations that are costly and time consuming without complaint, partly because they recognized changes were justified. However, they also believed to openly contest them would provoke an even greater reaction[26].

Animal rightists extended their activities (like bombers of abortion clinics) to violent attacks on research facilities. Despite their illegality, they were effective in disrupting the functioning of these laboratories. This disruption resulted not only from the damage done but also from subsequent government suspension of funds in some instances. The latter circumstance pertained when there was purported recognition that there had been some discrepancies from humane procedures and/or there was some question as to the importance of the research. However, the suspension of government funds in some instances was also a ransom paid by unduly frightened politicians and/or bureaucrats to appease the animal rightists whose violence was the same as that of the anti-abortionists and other terrorists. Many, if not most, of these attacks were by a group called the Animal Liberation Front, thought to be allied with a similar group in Britain. Despite illegal activity of this very small number of people over at least 6 years involving extensive sabotage in 26 different raids (including arsons costing up to $4,000,000 each), only one man had been charged in this entire time. Instead, in the view of one observer: "If the scope of the attacks continues to expand, it may mean the efforts to appease the movement will have to be broadened..."[27]!

Animal rights activists, recognizing that their issue alone was not sufficient to challenge research on legal grounds, joined environmentalists in their efforts to prevent construction of new research laboratories[28]. Indeed, lacking sufficient public support on the animal rights issue, they displayed "political savvy" by changing their tactic. They began pressing for their objective by exploiting the public's deep-seated fear of science and its big institutions, especially when the latter were in their immediate neighborhoods. As an example of how devious even fundamentalists can be, animal rightists exploited the public's suspicions of genetic engineering and nuclear and chemical radiations to delay (and make more expensive) new laboratories in the San Francisco Bay area.

The number of animals used in medical research is relatively insignificant compared with those used for food and clothing, yet the focus for the animal rightists appears to be the former. The obviousness to the general public of their need for food and clothing (and their sensitivity to increased costs of these items) as compared with the more remote benefits of research accounts for this strategy. Moreover, the increase in costs for research caused by animal rights activism is not a factor of immediate or self-evident concern to the public. Also, the save-the-various-species movements, based on no other reason than an *a priori* one, in some way is connected, and gives credence, to the animal rights movement.

Violent attacks by animal rightists were expanded in England, by 1989, to the fire bombing of fur stores and poisoning of meats for sale in markets. This displays that their objectives extend beyond halting only some research on some animals. Nevertheless, in Aspen, Colorado, where the question of the sale of furs as clothing was voted upon in 1989, the residents declared by a two to one margin that their city would not be a fur-free one. This is an indication that vivisection, like abortion, has the approval of the majority, but who only express themselves when the activities of the vocal minority actually could result in the prohibition, by law, of the exercise of their conviction.

Antivivisection societies arose in England over 100 years ago when only a modicum of animals were used for research - in 1885 less than 800 animals were so used in Great Britain[29]. Nevertheless their activities led to parliamentary action in a Cruelty to Animals Act in 1876. It was difficult "to understand how this relatively marginal Victorian social problem provoked such a furore". It was suggested that antivivisectionists then had, and the animal rights groups now have, a hidden agenda: anti-science[30]. This observer, president of Stanford University, believed their program has less to do with animals than it has to do with the control of science, which they fear. He gave cogent reasons for his opinion.

In 1986 over three and a quarter million animals were used in Britain for research and almost 20 million in the U.S. (according to the Department of Agriculture). Of the 20 million utilized in the U.S., 18 million were rodents and 1.7 million were: dogs (176,141), cats (54,126), primates (48,540), guinea pigs and hamsters. The 1.7 million animals above rodents on the evolutionary scale used in 1986, was down from the 2.1 million used in 1985.

The first World War seemed to put an end to the antivivisection movement for over a half century and it was in the inter-war period that the enormous increase in the use of animals in research occurred, an almost certain coincidence. Revival of the antivivisection movement (in a new form, as animal rightists) has been gaining momentum now for about two decades. It is being extended by a few extremists to the ending of hunting and to the ending of the raising of animals for food - with the purpose of making meat-eating illegal. There appears to be a distinct difference in the position between the previous antivivisectionists and contemporary animal rightists. Formerly the antivivisectionists were motivated by the principle of humaneness and the belief that harming animals degraded a person's humanity. Presently, those supporting animal rights believe in the equality of the species - perhaps a more religious orientation ("we are all God's creatures").

The concept of "rights" really is quite new, only arising in the past 300 years along with the increasing equality of opportunity for individuals, particularly in Western industrialized societies (see Chapter Two). The very success of such societies has enshrined the idea of "individual rights". Those whose concern for animals overwhelms them, have extended the concept of the possession of rights by individual humans, to individual animals. Some ask homeowners with rodent problems to use a device that catches mice alive. Lobsters have been "liberated" from restaurants and returned to the ocean. These groups consider any use of animals for food or research to be morally equivalent to human slavery.

Some animal rightists abhor the use of furs for clothing or leather for shoes, and others go so far as to believe it is wrong to use animals as a source of food[31]. There is a group called the Humane Farming Association that campaigns against eating veal. They attack the practice of confining calves in small pens and the withholding of solid food so as to get the higher prices of "milk-fed veal"[32]. A pre-medical student sued her college that refused to admit her to a biology course unless she agreed to dissect, or at least observe the dissection, of a frog. The student was described as not eating meat nor dairy products and refusing to wear leather[33].

Those opposed to animal experimentation have a variety of reasons for their position and they tend to become shrill about them. Some quote Bentham, who took the position that any animal that was sentient had the right not to suffer. Human beings are injured not merely if they are caused pain, but also can suffer if they are not allowed to live a worthwhile life "according to their nature". The same should be true for animals - surely they are capable of suffering in addition to feeling pain. Of course the recent contributions on the intelligence and social development of primates adds to the potency of these positions. I, too, can look back 45 years, and recall, all too well, the humanness of chimpanzees, and even macaques, in a primate "colony", and how little was thought about their confinement and use for experimentation, other than they be kept clean and healthy.

An Australian philosopher, Peter Singer, denied that there are any characteristics unique to humans: "animals may have no language or culture, but neither do small babies. The counter argument, that babies have 'potential' to develop, is answered by reference to severely mentally handicapped people - why don't we use them for all of our experiments?"[34] Animal rightists adopt this reasoning and use it together with the argument that "the ends do not always justify the means". They equate sentient animals with severe mental defectives on whom, certainly, no one would tolerate the inflicting of pain, no matter what good would come from the experiment. Indeed, some believe it is more moral to use humans, rather than another species, for research that only benefits humans. In opposition to using animals for research it glibly can be asked: "Would they justify research on unwilling humans for the benefit of other humans?"[35]

Those of a theological bent proclaim animals are as much God's creatures as is man and, therefore, morally, deserve the same consideration. Others, even if not religiously oriented, use *a priori* reasoning, derived from their feelings, to announce their reverence for life in all forms and condemn vivisection. They attribute the same rights to animals as is possessed by humans, and therefore the use of animals for research should be prohibited[36,37]. Many antivivisectionists cite appalling instances of so-called research to strengthen their position: experiments done on animals without anesthesia; constant shocking of monkeys to study epileptic fits; blocking the birth canals of pregnant animals until the uterus ruptures; animals starved to 80% of their body weights; animals melted down with irradiation; otherwise peaceable animals forced to fight to the death to study aggression; etc.

It is claimed that the enormous number of animals used in research is contributing to the extinction of certain species. The chimpanzee is cited as the principal example. The U.S. Office of Technology Assessment and a Physicians' Committee for Responsible Medicine recently surveyed the use of animals for teaching in medical schools. They found great variation in this practice. It was concluded by both that since all subjects for which dog laboratories are used are also taught successfully at other schools without the use of dogs, dog laboratories are not necessary and should be replaced by other teaching methods[38].

Investigators admit that there have been derelictions in the use of animals in research, and that the antivivisectionists have performed a service to bring them into focus. Doctors and medical institutions often are aggressive in pursuing research even if it be with projects that on proper scrutiny would not be rewarding. The very mass of investigation in the last decades, encouraged by the huge sums of money made available for it, was bound to create a cavalier attitude, in some investigators, to the use of animals. One example that was particularly reprehensible was macaque monkeys in which the sensory nerves to their upper extremities had been severed[39]. The vain hope of the investigator was that he might gain some insight into the problems of patients with spinal cord injury and strokes. The care of these severely disabled monkeys has been a constant problem for the National Institutes of Health which took over their custody. Their final dilemma was how to satisfy all parties when a recommendation was made to sacrifice, on humane grounds, 8 of the surviving 14 disabled animals. This was unacceptable to animal rights groups and a member of congress. No resolution had been arrived at by 1989, and the N.I.H. was continuing to look for a politically acceptable answer while spending $30,000 per year to maintain the monkeys.

The need for research to be relevant, especially when involving animal subjects, was highlighted by the activities of a new (1987) animal-rights group, Trans-Species Unlimited. Their announced tactic was to target research programs for attack, not on the basis of the mishandling of, or cruelty to, animals, but rather on the irrelevance of the project[40]. The first program singled out (after a computer search and consultation with three veterinarians and a clinical psychologist) had been going on for 14 years at Cornell Medical College and involved cats in the study of the basis for barbiturate addiction. Several hundred demonstrators were mobilized on April 27, 1987 and thereafter the College was picketed for four months. In addition, they conducted a national campaign and gained the attention of several legislators. The College wrote a letter in response to this pressure stating that the program was winding down and that future studies would not use cats. Nevertheless, in July 1988 the grant was renewed by the National Institute on Drug Abuse for several hundred thousand dollars over three more years. Then in September

1988 the College announced that the project had been terminated, believing they could not go back on their "unfortunate" letter and maintain their credibility. Peer review committees had given the program high marks on the conduct and methods of the research, but its relevance, after 14 years of effort, was less clearly stated.

Under the attacks of the antivivisectionists, research committees were being more scrupulous in their approval of projects involving animal research. They were being more careful not only as to the value of the investigation but also with regard to the number of animals used, their care and their position on the evolutionary scale. Review agencies (FDA, EPA etc.) and companies were reducing the number of animals necessary to test the safety of chemical, drug and consumer products. The increasing cost of animals was another factor in these reductions.

Nevertheless, the continuing demands of the government regulating agencies, the ever increasing volume of products, and the evolving of perceived environmental and medical dangers created the necessity for the continued use of massive numbers and varieties of animals in testing. This remained true despite the development of computer models simulating biologic effects; and new techniques using tissue cultures and bacteria and single cell organisms to replace the 50% lethal dosage criteria (the dose at which 50% of the test animals die); and the Draize test (in which rabbits' eyes are dosed with materials to evaluate their irritability) being replaced by a membrane from a fertilized chick egg as the test object. But even the latter did not pass muster for the Animal Liberation Front, because it considered such eggs as living things entitled to better treatment.

Clinical investigators contested the position of the anti-vivisectionists on the philosophical grounds that animals, not being persons and lacking free-will, are not members of the moral community and therefore have no rights. Obviously animals, even the primates, are incapable of accepting duties. On these grounds it is wrong to equate speciesism with racism. To those who believe that the pains of all animate creatures count equally in any utilitarian equation assessing the morality of an action, it was answered that the prevention of great human suffering by animal research must be counted too. Further, it was stated that the position of animal activists is an emotional response and is irrational - they view all animals only as they do their pets. Their activities slow the progress and increase the cost of research, thus doing harm to humans.

Data from the Association of Biomedical Research showed that the cost of animal care in research laboratories had been doubled by the new U.S. Government regulations, an increase in costs estimated in 1987 to be $1 billion nationwide[41]. The Department of Agriculture had turned over to the Office of Management and Budget for review, regulations on exercise for dogs and on the psychological well-being of primates to complete implementation of the 1985 additions to the Animal Welfare Act. These regulations were to be released before the end of 1988. The Agriculture Department estimated they would cost research institutions $111 million in capital expenditures on primate facilities and $138 million for dog facilities. The total cost of all varied parts of the new regulations would be $885 million in initial outlays and another $207 million a year in additional operating expenses. Compliance costs for facilities run by the federal government would be another $100 million. The source for these new funds was an unanswered question, as was any estimate on the overall effect of the new regulations on the nation's research efforts[42]. Indeed, considerable research still was required to determine what measures would produce the maximum in captive primate well-being (as the law demands), and there was no telling what further financial commitment this would entail[43].

It is of interest that recent studies revealed that exercise was not what made dogs happy and fit, but that socialization was what made them feel good[44]. Human contact was the single most consistent and important factor in encouraging dogs to be active. As a result of these studies the Animal and Plant Health Inspection Service of the Department of Agriculture, instead of specifying in excruciating detail design standards such as cage sizes and exercise regimens, appeared to be moving toward a more flexible approach leaving more to the discretion of institutions. The trend was toward keeping research dogs in groups in runs or pens, rather than in single cages.

Another way animal-rights groups increased costs was by their interference with the use of pound dogs for research. They had been successful in having this practice banned in six states, and in having a bill introduced into the National Congress for this purpose[45]. Pounds shelter seven million abandoned dogs each year and, after

28% are adopted and 2% are sold or donated to research institutions, 5 million (71%) have to be killed. It was stated that it was morally better to use expensive laboratory bred animals than pound animals because to use the latter encouraged the abrogation of the responsibility of shelters to provide a decent life and a humane death for animals[46]. It can be pointed out that the Nazis, while sanctioning medical experiments on "non-aryan" humans, had strict laws protecting animals from vivisection[47]. Actually, the U.S. Department of Agriculture has conducted an annual survey of research animal use. Their reports to congress stated that less than 1% of dogs and cats were subjected to painful experiments without being anesthetized, and then only because the anesthetic would have interfered with the purpose of the research. A majority (10) of local referendums (13) in the U.S. on the use of pound dogs for research had resulted in permission being granted by wide margins[48].

Certainly, drugs and new procedures require testing before their use on humans. Young surgeons, as well, need to make themselves skillful and, in many instances, this is best done by practice on animals, and a good example is training with the microscope for use in the operating room.

The problem in searching for a vaccine against AIDS highlighted a special dilemma. The only animal, other than man, that can be infected by the AIDS virus are chimpanzees and therefore they are necessary for experimentation in search of a vaccine. Chimpanzees can be infected with the viruses of hepatitis and AIDS but, unlike humans, they do not become ill with them. However, chimpanzees are distressingly close to man: they can be taught a primitive language of several hundred words; they can make primitive tools and cooperate in endeavors; they have a social life and can transmit cultural traits; etc. It has been said that, since children and senile or mentally disabled adults are lower in the "scale" than these primates, it would be more moral that they be used for research.

Chimpanzees are in short supply and no longer can be imported from their natural habitat in Africa, where they are regarded as an endangered species. Farming, mining and timber harvesting are gobbling up the jungles of Africa, reducing their numbers there. Medical scientists are dependent upon the ones bred in captivity, and while hundreds have been so produced, it is increasingly more difficult to accumulate an adequate supply. In the first place, animals bred in captivity are inept in mating and child rearing as the result of being psychologically wounded[49]. Secondly, many of the animals are used in experiments with a form of viral hepatitis, non-A non-B, that leaves them and their offsprings permanently infectious. Since there are no tests to determine which of the exposed chimpanzees are infected, large numbers of animals bred in captivity are not available for other kinds of research. Another important item is that the cost of maintaining a chimpanzee over its lifetime of 30 to 50 years ranges from $150,000 to $250,000 (as of 1988).

Some believe it is wrong to use these primates at all for research; Jane Goodall declared the shipment of chimpanzees from Africa for biomedical research is akin to the slave trade[50]. She, and others (World Wildlife Fund and the Humane Society), wish the chimpanzee be placed on the endangered list world-wide, which would stop their use for experimentation totally. More believe it is wrong to sacrifice these animals when they have been made infected and are no longer suitable for research, just to save money. Euthanasia of chimpanzees is not an option as a result of the influence of animal rights activists on governmental agencies which supply, by far, the greatest amount of funds for their use in research.

Researchers in viral diseases and immunology stated the need for chimpanzees in their investigations is irreplaceable. In December 1986 four baby chimpanzees were stolen from a private research laboratory funded by the National Institutes of Health and routinely inspected by the Department of Agriculture. They were stolen by a group called True Friends, spoken for by another group called People for Ethical Treatment of Animals who said the animals were slated to be used for AIDS and hepatitis research and were not being given proper care.

In 1989 the Southwest Foundation for Biomedical Research, a leading facility conducting AIDS and hepatitis research, announced that it was establishing a pension plan for "retired" chimpanzees[51]. The chimpanzees are ones infected with HIV or hepatitis and are no longer useful. It had put aside $700,000 for the fund and planned to increase the fund to $1.7 million over the next 10 years and, with investment returns, the fund should total $3 million by the year 2000. It was planned that the chimpanzees would live to 2025, and they would need care in groups of three housed in indoor-outdoor facilities costing $60,000 each.

An interesting recent discovery is that chimpanzees are closer to humans genetically than they are to other primates. This means that humans and chimpanzees came from the same branch of the evolutionary "tree", and all other primates (baboons, orangoutangs, etc.) descended from another branch. Nevertheless, recently it has been discovered that aging female baboons suffer with osteoporosis, the only animal other than man known to develop such an affliction[52].

A corollary to the animal rights movement is the even more widely supported sentiment to "save *a* species", and is mentioned to illustrate the depth of feeling evoked by any thought relating to the lives of animals. The mention of endangerment to any single species causes an immediate response to protect it, and, typically, no explanation is offered or requested. Presumably the reasoning involved is *prima facie* and is widely accepted. Of course, the closer to man the species is, the greater the response. Should an explanation be offered, and it rarely is, it is implied that the species in question is important to the food chain and/or biosphere, with a further implication that other species, and even man, will become endangered, if this "particular species is not preserved. This is a typical example of "slippery slope" reasoning, which seldom yields proper deductions anyway, and the conclusions reached in its use in instances of endangered species, are certainly almost never true. This paragraph is addressed to activism in behalf of single-species-preservation as opposed to efforts to maintain the bio-diversity of the species of our planet. The latter concerns are related to the possibilities for an imminent mass extinction of species as the result of the loss of forests, the use of fossil fuels for energy and other activities of man that degrade the environment.

On the other hand, farmers and animal domesticators and mankind in less advanced civilizations than ours frequently feel economically and physically threatened by some single species and try to diminish or eliminate them. It is never mentioned that the success of one species will most often threaten others, and that the normal biologic evolutionary flow over the eons, in addition to creation of species, included the extinction of even greater numbers of them, and this is ongoing.

The matter of protecting whales currently is causing serious diplomatic tensions between the U.S. and Japan. Japan sees the hunting of whales as an important industry and significant to their way of life; Congress has passed a law to protect whales but does not state, nor do articles on this controversy explain, why it is important to protect whales. There is little question that whales are appealing creatures: they are mammals, they are the largest animals in the world, they are purported to be relatively bright, they do not threaten us, etc. These are sufficient reasons apparently for our democratically elected government to side with "single-species-preservationists" and pursue an international dispute with an allied capitalist nation.

An evolutionary view on the origin of ethics and rights offers a reasonable justification for the use of animals, even primates, in research. In fact, in no other circumstance is its application more appropriate. There are numerous examples in nature of one species using another for its own benefit - predators are amply represented among the fauna and even the flora of the earth. There can be little question that the contributions made by the medical sciences, largely achieved through animal experimentation, have been a principal cause of the population explosion of *Homo sapiens*. This is a basic expression of the evolutionary purpose and is an empirical fact.

Other philosophical explanations on the use of animals for research, either pro or con, are really in the realm of speculation or metaphysics. For instance, man in his primitive and, possibly most natural, state was a hunter-gatherer and to advocate that this species be only a gatherer and give up eating meat, can only be a specious extrapolation of an emotional reaction. Philosophers who have tried to find justification for the position of single-species-preservationists and antivivisectionists utilize reasoning based on deontologic and/or utilitarian ethical principles[53,54]. Another resorts to human intuition, *a la* George Moore, as to what is "good"[55]. Although obviously familiar with Darwinian evolution, they do not appear to have ever heard of evolutionary ethics.

The editor of Science, perhaps unknowingly, thoroughly endorsed evolutionary ethics and an evolutionary origin of rights, and put into perspective the relationship of the species[56]. "The ecology world is one in which there is only one standard of ethics: survival.

Species that can put together the smartest programs are going to survive, often at the expense of others. Ivory-tower critics may talk about animal rights or plant rights, but the mosquito is not worried about infiltrating across a border, nor does the malaria parasite have fits of conscience because it may be a stowaway in the illegal action. Nor is the swatter of the mosquito particularly distressed by intruding on the reproductive cycle of this interesting species."..."Curiously the animal rightists and anti-evolutionists think in parallel in regard to the exalted status of man. Animal rightists suggest we have no right to attack other species. Anti-evolutionists say we are so different that we cannot learn from the behavior of lower species. Both are partly wrong and partly right. Evolution makes no case for gifts of rights to other species, and we have learned much about human behavior from studies of less complex species. But ecological studies also reveal that species adapt to threats to their own survival, and symbiosis is one of nature's prize stratagems." He went on to point out that man has to modify his behavior in destroying the habitat for so many species, or he will soon destroy the environment for himself.

What spurs the animal rightists and single-species-preservationists to their "activist" roles? It is clear they express a feeling for the preservation of the lives of non-human creatures, and also the closer the animals are to humans the greater is the sympathy elicited. The term that best describes the reaction elicited is altruism. Altruism, an unselfish concern for others, has been shown by ethologists and sociobiologists to be widespread in the animal kingdom, and particularly is observable in the behavior of the social animals. Man, of course, is a social animal and it may be presumed that altruism is an evolutionary characteristic that is preserved as a template in the circuitry of the human brain.

As has been discussed previously, altruism is "hard-wired" into the brains of the social insects and their behavior is inflexible, come what may. Human behavior is more flexible and, while it may be less efficient for a specific task that is hard-wired into a lower animal, it is more adaptable to changing circumstance and, therefore, overall, better for the individual, and, in the aggregate, for the species. A good way to conceive of some human behaviors, such as altruism, that are good for the preservation of the species, is that brain circuitry has been selected by the evolutionary process to be inherited as a template to make expression of that beneficial behavior an easy one, under most circumstances. The strongest expression of altruism is a mother's concern for her off-spring. Only the most perverse of circumstance can suppress it, and then the mother who foregoes her child is viewed as being sick. It is well recognized that individuals will demonstrate altruism for their relations, and the closer the kinship the stronger will be the expression of altruism. However, altruism to lesser degrees will be extended as far out as to members of the same nation, and then it is called patriotism. The value of altruism in all these circumstances to the well-being and/or benefit of the persons or groups involved is obvious.

The existence of this template for altruism in the human brain makes it easy to extend altruism to animals. The more the species of animals are like humans, the easier human altruism is aroused. Also, the younger an animal, that is the more they remind us of our children, the easier the altruistic response is stimulated.

Individual circumstance determines the strength of expression of the universal human sympathy for living creatures. Respect for life is a tenet of almost all religions and can culminate in the making of *all* animal life sacred, as in some eastern sects. Thus a religious bent in an individual will remarkably strengthen any altruistic sentiment toward animals, and it will be justified as "respect for life". Also, all individuals have ego, another strong human trait of obvious evolutionary value, and ego can be involved in one's opinions to a greater or less extent. An individual's ego can strengthen his or her altruism for an animal, and lead to the desire of forcing that opinion on others. Such concern for the survival of animals can become a focus for the lives of some. The attendant publicity can be ego-satisfying and fuel the desire for more of it. A confluence of some, or all, of these sentiments may result in a person becoming an "unrestrained activist". Perhaps a biological manner of describing "unrestrained activists" is to point out that their actions are governed by the circuitry of the phylogenetically old brain, from which arise human emotions, and which overwhelms (or is uninhibited by) the reasoning capability of their neocortex (or phylogenetically new brain).

"Unrestrained activists" are ones who take the lead in furthering a cause by use of undue pressure in the persuasion of others, and are so certain that their opinion is correct that they are contemptuous of opposing points of view. One cornerstone of a democracy is freedom of expression, therefore why should "unrestrained activists" be condemned for pursuing their objectives? It is when their tactics become undue pressure that they warrant exposure. Almost everyone agrees that when they break the law by using violence in an effort to intimidate their opponents - that is undue pressure.

Their organization of efforts to persuade legislators and administrators to rule in their favor should be viewed as a more subtle form of undue pressure. That is so because the vast majority of persons are far less aggressive, and could even be labeled passive, especially when they sense, in a democracy, that they are in the majority. In all probability lobbying should be severely controlled so that it only informs legislators and administrators, and does not become "undue pressure". Undue pressure lobbying, when it subverts the opinion of a passive majority on any particular question, should be viewed as perverting the democratic process. "Unrestrained activists" often achieve a similar result by excessive litigation, utilizing technicalities in the legal system. The view of a passive majority should never be permitted to be over-ridden by an aggressive minority. In all probability, the preservation of democracy warrants interference of activists when they pursue their objectives with "undue pressure". This is true even though a long view of history demonstrates that, even if delayed, the perceptions of the majority will eventually triumph if their perceptions are truly to the benefit of society.

The objection to "unrestrained activists", or fundamentalists of any persuasion, is that their sense of righteousness permits them to be a disruptive force to the equanimity of a society, even if their cause actually be right. The rightness or wrongness of a cause most often needs time and reasonable discussion, which a loss of societal equanimity will preclude. This well could be the motivation for President Bush calling for "a kinder and gentler" society, after his bitter election campaign in which he appeared to be a candidate responding to "unrestrained activists".

No one could seem better motivated than anti-nuclear activists, willing not only to be arrested for their actions but also willing to risk their limbs and even their lives. Certainly their cause seems to be irreproachable: to protect their fellow beings from the extermination of nuclear war, or the ravages of nuclear plant accidents, or from radioactive wastes. Yet, might they be wrong?

Could nuclear arms be preventing major wars (because leaders are as exposed to death as are ordinary soldiers, and/or they realize it would be the end of our world) ? Might nuclear power be necessary to preserve civilization when fossil fuels run out; or preserve the environment by circumventing use of fossil fuels right now? Might not their undue anti-nuclear activism preclude "a warmer and gentler" society from having a civilized discussion on the subject?

"Unrestrained activists" do not prevent the achievement of correct answers - those answers that are in the best interests of a society or, in some matters, of the species. The evolutionary process, which governs cultural as well as biologic development, guarantees correct answers will be arrived upon, eventually. However, "unrestrained activists" (or fundamentalists on either side of the political spectrum) can delay, even inordinately delay, the achievement of correct solutions.

Obviously "unrestrained activists", as defined above, pay no attention to Aristotle's advice to take a moderate position on all issues in the political affairs of man - the Aristotelian mean. Some of them, those who regard themselves as progressives, need to be informed that the posture of moderation is the most identifying of all the attributes of the true liberal.

Complimenting an evolutionary justification for man's use of other species for research is the requirement that this use be as humane as possible. The observation of the behavior of other predators shows that their use of other species does not extend beyond their need. In research, to sacrifice more animals beyond useful need, or inflict suffering upon them, serves no purpose, evolutionary or otherwise. It is likely the use of animals for testing cosmetics and toiletries (perhaps 10 to 15% of all those used in research) does not fall into the category of "necessary research",and from an evolutionary ethical point of view should not be defended. Physicians are expected to be sensitive to pain and suffering, and indifference to these feelings when dealing with animals is poor preparation for the practice of medicine. This is not "slippery slope" logic, which depends upon reasoning by analogy and which, in turn, too often can be unrewarding in ascertaining truth - analogous situations are seldom precisely congruent. Rather, it is that the maintaining of high standards of sensitivity to the pain and suffering of animals used in research can help weed out from medical practice individuals lacking such awareness. This should apply also to another desirable virtue for a physician, respect for life. This can be emphasized by insistence that research protocols specify the use of the minimal number of animals necessary to attain an objective, and that the objective be clearly relevant - and not mainly for the aggrandizement or financial benefit of the investigator or an institution.

3. Biotechnology (Genetic Engineering)

Advances in molecular biology have resulted in the ability to alter the inheritance pattern of living things. To do so is called biotechnology, or genetic engineering, or recombinant DNA technology. These achievements have been accompanied by constantly broadening discussions on its dangers and/or morality. As the rapid advances involved life forms higher and higher on the evolutionary scale, different groups of people felt it necessary to enter the controversy. When at first the technique only was capable of altering bacteria, the scientists involved were concerned about the consequences of such bacteria getting loose from laboratories and killing large numbers of humans having no resistance to them. When the capability to alter plants and animals came about, religious and animal rights groups attacked biotechnology as altering God's work or being unfair to animals. Finally, when changes in plants and animals, or the development of genetically engineered drugs or hormones (like bovine somatotropin increasing milk production when given to cows), promised to have an effect on food and raw materials production, farmers and other groups felt a threat to their economic interests and then added their political strength to that of the "activists" who were against all of biotechnology[57].

All these groups of people were discussing the questions of whether biotechnology should be allowed to proceed at all and, if so, under what conditions? The increasing public fear of science, caused by threats of world annihilation with atomic bombs or of a widespread disaster from an accident in the use of nuclear power adds to the credibility of critics of the science of genetic engineering, in the minds of the fearful. Also, a perceived threat to the environment from genetically altered bacteria, insects or plants further arouses those already skeptical of the scientific advances of our civilization that degrade the environment. Proposals by the Department of Defense, in its Biological Defense Program, to produce potentially lethal agents by genetic engineering of organisms add to the concern, not only of those opposed to biotechnology, but also of many in the scientific community[58].

The discussion starts with a debate as to whether the right to freedom of inquiry can be aborted. The defenders of this principle make an analogy to the freedom of speech, and if it be terminated, the deleterious effect that would have to the seeking of truth. Ever since Galileo, scientists have found it difficult to conceive that there are matters best left unknown. They, and others, feel knowledge is good and, therefore, there is an absolute right to free inquiry. Opponents to this principle say that it was alright in premodern times when knowledge only concerned theory without practical consequences. But in modern times theoretical inquiry is quickly translated into action affecting everyone and therefore it is correct to regulate science[59]. They add to their thesis, that it is wrong to permit investigation to go unfettered, by giving examples of horrendous scientific investigation in the past.

Another approach is the construction of an utilitarian equation on the possible gains versus the possible losses to society from genetic engineering. Proponents cite the already realized ability to make bacteria into biochemical factories manufacturing in quantity - hormones, antibodies, enzymes and other biological products. The U.S. Patent Office recognized the economic value of such genetically engineered bacteria and made them patentable in 1976. Plants, in all probability, will have the genes of viruses and bacteria placed in them to enable them to produce their own insecticides and fertilizers. In 1986 genetically engineered plants became patentable. The use of genetically altered viruses as insecticides was a particularly exciting development, insofar as they gave promise of replacing chemical insecticides (being safer, and environmentally and ecologically more desirable)[60]. In the not distant future it was believed that cows could be genetically altered so as to produce far greater amounts of milk, pigs to have more and leaner meat, and animals to be more resistant to disease. There was also the possibility that biotechnology would produce remedies for incurable hereditary diseases: the most promising one in 1989 was hereditary emphysema, an autosomal recessive disorder due to a lack of a gene that leads to an alpha-one antitrypsin deficiency affecting from 20,000 to 40,000 persons in the U.S.[61]

In anticipation that animals would be genetically altered, the patent office, on April 1, 1987, agreed that such animals would be patentable. One year later, Harvard University was awarded a U.S. patent on a mouse that had been genetically altered through the insertion of an artificial cancer gene. The U.S. Congress in the spring of 1988, under pressure from a loose coalition of religious, environmental, animal welfare and farming groups, was considering legislation to rescind the patenting of transgenic animals (animals with genetic material from other species inserted into their cells giving them foreign traits). The European Patent Office rejected an application for a European patent on the same mouse. This first application for a patent on a transgenic animal was rejected in Europe pending the broad discussion on the subject that was just beginning in 1989 in the various organizations of the European Economic Community (EEC) (its Commission, Council of Ministers and its European Parliament). The pressure on the representatives in these organizations - from the scientists on one side and animal rightists and, so-called, conservationists and environmentalists on the other - from the twelve countries of the EEC was intense, and there was no clear indication what decision would be reached. Molecular biologists and biotechnology companies on both sides of the Atlantic were watching closely the course of the debate.

Opponents of biotechnology cited the dangers of micro-organisms getting loose from the laboratory and causing uncontrollable damage. It was said that the tropical forests and wildlands and its numerous insect and animal species still existed because heretofore there have been no organisms capable of converting these lands to profitable agriculture and animal husbandry. All this would change with continued genetic engineering. The possibility was evoked that feral animals or uncontrollable weeds (which would decimate food crops) would be produced. Skeptics feared that something highly undesirable would be passed on to those who ate genetically altered food.

Genetic engineering evokes a moral discussion, particularly when it is capable of being carried out at the animal level. A spokesman for the National Council of Churches stated that the gift of life was from God and not subject to genetic alteration and certainly not patentable for economic profit[62]. Animal rightists maintain tampering with an animal's natural characteristics is cruel and invasive of their innate dignity[63]; these are often the same people who see nothing wrong with zoo's. They go on to claim that transgenic animals will suffer because they will be weakened and made more vulnerable to disease.

There are those who have no objection to genetic engineering in animals but believe it is wrong to tamper with the human genome. It is wrong to try to "normalize" individuals or work to the "perfectibility" of the human species[64]. In this connection it should be understood that only changes made in the germ cells (ova or sperm) are those that would be carried from generation to generation; changes made in somatic cells affect only the individual so altered. A physician wondered why there should be any objection to manipulating the genome of somatic cells to provide recipients with what they perceive as a highly desirable quality - taller, handsomer, cleverer, etc.[65] He remarked that self-improvement is a highly valued social attribute: people exercise, use diets and take other measures to improve their health. Why should they be denied other treatments for their well-being just because it involves bio-technology? Some might find it distasteful for others to use gene therapy to improve themselves, but it is their democratic right, as long as no harm is caused someone else. "Is there any difference from cosmetic surgery?"

From the viewpoint of a beneficent physician, patients should not be denied the benefits of biotechnology to cure, or relieve, disease. However, the same criteria should be applied to cosmetic surgery - to be used to relieve disease, or distortion so severe as to be ranked with disease; but beneficence would dictate that either used for beautification is, and would be, unsound. Unsound because it is, and would be, taking risks with procedures that place emphasis on the wrong personal attributes of the individual, for a society to be a successful one. Also, cosmetic surgery and gene therapy of the latter variety, if paid for by insurance or taxes for all the autonomous patients who demanded them, would not be economically affordable and thus would be detrimental to the entire community.

In a poll conducted in 1986 by Lou Harris & Associates for Congress's Office of Technology Assessment, 60% of people believed genetic engineering would make their lives better and 22% thought life would be worsened[66]. Plant and animal bio-engineering were broadly approved, but 42% of those polled looked upon genetic tampering with humans as morally wrong. Despite this amount of negative sentiment in the abstract, 80% would permit alteration of their genes to treat a serious or fatal disease in themselves. A large portion of those opposed to biotechnology did so on moral grounds and tended to be less educated, or more religious, or both[67]. The perceived probability of danger also declined, the more educated was the person surveyed.

Despite the U.S. having been in the forefront in introducing these innovative techniques, by 1988 it was distinctly trailing in the world-wide expertise in biotechnology as applied to agriculture[40]. This was because funds allocated to basic research in plant biology had been meager, because of the impedance of regulatory processes, and by legal actions of those opposed to biotechnology. Jeremy Rifkin, an "activist", had been the leading figure in initiating this litigation in the U.S. - this was besides his efforts on other issues such as biological warfare, the global climate and surrogate motherhood. Expertise in agricultural biotechnology was worldwide - average yields of wheat per hectare in the Netherlands and the U.K. were more than twice those in the U.S. The amount on the positive side in the balance in the U.S. trade in agriculture had dwindled. "The United States can persist in a policy of starving agricultural basic research and of over-regulating biotechnology. Others may not follow such a path."

A committee of the Ecological Society of America refuted the claim that crop and animal breeding in the past had proven that genetic engineering was safe, because molecular techniques provide the ability to transfer traits among very different species. This made possible the creation of combinations that could not arise from traditional breeding. The committee also said that the introduction of a modified species was not always safe just because the species altered was a native one, rather than non-native from a distant area. Both native and non-native species can become pests, said the committee.

Nevertheless, throughout history foreign species had been introduced into alien environments, often decimating local species. The migration of Polynesians to Hawaii[69] and, in prehistoric time, neolithic colonization of the Mediterranean islands[70] were recently described examples of this process. Obviously the introduction of alien species into an environment is not a new phenomenon as the anti-biotechnology forces would have the public believe. Further, transplants of marrow and organs introduce foreign tissues with genetic material into people, and x-ray treatments and certain drugs cause alterations in genes without serious objections being aroused. It is difficult to understand how anyone could object to the use of biotechnology to cure disabling genetic diseases.

In the last decade venture capitalists recognized the commercial potential of these new techniques and established companies which have quickened the pace of research. In 1986 a national law was enacted in the U.S. giving comprehensive rules, guidelines and definitions to regulate this new industry. The rules determined how the five federal agencies involved will assess risks and benefits of bio-engineered products. Opponents of biotechnology claimed the regulations were too weak to prevent the release of possibly dangerous organisms. Researchers believed the regulations were too inclusive and often incomprehensible. Yet other molecular biologists believed that the failure to place "regulator genes" in the oversight program was a mistake[71]. These regulator genes are powerful, acting to increase or decrease the function of other genes, and these scientists asserted their use also ought to be the subject of rigorous review.

An interesting legal question had been raised by a lawsuit brought by a man cured of leukemia and whose spleen was used to produce a cell-line used in making a new drug (by biotechnological methods) that controlled the number of white blood cells in the blood[72]. This new drug could be useful in treating leukemia and possibly AIDS. The question was whether patients retained commercial property rights to their tissues after removal from their bodies. Such tissues are blood, other tissues removed because they are cancerous, or are excreta (urine) - all these are used in medical biotechnology. The defense for the scientist and the University, both having made millions of dollars in the twelve years after treating the plaintiff, was that the blood-line used came from the spleen which the patient had "abandoned" in the course of surgery. The defendants also claimed that if the plaintiff prevailed, research could be hindered by still more bureaucratic obstacles. While the problem had every appearance of being only a legal one, nevertheless, an oft-quoted ethicist posed questions to make it an ethical dilemma (again without offering a solution, or even how to go about deriving a solution): "We are on the edge of a biotechnology revolution. This decision is going to set the framework within which that revolution is going to occur. Are we going to view body parts as somewhat sacred, beyond the realm of the market? What, as a matter of public policy is the appropriate stance, to facilitate the growth of biotechnology? This case is sitting in the middle of a critical topic."

Later, the California Court of Appeal, in a two to one decision, overturned a lower California court's judgment in the above case and ruled that researchers must get permission from patients before using tissues and body fluids obtained in the delivery of health care[73]. The Appeal Court also indicated that if research revealed that a patient's tissues could yield products of commercial value, the donor had a right to some compensation unless any financial interest had been specifically relinquished. (In July 1990, the California Supreme Court overruled the above Appeal Court's decision, deciding that a patient does not have property rights over body tissues that may be used to develop new drugs or medicines. However, a physician did have the "fiduciary" duty to tell a patient if researchers have an economic or personal in using or studying such tissues.)

The National Academy of Science in 1987 issued a panel report stating: "There is adequate knowledge of the relevant scientific principles, as well as sufficient experience with recombinant DNA techniques, to guide the safe and prudent use of such organisms outside research laboratories."[74] The panel also concluded recombinant DNA microbes posed no special hazards compared to organisms modified by other genetic methods (by irradiation, breeding, etc.) which are far less strictly regulated. The properties of a particular organism, not the method by which it was made, should be the basis for evaluating its environmental risks. The unfortunate consequences of introducing *naturally* occurring species such as the gypsy moth and killer bees into foreign environments could have been cited.

The National Academy of Science did not believe that strict and rigid control for releasing all biotechnological products was justified. This was not to say there was no danger: the panel warned that some experiments could be risky if they involve potential weeds or pathogens or organisms alien to the environment into which they are introduced. It is the nature of the redesigned organism and the environment into which it is to be released that determine the risk. There is far more risk in working with a potential pest than with a slightly altered corn plant. What is needed is a scientifically sound hierarchy of categories defining the degree of risk for different types of experiment. This should be done as soon as possible and "it is unhelpful to clamor either for stricter indiscriminate control or for giving free rein to experimenters."[75]

In late 1989 a panel of the American National Academy of Science updated its report and reiterated that field testing of genetically modified plants and microorganisms "will not pose any hazard" to the environment if done carefully under laws existing at that time. They pointed out that eighty modified plants and microbes had been tested in the environment without accident, by the time of their report. Nonetheless, by May 1990, the availability of crop plants genetically engineered to resist plant pathogens and herbicides still were being held up because of lack of agreement among U.S. federal agencies on what should be the regulations for their outdoor testing[76].

A German Parliamentary Commission in early 1987, on the other hand, recommended a five year moratorium on all experiments involving the release into the environment of genetically engineered viruses and bacteria, to allow time for further research on potential ecological side effects[77]. They also suggested a ban on genetic screening of newborns for diseases that cannot be treated, although it welcomed prenatal screening for diseases where medical intervention could be helpful. The commission's broad conclusion was that the potential benefits of biotechnology were likely to outweigh its social or environmental risks. This broad endorsement was rejected by one Commission member, a representative of the Greens, an environmentalist party that had recently been making strong political gains in Germany. The influence of the Greens, many of whom could be classified as zealots or fundamentalists, undoubtedly influenced other members of the German Commission to issue the relatively conservative report on biotechnology. The hostile atmosphere to biotechnology in Germany was causing German biotechnology firms to open laboratories abroad to protect their interests[78]. In England, approval was given in 1986 to release a caterpillar infected with a genetically marked virus into a cabbage patch.

This variation among nations in their attitude to safety guidelines for the release of genetically altered micro-organisms into the environment was reported to be the biggest outstanding issue in Europe in the overall regulation of biotechnology[79]. There was an effort being made by a commission of the European Economic Community to reconcile the differences of its various component countries on this question. There was great pressure from financial circles, and others, to reach a prompt consensus so that Europe would not fall behind in the international race to develop the biotechnology industry.

In January 1988 the New Jersey Legislature rejected a measure that would have established the first state regulations to control genetically altered bacteria.

In the less than two decades since the first report of a successful recombinant DNA experiment in bacteria, the discussions on the use of biotechnology are encouraging to anyone who is optimistic that the human species will continue to follow its evolutionary destiny and believes in the beneficence of our scientists. Biologists themselves in 1975 were sufficiently concerned about the potential of the new technique to ask for a moratorium on its use. Reacting to this warning, the National Institutes of Health formed a committee to monitor biotechnology research and formulate new research rules. Since then confidence has been gained in the ability to use recombinant DNA techniques safely. This has come from increased knowledge of the events that lead to uncontrolled growth of cells and the recognition that genetic engineering has been going on in nature for eons without catastrophic consequences, albeit more slowly[80]. Moreover, animals and plants have been manipulated for centuries by man - domestication and breeding have produced animals such as overproductive dairy cows that never could survive in the wild.

Advances in biotechnology raise the possibility that certain genetic defects in man might be corrected. These possibilities were so advanced by 1988 that research councils of Europe felt compelled to issue a joint statement on the subject[81]. The scope of their statement was limited to the correction of specific genetic defects in individual patients. This treatment was to be distinguished from the application of gene therapy for the enhancement of human characteristics such as physical appearance or intelligence. The latter, in their view, raised profound ethical problems and should not be contemplated. This part of the statement was in recognition that treatment of genetic defects could be done by insertion of foreign genes into somatic cells or germ cells. Since the latter (germline gene therapy) would cause the foreign gene to be passed on to offsprings, it was not to be contemplated. To the contrary, insertion of genetic material into somatic cells and their subsequent transplantation is the same as any organ transplantation or blood transfusion.

They predicted that only single gene defects would be amenable to treatment for the foreseeable future, and they gave some details of those which they believed first ought to be investigated. They endorsed the use of retroviruses for these purposes, pointing out that modern production techniques assured that they would not subsequently replicate. Safety was emphasized - there must be no possibility of producing active, possibly cancer inducing, helper or vector viruses; nor the possibility of the inserted gene inducing cancer or cause other harmful disturbances of cell regulation or function.

In the fall of 1988 the Recombinant Advisory Committee of the U.S. National Institutes of Health, in a 16-5 vote, gave approval to the National Cancer Institute to insert a bacterial gene into white blood cells of human patients with melanoma. The purpose was to better track enhanced white cells that previously had given promise in the treatment of melanomas. The approval of the Director of NIH and the Federal Drug Administration were necessary before the experiments could proceed. This approval was delayed because it was disclosed that some of the accumulated data on the project had been withheld[82]. The reason given for the withholding of data was that the scientists involved had some concern that otherwise their chances for publication of papers in scientific journals would be jeopardized. The jeopardy would be that the wide pre-publication dissemination of the data would cause journals to refuse papers subsequently submitted. The Editor of Science admitted the fear was a real one, but said he never refused to allow authors to give data to governmental agencies.

Finally, by January 1989 all necessary review committees, the Director of NIH and the FDA had given their approvals and the experiments were authorized to proceed. Immediately an "activist" began efforts to halt the experiments by suing in the Federal District Court on the ground the NIH review panel had failed to follow proper procedure. This "activist" had previously been quoted as opposing biotechnology research in general, chemical and bacterial warfare research by the army, surrogate motherhood, etc. His claim was the fundamentalist one, that it is wrong to tamper with the human chemical blueprint (the DNA) and that, secondly, it was dangerous. In support of the latter argument the "slippery slope" was cited: crossing the threshold into direct genetic manipulation may lead to outcomes which cannot be controlled - workers may be "engineered" to render them less susceptible to chemical carcinogens in lieu of cleaning up the workplace. He called for a moratorium on all human gene therapy research until the NIH established an "Advisory Committee on Human Eugenics" to review the social and ethical implications of human genetic engineering. "The NIH took obvious offense at Rifkin's use of 'eugenics' and turned down his proposal, saying that current mechanisms are sufficient"[83], and the experiment proceeded.

The first argument offered above against human gene therapy, the fundamentalist one, is dismissed by the vast, although usually less vocal, majority as merely a personal opinion; the second argument, that bio-engineering is dangerous, has been discussed and answered above, and the fallacy in using the slippery-slope approach also has been amply explained previously. To repeat, the NIH did agree that there are ethical problems associated with gene therapy, but that these could be resolved by its Recombinant DNA Advisory Committee and that the Eugenics Committee suggested by the activist, Rifkin, was not only unnecessary, but also was a trap.

In early 1990, a National Institute of Health panel, the Institutional Biosafety Committee, approved a proposal to treat children suffering with adenosine deaminase (ADA) deficiency by inserting new genes into their blood cells. ADA deficiency is a genetic disorder that permits the build-up of a toxic chemical in the body that destroys the immune system and requires the child to live in a sterile enclosure to protect against infection (as the highly publicized "bubble boy"). It was proposed that T-cells be isolated from a

patient's blood and they be infected with a genetically engineered
mouse retro-virus containing the gene to make ADA enzyme. The
infected T-cells will then be transfused back into the patient. The
mouse retro-virus was so designed that it could not cause disease in
humans. Before this experiment could proceed the approval of six
other federal regulatory panels was required, which would take, at
least, the better part of a year. Other genetic-defect diseases that
were believed to be amenable to similar treatment were cystic
fibrosis, familial cholesterol disorders, metabolic deficiencies of the
liver, etc.

4. The Human Genome

It is almost certain that the human genome (the complete set of
hereditary factors - 3 to 3.5 billion base pairs) will be fully mapped
and its DNA sequenced in the not distant future. Following upon
this, it is believed that it will be possible to identify individuals prone
to diseases that result from multi-genetic characteristics. The diseases
thought to result from the interaction of a number of genetic
peculiarities are arteriosclerosis and early heart attacks, hypertension,
susceptibility to a variety of cancers, major psychiatric disorders,
diabetes, arthritis, emphysema, alcoholism, etc. If in fact, as seems
likely, genetic predisposition to various chronic diseases becomes
predictable, then individuals could avoid lifestyles and/or
environmental conditions that would be of specific hazard to them.
This is visualized as a monumental advance for preventive medical
care, enhancing the quality of life for all and reducing the present
enormous costs of therapeutic medical care.

Mapping the human genome means locating one of the
estimated 50,000 to 100,000 genes at a particular place on one of
the 46 human chromosomes (23 pairs, one from each parent).
Sequencing means identifying the order of the chemical sub-units of
DNA in any segment of a gene. A single sequence of DNA in the
gene, the arrangement of the four chemical subunits (amino-acids)
involved together with that on the adjacent other strand of the
double helix, is called a base-pair. Together these factors, mapping
and sequencing, allow the pinpointing of the location of genes and
a knowledge of their chemistry, which would permit an understanding
of their functions in every aspect of human life. It was believed, in

1989, that it would take 5 years to map the chromosomes and perhaps 15 years to complete the sequencing.

The down-side of defining the human genome would be the serious threat to the insurability or employment prospects of many individuals. It is foreseen[84] that employers would demand genetic screening of prospective employees to weed out those susceptible to their environment or likely to be financial risks in the future because of poor health or even as a threat to being disruptive to the work force. The ability to determine the genetic composition of all individuals will bring the conflict between individual rights and the rights of society and companies into the sharpest focus.

Another aspect of the rapid advance in the science of genetics is the assessment of the effect of it possibly making the results of human mating more predictable. Some might fear it would lead to a renewed effort to revive previously debunked eugenic programs to improve the species or even to create a "master race". Some might fear it would reduce the uncertainty of life - making it duller, less interesting and less "romantic".

Others say that the ethical questions associated with eugenics and genetic screening already confront us and merely would be heightened by knowledge of the entire sequence, and thus the project would not "diminish our dignity, and interfere with the moral standing of human kind." They believe the biologic benefit to the species will outweigh all objections. Perhaps in a strong democracy the emphasis on individual freedom can preclude over-regimentation that otherwise could follow upon the complete elucidation of the human genome - and even if it required the sacrifice of some health goals. An important opinion was expressed by the Editor of Science: "There are immoralities of commission that we must avoid. But there is also the immorality of omission - the failure to apply a great new technology to aid the poor, the infirm, and the underprivileged."[85]

However, the fear that elucidation of the human genome will lead to eugenic manipulations that would favor desirable human characteristics - such as intelligence, appearance or even altruism - seem far-fetched. Such characteristics are determined by the interactions of the effect of multiple genes, probably together with the participation of the environment. Steven Rose, a neurobiologist and a well-known critic of "biological determinism", believes that biology cannot be reduced to the additive effects of individual DNA strands and that the outcomes of genes functioning in a multi-determined environment, in developmental and evolutionary terms, are unpredictable from a simple knowledge of their sequences[86]. Moreover, the possibility of changing the DNA of an individual so as to modify complex characteristics are extremely remote. It cannot even be certain that simple single-gene disorders will ever be overcome by bio-engineering, no matter how desirable is such a goal.

That there are ethical problems sure to arise with the mapping of genes responsible for characteristics other than those of medical importance already was revealed in 1989, before the genome program had even gotten underway[87]. One investigator, in the course of charting the lipoprotein genes of patients, came up with data on their color blindness. He did not inform those patients of this data and when asked why, he replied: "I didn't want to worry them." A colleague retorted: "Don't you think you were obliged to pass on your findings? They might explain a lot of traffic accidents."

The complete definition of the human genome provoked a controversy at another level. The Department of Energy, because of its interest in the genetic mutations caused by nuclear radiation, expressed the desire to sponsor the project. This prompted the National Institutes of Health to fear that the Department of Energy would dominate a project more familiar and more pertinent to their personnel and to their interests. The dispute was resolved late in 1988 with the project handed over to a new "Office for Human Genome Research" in the NIH, to be headed by a discoverer of the DNA double helix, James Watson.

With the technology available, the project was estimated to require at least $3 billion over 15 years. This huge cost could well result in long delays in getting on with the undertaking in the U.S., because of the difficulty in obtaining appropriations in an era of severe governmental budget deficits. However, the Japanese and the Russians were working on the project, and the Europeans, with their smaller resources, were doing what they could.

The cost of the genome project, nevertheless, is much smaller than the cost of a supercollider or a space station, and it is a cooperative enterprise of many laboratories, not a massive assembly line production as are these other "big science" projects. Another manner of viewing costs is to compare amounts spent on single diseases with the cost of the human genome project. The various foundations, such as those for cystic fibrosis, multiple sclerosis, etc., plus the Federal Government spend hundreds of millions of dollars each, as compared with the $200 million yearly cost of the genome project. The markedly greater number of individuals benefited by the latter as compared with the former makes the genome endeavor a remarkably cost-efficient one.

It is envisioned by some in the U.S. that a private corporation, with venture capital, could complete the project in several years and be able to sell the information around the world for a fine profit. Ethicists, and even a business man, are quoted that the project on the human genome should be a national one since it is entwined with many ethical questions, and it would be unseemly to leave it in the hands of Wall Street[88].

Another perception on the value of complete sequencing of the human genome recently had been expressed[89]. It was agreed that a mountain of data would result, but it was argued that most of it would be meaningless. It would be the mapping of specific traits to specific genes that should be helpful, but sequencing would have only a marginal effect. In the opinion of this scientist: "those who fret about the sanctity of the human genome needn't worry - we may understand less about ourselves at the end of this project than when we began."

It rarely takes more than 5000 base pairs to describe a protein and the number of proteins is probably less than 100,000. So only 500 million base pairs are truly informative, less than 2% of the genome. The remaining 98% of the genome is probably meaningless junk, punctuated by hulks of useless genes evolution had bypassed. However, developing technology might soon be able to look around the meaningless junk to the genes and thus speed the process of deciphering the genome.

A National Academy of Science committee reported in February 1988 that, despite the above opinion, they favored sequencing the entire human genome[90]. They said early efforts should focus on regions of particular interest, and by the time sequencing begins on a massive scale technical advances will make it easier and cheaper to sequence whole blocks without attempting to discriminate among them. In addition, they believe many of the apparently uninteresting stretches will undoubtedly prove to be otherwise.

A world-wide conference held in Valencia in October 1988 called for international collaboration on the genome project so as to save resources by avoiding duplication of efforts. However, the lack of actions taken, and the general atmosphere of the meeting, bespoke more for competition between nations than collaboration[91].

The Commission of the European Economic Community (EEC) in early 1989 proposed a 3-year $19 million program to increase cooperation among the genome efforts of their various nations, and to find ways to integrate European efforts into any future collaborative project with U.S. scientists. A few critics from the European Parliament of the EEC, led by a member of the German Green party, argued that the attention of the EEC first should be on social and ethical aspects of the research before it is allowed to proceed. This led to amendments being added to the proposal which stipulated the program be broadened to study "the history of and current trends in eugenics" and for the preparation of a list of "possible and desirable measures to prevent the misuse of scientific knowledge of the human genome."[92] Also, that there be a clear legal agreement with individuals whose DNA was being studied, covering the nature of the use and study of their DNA and the rights of those concerned in respect to the use of the research results. There were forty families already being studied in France by French scientists in collaboration with the U.S. Howard Hughes Medical Institute. Most of the European nations were opposed to the restrictive amendments, but the German Bundestag had already given qualified approval to them. Some observers attributed the German attitude to a lack of centralized medical research policy in West Germany and to a continuing national guilt complex about Nazi atrocities based on "eugenics".

In February 1989, the Parliament of the EEC extended their debate on the EEC Commission's proposal to study the human genome. Their conclusion at that time was that they would approve the program only if some of the money was to be used to finance items such as studies of the history of eugenics movements and/or for public information campaigns emphasizing both the potential benefits and hazards of human gene analysis and therapy. As a result of the fierce Parliamentary debate the Commission decided to delay the start of the new program, which was to have been back-dated to January 1, 1989. As of April 1989, when the EEC Research

Commissioner called a halt to the program until a professional and ethical code could be agreed by the twelve members of the council of Research Ministers, it was not certain that the program would ever begin[93].

It may be concluded that biotechnology is making contributions to the well-being of the human species, and there is every promise of it continuing to do so in the future. This is contested by fundamental activists, who seem always to need a "cause", and who have decided to try to stop genetic engineering for fear, vaguely and incorrectly reasoned, that it will contaminate the world. There are other categories of individuals, such as animal welfare and religious groups, who perceive their sentiments threatened by biotechnology. Despite all this opposition, the rational basis of the contribution that genetic engineering can make to the welfare of society was broadly comprehended and it was being pursued worldwide. This is the major factor that must overwhelm those attempting to halt the pursuit of biotechnology. (Could anti-biotechnology activists be labeled unpatriotic?) Even if biotechnology is slowed down in various places, to the despair of the scientists therein located, competition from progress elsewhere in the world will force resumption of its pursuit.

A report to the 1988 meeting of the American Association for the Advancement of Science on the state of Soviet Science reveals that the U.S. leads in biotechnology, "although not distantly,"[94]. Another report noted that Japan was spending $200 million a year for research on rice genetics and European governments were supporting gene mapping on grains and vegetables, as well as other forms of bio-engineering. Competition among nations in the past forced development of scientific advances that appeared to be even less promising for the welfare of the species, such as the atom bomb.

CHAPTER EIGHT. PROBLEMS OF REPRODUCTION - ABORTION
(with notes on contraception)

Reading the contributions to the literature on the abortion controversy is most illustrative of the current impasse in many bioethical discussions. The positions of writers, on either side, arise from motivations that appear to them to be correct *a priori*. Their points of view are then supported by analogies, more or less cleverly constructed. The arguments center about: one, is abortion ever justified?, and second, if ever justified, are there limitations? A negative answer to the first question generally is based on straight-forward reasoning from a religious conviction that the reproductive process is sacred and should not be tampered with.

In answering the second question all persons, except the religious fundamentalists, believe that if conception is occasioned by rape or incest, abortion is justified. In instances of a pregnancy threatening the life of a mother, more people would favor saving the mother than preserving the fetus. Malformation of the fetus, promising a difficult life ahead for the child and the parents, is regarded by many as justification for abortion. Indeed, many regard it to be ethically deficient not to test as far as possible to be certain the fetus is healthy. A final consideration, if it is agreed abortion is ever permissible, is when (and what factors determine when) in the course of pregnancy abortion might be performed.

If abortion is to be done, the earlier in pregnancy it is done the safer it is for the woman, and as the pregnancy advances the more dangerous it becomes. Even after only 14 weeks there is one chance in 5900 of a fatality in the woman as compared with a case mortality of 0.5/100,000 for all stages of pregnancy combined.

When abortion is sought for the convenience of the parents, principally because they are unmarried, or as a measure for birth control, most often the controversy is about when, in the reproductive process, new life begins. This is believed to be important to determine when the rights assigned to an individual start and the duty of the state to protect those rights arises. The considerations used by varying individuals, or groups, as a dividing point before which abortion is permissible and after which it is wrong are: the time when the fetus becomes viable outside the womb, or becomes sentient, or acquires a soul; or when the fetus becomes a person, or whether only the potential for personhood is significant.

The beginning of life cannot be determined since, in reality, *it is a continuum* of living cells from one generation to another. Nevertheless, some suggest life begins at fertilization and others when the embryo implants itself into the wall of the uterus (14 - 17 days after fertilization). The reason given for the latter event to be the "beginning of life" is that at least 60% of fertilized human egg cells fail to implant themselves and are lost. Others believe life should be regarded as begun when the embryo takes on human form and becomes a fetus, at 7 or 8 weeks of pregnancy and after this, abortion could be called a killing. Roman Catholic dogma is driven by its own logic to the position that ensoulment takes place at fertilization. In this regard, the attitude toward the development of vaccines against conception is revealing. Such vaccines are feasible either to be given the woman so she would abort spontaneously immediately after conception, or given the man so that the sperm be prevented from fertilizing the ovum. More people regard the latter type of vaccine to be more acceptable, because "life" never is begun[1].

It is agreed, medically, that viability of a fetus (able to survive outside the womb) occurs at 24 to 26 weeks of pregnancy (down from 28 weeks in 1973), but it is unlikely ever to go below 23 weeks since before then the lungs are not mature enough to function even if ventilated. By 1987, at 25 weeks one premature baby in two could be saved; at 24 weeks one in five. Below 22 weeks of gestation there is no prospect of keeping a premature baby alive.

Still others would designate 12 weeks from the first day of the mother's last period as the time limit for abortion because that is the earliest point, in the development of the human brain and nervous system, that sensation of the fetus is first possible. On this basis a more reasonable cut-off time for abortion is 18 weeks, because after that time the fetus possesses a distinctly formed brain that reasonably can be regarded as functional. It is believed by some the development of the brain marks the beginning of life because it is the organ for thinking and feeling (sentience) and marks when the fetus becomes a person. Another reason to focus on the appearance of the brain as the beginning of life is that it is agreed widely, now, that its death is the point at which life ends.

Actually in 1986 there were a total of 4594 abortions done on women living in England and Wales after 18 weeks of pregnancy (3% of the total number of abortions that year). Of these late abortions 14% were for fetal abnormalities, and 40% were in women under the age of 20 with 6% under the age of 16[2]. The point of this latter report was that most of these late abortions were the result of delays in the system and not on the part of the women. Some delays resulted from practitioners being morally opposed to the procedure, and it was stressed that the ethical guidelines of the British Medical Association stated that such a doctor had the duty to refer the patient promptly to another physician.

Another British report[3] concluded that limiting the gestational age at which abortion can be done to 18 weeks would seriously disadvantage women most in need of abortion. In 1985, 323 women of England and Wales had legal abortions at the gestational age of 20 or more weeks because of risk of the child being born handicapped. In 1986 this number had risen to 648. If these abortions would have been prevented by law, in addition to the suffering and burden the resulting children would have been to themselves, their mothers and families, they would have posed an estimated financial burden of at least $50 million to their families and/or the state over the course of their lives.

The conservative advocate denies abortion is ever permissible, the liberal believes it is always permissible, while the moderate believes it is allowable before either viability, sentience or the potential for personhood of the fetus is attained. These varied positions are defended, or attacked, also, according to how the rights of the mother and fetus are viewed. As an example, a legal controversy raged in California (and could still be going on) over the criminal prosecution of a woman for allegedly not providing adequate medical care for her fetus. One contending side claimed the rights of the fetus were compromised, as well as those of the father; the other side (supported by the A.C.L.U.) argued that the rights of women were being ignored, and the woman was being subjected to sexual discrimination. Both sides agreed that an important issue was the determination of when the fetus became viable[4].

Another aspect of the conflict between the perceived rights of the mother and fetus arises at the time of delivery. In the event that a Caesarean delivery is thought necessary by an attending obstetrician (or obstetricians) to protect the fetus, can the mother refuse? The courts have been appealed to on 21 similar occasions since 1981[4] and in all but three instances the judges issued court orders to hospitals to go against the will of the pregnant woman. Their decision was based on the opinion that they "could not indulge the desires of the parents when there is substantial risk to the unborn infant".

Indeed the court even over-ruled the opinions of attending physicians not to intervene in the case of a woman who was 26 weeks pregnant and dying of cancer, granting a petition of the hospital to do a Caesarean section in an attempt to save the fetus (which probably was not yet viable). This was over the objections of both parents to the operation. The woman and the baby both died shortly after the operation. Thereafter the District of Columbia Court of Appeals affirmed the order, three judges ruling that since the woman had "at the best only two days left of sedated life" the lower court was correct to place the interests of the unborn child over the mother's right to avoid bodily intrusion. However in March 1988, when this case was reappealed to the same court by the American Civil Liberties Union and 39 other organizations including the American Medical Association, eight judges set aside the above three-judge ruling without elaboration, but said the entire court would hear new arguments in the case later in the spring of 1988. The organizations had argued that there was no legal precedent for requiring one person to submit to medical treatment for the sake of another, and that the reasoning of the three-judge panel suggested that the wishes of ill or disabled individuals should count for less than those of healthy people.

Finally, on April 26, 1990 the entire Appeals Court of the District of Columbia ruled in a 7-to-1 decision on the above case that the pregnant woman should not have been forced to undergo the Caesarean delivery against her will. The majority opinion noted that courts had uniformly refused to require people to donate organs or undergo other forms of "significant intrusion" for the medical benefit of others. A fetus cannot have rights in this respect superior to those of a person who has already been born, the opinion stated. Also: "The right of bodily integrity belongs equally to persons who are competent and persons who are not," and "it matters not what the quality of a patient's life may be; the right of bodily integrity is not extinguished simply because someone is ill, or even at death's door." This was the first appellate decision in the U.S. to address any version of this issue on the basis of full briefing and arguments, and was expected to have broad influence despite the ruling being binding only in the District of Columbia.

Another judge in another case refused to grant a petition to do a Caesarean section against a woman's will, reasoning from the analogy that a judge has no right to force a man to risk surgery to donate a kidney to his child. It is ironic that a few hours after this judge's decision the woman delivered a healthy child despite the pre-delivery opinion this was not possible because of the umbilical cord being wrapped around the infant's neck.

In England, in January 1988, a local authority petitioned the court to make a fetus its ward, fearing that the mother's way of life was endangering it. The court, upheld by an appeals court, ruled it would be infringing on the mother's rights to grant the petition. This decision, which was contrary to most decisions in similar cases in the U.S., was supported by the English press[5].

It would seem that in instances which pit the health or habits (use of illicit drugs, alcohol, tobacco, etc.) of the mother against the health of an unborn fetus, a principle that might well be labeled proportionality ought come into play. That is the risk to the mother should be weighed against that to the fetus, both determined empirically, and one should overwhelm the other before a decision to act is made.

One medical ethicist expressed the opinion that forced Caesarean sections usually arise in cases involving poor women, foreign women, or women that have religious beliefs the doctors do not share[6]. He said: "What I think happens is that a lot of doctors identify more with the fetus than with a woman who is different from them." He did not believe the doctors were practicing defensive medicine for fear of getting sued if the baby was left to deliver naturally and was not perfect. To a physician, this was an amazing interpretation, particularly when it is well-known that obstetricians are in the forefront in taking the brunt of the onslaught of malpractice suits, in suits most often based on this very issue.

The controversy in these cases rages on, by doctors, lawyers and ethicists with no resolution in sight. One view was that, *a priori*, the autonomy of pregnant women always should supersede the beneficence of physicians (to mothers and to their fetuses) in these disputes[7]. This was a further pursuit of the recent emphasis on autonomy over beneficence by medical ethicists. Moreover, these authors believed that a physician's fear of civil and/or criminal liability, for either honoring or disregarding a competent woman's wishes, was misplaced. They gave valid legal explanations that this should be so, but failed to summarize actual court experiences to prove their point. Practical results all too often vary from what ought to happen theoretically according to ethicists, especially if it depends upon how juries interpret facts.

An evolutionary ethical approach might well assume that all potential mothers have a common instinct to protect their fetuses and for a woman to go against this instinct must be an aberration, and especially so if it is against the advice of medical experts. The majority of judges obviously make decisions in accord with this principle - unknowingly, but, again, perhaps instinctively. A vital criterion, the origin of rights (see Chapter Two for the proposal for an evolutionary origin), is not discussed by those participating in the abortion controversy. It appears that the attitude of both sides is that the existence of rights is obvious, and reasoning by analogy will explain their relationships and priorities. Similarly, moral principles are frequently cited, but where these originate is not defined. Indeed, one writer[8] gives credence to her view because it arises from her intuition, and believes positions on abortion opposing hers, are based merely on emotion!

The position of conservatives against abortion (and they are usually against contraception) is easiest to understand. It is stated simply: life is a gift from God, therefore sacred, and interference with it cannot be tolerated. Those opposed to this position give numerous arguments along the lines described above, but they never attack the basic conservative premise publicly; theism is never identified as a hypothesis and can be, therefore, only conjectural.

Such is the continuing power of religion in moral debates, despite its weakening over the last 300 years (as discussed in Chapter One). An anti-abortionist with a more subtle philosophical mind but nevertheless intrigued by the "...emergence of life, and especially of mind, are mysteries which we cannot explain" concluded that life should not be manipulated without fully understanding its special (mystical) properties[9]. Other anti-abortionists who would deny they are theists nevertheless base their position on a "reverence for life".

The fundamental anti-abortionists do make a telling point: infanticide, at present, is condemned universally because we all have an intuitive feeling that newborns are of the same moral importance as the rest of us. Since the infant is no more of a person than a fetus, those who justify abortion on this basis, to be logical, must condone infanticide. The rejoinder of a pro-abortionist is that infants, unlike fetuses, are in demand for adoption and in any event the public loves infants and is willing to support them in orphanages or otherwise provide for their care[8]. It is further argued that: "so long as the fetus is unborn, its preservation, contrary to the wishes of the pregnant woman, violates her rights to freedom, happiness, and self-determination." It would seem a stronger reply would be that any reference to personhood is fallacious since not even a baby is truly a person. Personhood has been variously characterized as: a rational, willing agent (Kant); a thinking, intelligent being (Locke); a being that is self-aware and able to think (M. Tooley).

Those in favor of abortion, particularly physicians, list several items as justification for their opinion. First are the great number of fetal anomalies and severe complications of pregnancies that make abortion in such situations the treatment of choice for all concerned. Second is the enormous contribution abortion makes to the mental health and material welfare of many women. A third justification cited are the number of teen-agers whose lives are rescued from a ruinous destiny. Another point is: women who become pregnant against their wishes will have an abortion if it is legal or not; making it illegal will only drive them into the hands of "back-alley butchers". In addition, many social workers favor abortion because of their experiences with the unhappy fate of unwanted children.

In the closing days of his term (1989) President Reagan, whose anti-abortion views were well-known, requested a report from his Surgeon General on the effect of abortions on the health of women.

The Surgeon General, also well-known to be an anti-abortionist, replied that scientific data on this subject were inconclusive, and therefore he could not complete the report. This disappointed the Administration but, it was the best the Surgeon General could do, since specific investigations do indicate that abortion is of benefit to women's health. One might even say the evidence is overwhelming in this direction. In the first place there is solid data on the immediate physical effects: the death rate of women had dropped from 4 per 100,000 abortions in 1972 to 0.5 per 100,000 (0.0005%) in 1985, and thus the risk from abortion is down to a level seven times safer than that of natural childbirth[10]. This data had been collected by the Federal Centers for Disease Control of the Surgeon General's office. Data also indicated that there was no long term physical problems resulting from abortion. With regard to the emotional consequences of abortion, investigators said the evidence indicated that most women suffer no lasting damage. There was evidence of more emotional stress from unwanted pregnancies than from abortions. It had been found that the feelings of guilt, regret, or loss elicited by a legal abortion which arise in some women were generally temporary and appeared to be outweighed by their positive life changes and feelings of relief. There was no evidence of a response after abortion that even could compare to the prevalence and duration of postpartum depression, which affects 7% of mothers.

Furthermore, a review of methodologically sound studies of the psychological responses of U.S. women after they obtained legal, nonrestrictive abortions, published in April 1990 (but such studies were available prior to the Surgeon General's report to the President), determined that distress was generally greatest before the abortion and that the incidence of severe negative responses was low[11]. Most women (76%) reported relief and happiness after an abortion and only 17% reported feeling guilt. In a study of 360 adolescents seeking pregnancy tests which compared those not pregnant, those who were pregnant and had abortions, and those who carried to term. After two years "the abortion group showed, if anything, a more positive psychological profile than either of the other two groups." In aggregate, "severe negative reactions after abortion are rare and can be best understood in the framework of coping with a normal life stress."

Induced abortion, therapeutic or otherwise, is widely practiced and/or approved by the majority of people in most of the world. Even Portugal, an almost entirely Catholic country, enacted a law in 1984 permitting abortion under very limited circumstances, such as a threat to the life of the mother or after a rape, and only with a court's permission. A similar law was enacted in Spain in 1985. Ireland and Belgium had been the only countries in Europe to maintain a complete legal ban on abortion up until 1990. In March 1990 the Belgium Parliament approved a law allowing abortions to be done within the first 12 weeks of pregnancy for women in a "state of distress". The women of Ireland evade the ban by going abroad. In 1985 nearly 4,000 women giving Irish addresses were aborted in Britain; the total number of Irishwomen having abortions in England was thought to be nearly three times that number[12].

It was estimated that 30 to 55 million abortions worldwide are done yearly, with nations containing 40% of the world's population permitting it on request in the first trimester (e.g., U.S., the U.K., Italy, France, China, Tunisia, Scandinavian countries)[13]. In 1984, 12.8 abortions were done in England and Wales per each 1000 women aged 15-44; France 14.9; Sweden 17.7; Denmark 18.4; Italy 19.0; Israel 21.9; German Democratic Republic 26.6; USSR 181 (1982); U.S. 27.4[14].

Abortion is totally prohibited in countries containing only 10% of the world's population, as for example, Saudi Arabia or Afghanistan. Abortion of female fetuses had become a frequent practice in many other parts of Asia, often replacing female infanticide as authorities were enforcing laws against the latter[15]. In Bombay alone there were more than 500 "sex-detection" centers performing amniocenteses.

The practice of aborting healthy fetuses in order to obtain a child of a preferred sex was apparently spreading in the U.S.[16] An interesting side-light of this issue was an explanation offered by doctors when confronted with the possible ethical aberration of pre-natal determination of the sex of a healthy fetus that could lead to an abortion. They said their actions were in line with the growing disinclination of doctors to be paternalistic and an increasing tendency of their patients to request the test for the only purpose of determining the sex of the fetus. One doctor was quoted: "What we are talking about is a collision course which puts a patient's autonomy and the right to do what she wants with her own body against the broader issue of social responsibility."

Abortion is illegal on almost any basis in all of Latin America except Cuba. But it was estimated at least 10 to 12 million women each year put an end to unwanted pregnancies and, according to the Pan American Health Organization, abortion was the leading cause of pregnancy-related mortality in that area[17]. Probably 20 to 30% of pregnancies, from Mexico through to Argentina, are deliberately aborted. The vast number of complications that result are said to account for occupancy of 45% of the beds in maternity and gynecological wards of Latin American hospitals. These complications result in the deaths, or the sterilizing, or maiming of innumerable young women, and is illustrative of what happens when a safe procedure under legal circumstances, is outlawed. A corollary concern are the numerous unwanted and neglected children that roam the streets of many Latin American cities. It is to be recalled that the birth rate in Latin America is at least double that of the industrialized nations of the world. The wealthy women can have clandestine, but safe, abortions in private clinics; poor women must resort to dangerous self-induced or "back-street" methods. It was said that each year between 10 million and 12 million women all over the world are condemned to unwanted pregnancies because they have no means of preventing conception, and 200,000 die of unsafe abortions![18]

In the U.S. a poll done by the New York Times [19] in early 1986 revealed the majority (66%) favored abortion "in a bad situation". Abortion was sanctioned despite a majority (55%) responding that it was the "same as murdering a child". One opinion offered to explain this contradiction was that it represented a pragmatic approach to a very complicated moral argument, similar to one that upholds killing in wartime. People can imagine themselves in such a situation and know what they would do, but don't wish to impose their view on others. Another explanation was that many are taught abortion, morally or religiously, is murder. This teaching was in the abstract, but when the respondents considered a real-life problem, they fell back on their innate common sense for their answer[20]. 40% believed abortion should be legal, and it was significant that a majority of those who attended college (53%) and only a minority (34%) of the less well educated were in favor. The same discrepancy in opinion was found on the basis of income: those with higher incomes were less hostile to abortion than those with lower incomes.

A repeated national poll by the New York Times and CBS News in mid-April 1989 confirmed their above findings of 1986[21]. In addition, the 1989 poll showed that younger people (18-29) were more in favor of keeping abortion legal than are older people, and that those who knew someone who had an abortion are more favorable to keeping it legal than is the rest of the public. It was interpreted that these two latter trends in favor of abortion, for demographic and other reasons, would grow with the passage of time. Religious inclination was an important factor in the attitude to abortion: of those who responded that religion was very, or extremely, important in their lives only about 30% favored keeping abortion legal; while of others who described religion as less important to them 68% (Protestants) and 72% (Catholics) favored keeping abortion legal.

A California Poll in May 1986 found that 61% of Californians favored abortion on demand[22]. A national poll reported in 1988 confirmed this trend in the U.S.: 88% favored abortion rights in some form, while 10% opposed abortion under all circumstances; 39% supported abortion on demand and 49% would limit abortion to particular circumstances such as pregnancy resulting from rape or a pregnancy threatening the health of the woman[23].

In the general election of November 1986, voting on abortion-based issues revealed a general trend in favor, by the majority of the electorate in all parts of the nation. The pro-abortion movement picked up three senate seats (Georgia, North Carolina and South Dakota) and five in the House (all in the South and West), and no avowed pro-choice incumbent was defeated for any federal office. Nevertheless this election still left the majority of the House of Representatives pro-abortion and the Senate evenly divided on the issue[24]. The sharpest loss for the anti-abortion movement was defeat in three ballot-initiatives that would have restricted access to abortion. These occurred in the states of Oregon, Massachusetts and Rhode Island and in the latter state, the most heavily Roman Catholic one in the nation, the voters defeated the initiative by a 2-to-1 ratio.

However, in the November 1988 general election anti-abortion forces won referendums in Michigan and Colorado to ban public financing of abortions (by 58 to 42% in the former and 60 to 40% in the latter). Arkansas voters approved (by 52 to 48%) an amendment to their constitution defining life as beginning at conception, and banning the use of state funds for abortion. The latter results might have reflected people trying to protect their pocketbook. A New York Times/CBS News poll taken in October 1988 revealed that 42% of people were still in favor of abortion being legal, as it was at that time; 39% favored it being legal only in cases of rape, incest or to save the life of the mother; 14% believed it never should be done, and 6% had no opinion.

A principal criticism of the anti-abortionists is that they have no right to impose their opinion on others, and that they attempt to interfere, often by force, with the right of a woman to determine the fate of her own body. Similarly, it is an imposition on the rights of anti-abortionists to legislate payment for abortions with public funds, to which they, the anti-abortionists, have contributed with their taxes. If anti- abortionists would confine their opposition to public financing of abortions to this last issue, their position would be a strong one. However they base their aversion to public financing of abortion, or at least give the impression that they do, on the more fundamental issue that it condones murder. Pro-abortionists counter the attack on the use of public funds with the proposition that public financing of abortion is a measure to help the poor, and a step toward the equalizing of opportunity. Pragmatically, barring the use of public funds (Medicaid) for abortion results in a much larger expenditure by Medicaid for the delivery of health care to the increased number of children born into poverty[25].

In England an abortion before 28 weeks of pregnancy was legalized by parliament in 1967, if two doctors agreed that it was in the best interests of the mother and fetus; admittedly, it was practiced widely prior to legalization; even in 1989 it was not prosecuted if done after 28 weeks. In the 1960's when an abortion was a criminal act, it was a common cause of maternal death and gynecological morbidity; it was certainly the commonest cause of tubal blockage. Legalizing abortion caused the incidence of these complications to fall dramatically, and no maternal deaths from abortion occurred in the two year period 1985-1987[26]. A poll by a London newspaper recently confirmed that the majority continue to favor abortion. An anti-abortionist had introduced a bill in parliament to make abortion illegal after 18 weeks. This bill would not make exceptions for defective fetuses; the proposer of the bill, a Catholic bachelor, believed handicapped children can grow up to lead full lives[27]. In May 1988, procedural ploys and filibustering, apparently with government approval, prevented a vote on this bill, and it is unlikely to come up in Commons again in the foreseeable future. In April 1990, the House of Commons did decide (335 to 129) to lower the time limit on abortions from 28 weeks to 24 weeks (except when the life of the pregnant woman is at risk or when fetal abnormality is diagnosed too late for an earlier abortion). The result of this vote, taken free of party discipline, was interpreted as a bitter blow to anti-abortionists since they were campaigning to reduce the time limit to 18 or 20 weeks and, when this was not possible, had offered to compromise on 22 weeks.

The Canadian Supreme Court, in a 5 to 2 decision, with two Justices not taking part, on January 28, 1988, declared the then current Canadian law permitting only therapeutic abortion approved by hospital committees violated the fundamental justice guaranteed in Canada's Charter of Rights and Freedoms. The majority opinion said the abortion section of Canada's Criminal Code clearly interfered with a woman's physical and bodily integrity. "Forcing a woman by threat of criminal sanctions to carry a fetus to term unless she meets certain criteria unrelated to her own priorities and aspirations is a profound interference with a woman's body and thus an infringement of the security of the person." Prior to this ruling about 60,000 legal abortions a year had been done in Canada. The Court decision aroused the anti-abortionists and it was said that how much restraint on abortion should exist could well be an issue in the ensuing general election.

Abortion is available on demand in the Soviet Union and is the pre-eminent form of birth control in that nation. In 1978-79 the annual abortion rate was 102.4 per 1000 women of child-bearing age in Russia, compared with 11.4 per 1000 in Great Britain and 5.9 per 1000 in West Germany[28]. 6.4 million abortions were performed in 1987, almost a million more than the number of Soviet births that year. Almost one in ten Soviet women of childbearing age have had an abortion, compared with a rate of about 1 in 36 in the U.S. More abortions proportionally were done in the Russian Republic than in other areas of the Soviet Union. Because of falling birth rates among

Russian and Slavic women (particularly as compared with Moslem women in the Soviet Union), the Government had offered incentives to encourage such women to have more children, but without any effort being made to discourage abortion.

Abortion is allowed on demand in most European countries prior to viability of the fetus but it is forbidden thereafter, except in West Germany. In West Germany abortion is allowed on social or psychological grounds up to 12 weeks, on eugenic grounds up to 22 weeks, and at any time on medical grounds (principally if the life of the mother is endangered). In Bavaria, a mainly Roman Catholic area, certification is required from two doctors and an accredited counseling clinic before abortion may be performed. A national referendum in Switzerland in 1985 voted two to one in favor of keeping that country's liberal abortion law and against any restriction on available methods of contraception.

It is said that Vietnam, since 1985, has been coercive in having women use abortion in an effort to contain their population growth. Similar compulsion for similar purposes has been reported in China, and 10 million abortions were done there in 1987. The United Nations Population Fund had been trying to help China manufacture more effective contraceptives, such as copper T intrauterine device, condoms, pills and spermicides. These efforts were set back because the U.S., citing criticism of China's population control policies and its high abortion rate (even before 1987), reneged on a payment of $65 million to the fund[29].

Presently, about 1.5 million women, one of three pregnant women in the U.S., seek an abortion each year[30]; 90% are done in the first three months of pregnancy, and fewer than 1% are done at, or after, 21 weeks. In 1967, when abortion was generally illegal, it is believed probably no more than 135,000 were done (with about 235 deaths reported). It was suggested, from this data, that a woman's willingness to terminate an unwanted pregnancy largely depends on how difficult it is for her to have an abortion. In Pennsylvania, when Medicaid funding for abortions was denied in 1984, the births among poor women rose 25%. Despite the class inequity of this denial of funds (the abortion rate among richer women remained unchanged), an anti-abortionist legislator expressed great satisfaction with its effect and closed his ears to any report on the hardships it created. Anti-abortion "terrorism" can reach even into legislatures.

A large proportion of abortions are done upon unwed teen-agers, 40.5% of the 822,027 that became pregnant in 1983 (up from the 28.6% aborted in 1974)[31]. The pregnancy rate, both wanted and unwanted, of the 15- to 19-year old girls in the U.S. was 96 per 1000 in 1986. This was the highest rate for any of the western industrialized nations: for example, compared with 14 per 1000 in the Netherlands and 35 in Sweden[32]. This discrepancy was attributed, in part, to better access of teen-agers abroad to knowledge of contraception. The U.S. ranks with Portugal and Spain in the use of contraceptives, far behind the countries of northern Europe. Through the Public Health Service Act of 1970, the U.S. government did give $136 million in 1988 to family planning clinics that serve low-come women, 30% of whom were teen-agers. However, the Republican Administration since 1981 (and its presidential candidate in 1988) opposed giving contraceptives to minors without parental consent, a restriction that surely kept many teen-agers away from such clinics.

A joint report of leading world-wide health organizations cited the dangers of adolescent pregnancy to the health of both mother and child and disadvantages to a woman of early motherhood in terms of her social and educational status and development[33]. They went on to point out the continuing rise of unwanted teen-age pregnancies in 1989. They also stated that the main barrier to control this problem was the widespread lack of effective policies with programs for education and improving access to services promoting adolescent reproductive health (including the supplying of contraceptives).

Studies reported in 1990 revealed that pregnant teen-agers in the U.S. that chose abortion did better educationally and economically than those who had babies. One explanation offered was that the former had higher school grades and more options and greater aspirations for the future than those who chose to give birth[34]. Those choosing to have babies, since they had fewer options, did better for themselves by becoming tied into a more dependent status in their families.

Despite only 11% of Americans, according to one poll, having any moral or religious objections to birth control all three major television networks refused to broadcast paid ads on birth control. This was interpreted "as the effect of tyranny of the minority carrying more weight than the needs of public policy"[32]. An impetus to advertise on television in support of oral contraception was the wish to counteract erroneous beliefs of the public, revealed in a poll reporting that 76% were of the opinion that "the pill" is associated with serious health problems and 31% thought it caused cancer.

There are two principal reasons for promoting contraception: firstly, to prevent the personal anguish of unwanted pregnancy - half of the 1.5 million abortions in the U.S. result from contraceptive failure; secondly, to alleviate the perceived population explosion that otherwise will occur in the 21st century. In 1990 there were 5.3 billion people in the world, and this number could triple in the ensuing 100 years, due almost entirely to increases in unindustrialized nations (for the effects of such a growth see Chapter Nine). Nonetheless, in the U.S. as of 1990, it had been 30 years since a new type of contraceptive had become available and lawsuits had shrunk the number of companies doing contraceptive research from 17 to 1., Moreover, the politically conservative forces had succeeded in eliminating U.S. governmental contribution to family planning in developing countries.

Religious objection to the providing of contraceptive information to teen-agers is based, in part, on the belief that it will encourage their sexual activity. This opinion was expressed despite convincing research demonstrating that adolescents who are informed about, and with access to, contraception are no more sexually active than those left in ignorance[35]. Similarly, a Massachusetts law requiring doctors to obtain the consent of both her parents before aborting a minor reduced the number of abortions on minors, but it did not reduce the number of minors that became pregnant[36].

New data reported in 1988 by the Alan Guttmacher Institute of New York disclosed that the U.S. had fewer contraceptives approved and a greater number of unplanned pregnancies (except Greece and Ireland) and more abortions (except Italy) than other industrialized countries[37]. The same organization reported in October 1988 that the abortion rate in the U.S. was remaining constant at 3 per 100 women aged 15 to 44, despite the well publicized activities of the anti-abortionists[38]. The rate for hispanic women was 4.3 per 100, and for non-hispanic white women it was 2.3 per 100. The highest rate was in non-white women, most of whom were black: 5.3 per 100. The rate among Roman Catholic women was the same as the national average of 3 per 100, while the rates among women who described themselves as Protestant or Jewish were 30% below the national average. It is probable that these data correlated inversely with the use of contraception in the various groups.

The reports of this Institute went on to point out that taxpayers save $4.40 for every public dollar spent to provide birth control to women who might otherwise not have access to contraceptives. Their study showed that the publicly financed family-planning services used by 4.5 million American women prevented 1.2 million pregnancies a year. These pregnancies, if allowed to occur, would result in about 516,000 abortions and about 509,000 unwanted births. Those births, in turn, would require government spending on prenatal and obstetric care, pediatric care for the baby's first two years, welfare payments, food stamps and other mandated support programs. All told, it was estimated that in 1987 the $412 million in public funds spent for family planning services saved taxpayers $1.8 billion in short term costs alone.

Even though contraception is less practiced by poor people and less available in the third world, it steadily is becoming more widely utilized, especially with the introduction of "the pill" and improvement in sterilization techniques. In fact, sterilization had become increasingly popular as a major form of birth control for the married middle class everywhere[39]. In 1982, in the U.S., 26% of married women and 15% of married men had been sterilized, rising from 7% for the former and 5% for the latter in 1965. In fact in 1990, among married couples sterilization was the most common method of contraception in the U.S. and Britain, being used by almost 30% of couples of reproductive age. It was predicted that in the U.S. during the 1990's, three out of four couples will choose sterilization between their last wanted birth and the menopause[40]. Despite the cost of vasectomy (about $750 in 1989) being much less than for tubal ligations in women, as well as being a much safer procedure, it still was being done less than 50% as often as female sterilization in the U.S. in 1989. In England, the number of male sterilizations done in NHS hospitals in 1985 was 59,100[41]. The number of female sterilizations done that year were not exactly known, but a projection from previous data placed the number at about 72,000.

In 1990 voluntary sterilization was still the single most common form of fertility control world wide. 130 million women and 50 million men had been sterilized, and more couples were using sterilization than oral contraceptives and intrauterine devices combined[40]. For most women in India, up to 90%, birth control means sterilization, largely because health officials decided it was the easiest administrative method - no follow up, no need to teach illiterate women how to use pills or IUD's, no failures. But in India, sterilization is an assembly-line, unsanitary practice with many unnecessary complications and even deaths, so that many will not undertake it until they already have had six or more children.

The development and marketing of drugs and mechanical devices for contraception in the U.S. had made little progress in the decades after 1970[42]. At first it was the demand of feminists and legislators that the drugs and devices be absolutely safe before the Federal Drug Administration would permit them to be marketed. Later, it was the litigious climate in the U.S. that prevented progress: by 1989 only one large pharmaceutical company was doing any research and/or development in contraception, having dropped from 17 in 1970. European companies which had developed more advanced (lower and safer dosages) contraceptive "pills" had not introduced them into the U.S. because of potential liability exposure. Finally, it was the influence of ultra-conservatives and religious fundamentalists during the Reagan and Bush Administrations that deterred its financial support of contraception domestically (and worldwide).

A report of a panel of experts of the National Academy of Sciences in February 1990 confirmed that the above situation on contraceptive development and distribution in the U.S. was continuing at that time[43]. They said the contraceptive devices available in the U.S. did not match the needs of many people, particularly young women, who found the available methods inconvenient. 1.2 million to 3 million accidental pregnancies were occurring in the U.S. each year as a result of contraceptive failure (including use too difficult to maintain). Contraceptive failure accounted for half of all the 1.5 million annual abortions, and most sterilizations too, the report said. Women in Finland, Sweden and ten other countries were being protected against pregnancy for up to 5 years by a contraceptive implanted under the skin of the upper arm. The West Germans were marketing in 40 countries an injectable contraceptive that protected for two months. China and Mexico both were manufacturing their own 1- month contraceptives. All this while "U.S. couples were stuck with the old standbys: the Pill, condom, IUD, diaphragm, and surgical sterilization. Indeed, in the three decades since the Pill and IUD came on the market, no fundamentally new form of birth control has been introduced in the United States,".

An ethical problem for doctors is whether to honor a desire of a woman to have contraceptive advice over the objections of her husband. This problem was examined in the context of what the guidelines should be for family-planning clinics[44]. It was found that often it was assumed that spousal approval was necessary before advice was provided. In the opinion of these particular authors the requirement of spousal approval was an invasion of "human rights". The laws against discrimination on the basis of gender were cited in support of their opinion, as well as the proceedings of the UN Convention on the Elimination of All Forms of Discrimination against Women. The various articles of the latter require that any discrimination against women in the provision of family services should end. They conclude that it is the duty of health care providers to respect their patients' autonomy and to respond to their needs, rather than those of their spouses. Whether or not this has been tested in the courts is not known, however it would be circumspect for the health providers in the U.S. to be certain of their legal position when giving advice based on this point of view.

In the U.S. abortion was established as a constitutional right in 1973 by a decision of the Supreme Court in the now famous case of Roe versus Wade. The decision by a vote of 7 to 2 established that abortion prior to the viability of the fetus outside the womb could not be legislated against, because it would violate the due process clause of the Fourteenth Amendment. This clause forbids the deprivation of life, liberty or property without a court review or trial. The Justices in the majority obviously extended the concept of due process to the personal privacy of a mother in making a decision for abortion. This was an extension of the same reasoning that led the Supreme Court to strike down, in 1965, a ban on the prescription or use of contraceptives (Griswold v. Connecticut). That decision, on the use of contraceptives, was viewed as having created a constitutional right of privacy more general than anything specifically mentioned in the Bill of Rights. The Justices said right of privacy could not be found in any single constitutional amendment, but that it could be derived from the "emanations" that surrounded many separate clauses of the various amendments.

The decision did go on to say that "for the stage subsequent to viability the state, in promoting its interest in the potentiality of human life, may, if it chooses, regulate, and even proscribe, abortion except where it is necessary, in appropriate medical judgment, for the preservation of the life or health of the mother." Thus the state has an interest in protecting the life of the fetus only after the point of its viability out of the womb; after viability, that is after the beginning of the third trimester of pregnancy, the state can regulate abortion. Also, the state has an interest in maternal health particularly after that point in pregnancy when abortion becomes more hazardous than carrying pregnancy to term, generally after the beginning of the second trimester. Therefore with the onset of the second trimester the state has the right to regulate abortion in behalf of maternal health. This left the option for abortion solely with the woman only in the first trimester of pregnancy.

The reasoning behind the decision made clear that the majority of Justices did not view the effort to ban abortion to be an attempt to control illicit sexual activity, nor because it was believed to be a dangerous procedure. The Justices accepted that the state could have an interest, even a duty, to protect prenatal life. However the majority stated there was no legal precedent for this position and indeed prior legal interest focused on protecting the health of the woman rather than the preservation of the embryo or fetus. The compelling and over- riding argument for their decision was their interpretation that the concept of liberty in the Bill of Rights extended to a right to personal privacy. They also believed the right to personal privacy included activities related to marriage, procreation, contraception, family relationships and child-rearing and education.

The Court reviewed the question as to when life begins and agreed it was pertinent. It was concluded there was no agreement on the answer at that time, but historically it was generally thought to be at birth or, particularly in the English Common Law, at quickening. The Common Law did not regard abortion as a legal matter until after quickening, the moment the fetus could be felt moving in the womb. The majority of the Court was obviously impressed with the concept of viability of the fetus and the time at which it occurs, and used it as part of their decision as quoted above. The matter of personhood and fetuses was considered and rejected. It was agreed that if a fetus were a "person" it too would have a Constitutional right to protection; this was not proven by the anti-abortion lawyers to the satisfaction of the majority of Justices.

The dissenting Justices did not believe the Constitution extends any special right (of privacy) to pregnant mothers, and thus overrides any existing anti-abortion statutes of the various states. They felt the issue of abortion should be "left with the people and to the political processes the people have devised to govern their affairs." Both the majority and minority opinions in Roe v. Wade confirm the relationship of the law to ethical principles as discussed in Chapter Two: that the former is an expression of the latter, when the latter has been accepted by the (usually vast) majority of the people. The majority opinion of the Supreme Court reflected what those Justices discerned as the opinion of the vast majority of the people. At least the vast majority were thought to believe that at some stages of pregnancy it was a personal matter whether it should or should not be terminated; and that an individual should not be harassed by others (probably even if the "others" were in the majority). The Justices in the minority did not believe that an opinion on abortion had been expressed by a clear majority of the people, as yet, and recommended that it be returned to the democratic political process for settlement. At least they inferred this sentiment in the wording of their dissent.

The decision of the Supreme Court had at least two effects. First, abortions became safer and were done at earlier stages. In 1965, 235 deaths from abortion were reported in the U.S.; by 1976 there were only 13 in 10 times the number of abortions done. Second, it fueled the resolve of the anti-abortionists to limit access to abortion. Anti-abortion became a centerpiece of many fundamentalist Christian churches, who joined with Catholic groups in efforts to overthrow Roe vs. Wade.

The Supreme Court ruled by a vote of 6 to 3 in 1976 that it is unconstitutional for states to require that the only way a minor can obtain an abortion is with parental consent. The Court did agree parental consent laws would be permissible only as long as they provided an alternative source of permission, such as a court, in cases in which the girl did not want to approach her parents.

In 1983 the Supreme Court reaffirmed the essentials of their 1973 decision on abortion, but by a vote of 6 to 3 - the Chief Justice changing his position on the matter. Again the issue came before the Court in 1986 and again the basic position on abortion of the majority was upheld, but now the vote was reduced to the meager majority of 5 to 4[45]. A new appointee to the Court by President Reagan sided with the original two dissenters and with the President Judge, who had changed his position by 1983.

The 1986 case involved a Pennsylvania law that required doctors provide women seeking abortion with detailed information about the risks of, and alternatives to, abortion and keep detailed records of such interviews as well as other factors in each case. The law required that two doctors be present at late term abortions and that they use methods most likely to produce a live birth unless it would impose a significantly greater risk to the woman. The majority opinion of the Supreme Court said some of these provisions were designed to deter women from having abortions and others would require doctors to risk the health of pregnant women to save late-term fetuses - therefore the Pennsylvania law was unconstitutional.

The four dissenters said the provisions of the Pennsylvania law were consistent with the Court's 1973 decision which said states may regulate abortion in the second trimester of pregnancy to protect the health of women and, in the last trimester, to protect the state's compelling interest in keeping alive fetuses that could survive outside the womb. The dissent also reaffirmed the original opinion of the two dissenters in Roe v. Wade: that the interpretation of the Constitution by the majority of the Court "had done nothing more than impose its own controversial choices of value upon the people." The dissenters believed such a "hotly contested moral and political issue" should be resolved "by the will of the people,". It is disturbing that Justice Stevens wrote in concurrence with the majority: a woman's right to choose whether to continue her pregnancy was "more important than the will of a transient majority". All signs, as cited previously, indicated that the majority of people favor abortion. Is it possible that the shrillness of the anti-abortionists could mislead even a Supreme Court Justice (Stevens) into believing that anti-abortionists were in the majority?

Efforts to impair access to abortion continued to be rebuffed by the Federal Courts[46]. In September 1987 a three judge panel of the U.S. Court of Appeals for the Eighth Circuit struck down a 1981 Minnesota law requiring minors to notify both parents or receive a court's permission before getting abortions. In the same month a Federal District Judge barred Georgia from enforcing a similar law. In the Georgia case the judge said the requirement that an adult accompany a girl to a clinic was unconstitutional because it unduly burdens the minor's rights. He stated also that the Georgia law in its proscribed procedure was also an unconstitutional invasion of a juvenile's right to anonymity.

Nevertheless this line of attack on abortion continued. In October 1987, California became the 23rd state to pass legislation requiring some notification or consent of parents or a judge before a minor could obtain an abortion. In six of these 23 states enforcement was being withheld until the matter had been again reviewed by the Supreme Court. In almost all of these states a minor is anyone under the age of 18. In early August 1988 a Federal Appeals Court based in Minnesota, by 7 to 3, reversed a lower Federal Court's decision (v.s.) and upheld the Minnesota law that requires women under 18 who want abortions to notify both parents - even if divorced or the father has deserted his family - or get approval from a state judge. Six of the seven judges in the majority had been appointed by President Reagan. Within days after this Appeals Court decision in Minnesota an Ohio Federal Appeals Court upheld (3 to 0) a lower Federal Court's decision that a similar Ohio state law was unconstitutional. The Ohio law required the doctor to notify the parents of the minor, and this too was an objection, because it was a breech of confidentiality. The discrepancy in the decisions of the Appeal Courts was thought to result from the difference between the Reagan Administration and previous Democratic ones, the former appointing conservative judges and the latter more liberal ones[47].

Such restriction on abortion is effective and was attested to by the 38.6% jump in the birth rate among 15- and 16-year-olds in Minneapolis after such a law took effect in 1981. An argument about these laws centers on their effect on family life. Anti-abortionists favor such laws on the basis that they strengthen family bonds by insuring that the parents' greater maturity and experience, as well as their support, will be available to their daughter in making an important decision. Their opponents argue that this rosy picture of family life simply does not exist for many teen-agers and that a daughter's pregnancy often causes even further deterioration of an already poor situation. The same points of view are expressed with regard to contraception: the religious fundamentalist says contraception promotes sexual license and weakens the family; its proponents say it prevents worse social problems that ensue from sexual freedom, and the latter is a right. Those in favor of contraception being taught to teen-agers go on to remark that it strengthens the family by preventing economic and emotional problems that would otherwise occur from teen-age pregnancy.

In December 1987, with one seat vacant, the U.S. Supreme Court voted 4 to 4 and, therefore, left undisturbed lower court decisions striking down an Illinois state law restricting a minor's access to abortion. The Illinois law stated that the minor (under 18) had to notify both parents and then wait 24 hours before being aborted. Legal experts maintain the tie vote set no precedent for the 23 other states which had enacted analogous laws. A definitive ruling on the constitutionality of such laws would have to await another, similar case being argued before the Court. The ninth Justice was appointed by President Reagan in 1988 and pro-abortionists feared that the Court would vote 5 to 4 to upset lower court decisions holding restrictions on abortion (detailed above) to be unconstitutional.

In summary, by early 1989 14 states had parental consent laws for abortions in teen-agers, but in two they were not being enforced and in three others they were blocked by the courts. Twelve states had laws requiring parents only be notified of an abortion on a minor. But, in four of these states the notification law was not being enforced and in five others it had been blocked by the courts. The matter of parental consent for abortion by a minor was to be reviewed by the Supreme Court with a decision expected by the end of 1989.

(Actually, the Supreme Court handed down its decisions in June, 1990. It ruled, 6 to 3, to uphold the Ohio Law requiring unmarried young women under 18 years either to notify one parent or to get a judge's permission before terminating a pregnancy. This overturned the ruling by a Federal appeals court in Ohio, cited above. Then, in a 5-to-4 vote, the Court ruled that Minnesota's requirement of notification to both parents by unmarried women under 18 - the strictest such law in the country - was constitutional only because the state provides the alternative of a judicial hearing. This was in contrast to the Ohio decision in which the Court did not rule on whether the Constitution compels the availability of a "judicial bypass" when notice to only one parent is required. The 1981 Minnesota law requires notification even of a parent who has never lived with the teen-ager or does not have legal custody of her.)

Early in 1988 the Reagan Administration issued a regulation that family-planning organizations receiving Federal funds may not provide abortion counseling, may not refer women to abortion providers and may not engage in lobbying or legal action to increase the availability of abortion. Immediate legal challenges to this ruling, on constitutional grounds, were begun. This ruling of the Administration also applied to all family-planning agencies overseas receiving funds from the U.S. Government.

The Reagan Administration then extended its opposition to abortion by even banning federal financing of research on the transplantation of fetal tissue, for fear such research would promote abortions. To appease its anti-abortion supporters, this policy was continued by the Bush Administration (see Chapter Eleven).

The Supreme Court by July 1989, with the addition of the Reagan appointees, had a majority of Justices who reasoned to constrain the previous broad rulings of the Court easing the access of women to obtain an abortion. Their 5 to 4 decision in that month upheld a 1986 Missouri Law that restricted the performance of abortions. This Law had been declared unconstitutional by the local Federal District Court and Federal Appeals Court.

The Missouri law banned public hospitals or other tax-payer-supported facilities from being used to perform abortions not necessary to save the mother's life, even if no public funds were expended; it prohibited public employees, including doctors, nurses or other health-care providers, from performing or assisting in abortions not necessary to preserve a woman's life; it required doctors to perform tests to be sure the fetus is not viable in any women they believed to be at least 20 weeks pregnant and for whom they planned an abortion. (A previous Missouri Law banned abortion of a viable fetus, but since such a ban was not part of the Law under review, the Justices did not address themselves to the issue as to when viability occurred.)

The majority opinion (by Chief Justice Rehnquist) reasoned that the state's interest in protecting potential human life did not start only at the point of fetal viability (as stated in Roe v. Wade) and therefore the state could restrict abortion at any time, even before fetal viability. Associate Justice O'Connor, while voting with the majority to uphold the Missouri Law, disagreed with the reasoning in the previous sentence on the grounds that the point as to when the state had a stake in the potentiality for life of a fetus was not at issue in the Missouri case. This equivocal position of Justice O'Connor, together with the firm one of the four other Justices (in minority), makes it uncertain whether the Court will ever overthrow Roe v. Wade when the issue of viability is addressed specifically in subsequent cases. To reiterate, Roe v. Wade established a principle that the state can never have sufficient interest in a potential life of a fetus prior to viability, sufficient to intrude into the privacy of a woman.

The upholding of the Missouri Law, while not forbidding abortion, did have the impact of making it more expensive for some Missouri women and virtually impossible to obtain in a Missouri hospital. The availability of early abortion obtained in private clinics or doctors' offices was not restricted. With regard to "tests for fetal viability", such tests could only be those that determine the fetal age by ultrasound measurement of size, with extrapolation from this to the data extant on viability at a given fetal age. The estimate of fetal age from its size in up to 12 weeks of pregnancy is only accurate to within a range of 6 days; and the range at 20 weeks is about 10 days. The Court mentioned lung maturity as a test of viability, but such tests are not applicable until well after 26 weeks of pregnancy, and certainly not at 20 weeks. Therefore the requirement to test for fetal viability at what only can be estimated to be 20 weeks of pregnancy, as a practical matter, is a most uncertain directive.

The perceived threat to freedom of abortion from this Supreme Court decision allowing states to put limits on abortions, led to an activation of the pro-abortion forces (mostly women organizations). The first results were un-expected victories of underdog, pro-choice congressional candidates in all the special elections held during the summer of 1989 (California, Texas, South Carolina).

Early in October 1989, the Florida Supreme Court, in a 6 to 1 decision, struck down a law requiring teen-age girls to have a parent's consent for an abortion. The Court said such a law violated a clause of the Florida Constitution that guaranteed a citizen "the right to be let alone and free from governmental intrusion into his private life." This decision was not appealable to the U.S. Supreme Court and cannot be affected by any action that might be taken by that Court limiting abortion rights. The privacy clause had been put into the Florida Constitution after having been overwhelmingly approved by voters in 1980. At least five other states had explicit statements in their constitutions similarly guaranteeing the right to privacy. When the anti-abortionist Governor called a special session of the Florida legislature to reverse the effect of the above court decision, to everyone's surprise, the legislature rebuffed his purpose.

Another evidence of the increased activity of the pro-abortion forces was in the policy reversal of the House of Representatives. In October 1989 they voted to permit the Federal Government to pay for abortions for poor women whose pregnancy resulted from rape or incest, reversing their position voted in 1981. This followed upon a vote, a few weeks previously, which had lifted their former ban on the District of Columbia spending its own money to pay for abortions. However, President Bush vetoed both legislations, and the House of Representatives failed to achieve the two-thirds vote necessary to overturn the veto of the Act to let Medicaid pay for abortions resulting from rape or incest. Nevertheless, the vote of 231 to 191 to overturn was 15 more than the measure had received when passed two weeks previously, and its supporters were vehement in pledging not to give up the effort. However, several weeks later the House of Representatives capitulated to President Bush (knowing they did not have the two-thirds majority votes needed to override vetoes) and approved two bills that barred federal financing of abortion for victims of rape and incest. These were appropriation bills to which the anti-abortion amendments had been attached.

In the November 1989 election, two men were elected governors of New Jersey and Virginia and a third became mayor of New York City, all with clear pro-abortion stands.

To the contrary, Pennsylvania enacted a strong anti-abortion law in November, 1989. Its provisions provided for a ban on most abortions in public hospitals; prohibited all abortions after 24 weeks, except to save the life or maiming of the mother; prohibited abortion on the basis of the sex of the fetus; the woman intending abortion must notify her husband of her plans, must be informed by a physician of the fetus's development and alternatives to abortion, and must wait 24 hours before the abortion can be done. Medical personnel who violated the restrictions would be subject to criminal charges. In January 1990, at the request of various pro-choice groups, a federal district judge issued an injunction against all the provisions of the bill except the bans on non-emergency abortion after 6 months of gestation and abortion for the choice of sex. Planned Parenthood did not ask the court to enjoin the latter provisions, which it said did not have any impact on women. The court, in granting this preliminary injunction, amended it onto the pending legal challenge of the State's Abortion Control Act of 1988, which contained a provision requiring minors to obtain parental consent before having an abortion. That law had been enjoined in 1988.

On the other hand, at about the same time the State of Illinois dropped its effort to severely restrict abortion clinics. Its Attorney-General settled, out of court, a case on this issue just before it was to reach the Supreme Court. It was widely regarded that this case offered that Court its best chance to overturn or eviscerate the 1973 Wade v. Roe ruling that established abortion as a constitutional right.

It would appear that the majority who favored abortion, as long as access was relatively unrestricted, remained quiescent and permitted the overt activity of the anti-abortionists to intimidate politicians. But as soon as their position became legally threatened, the pro-abortionists began to exert themselves, particularly at the ballot box. It may be predicted, now in 1989, that the eventual outcome, despite the extreme activity of the "right-to-life" fundamentalists, will be in favor of the "pro-choice" majority.

A twist in the abortion dilemma has come about as a result of innovations in the treatment of infertility[48]. The taking of fertility drugs or the implantation of multiple embryos produced by *in vitro* fertilization has resulted, in some instances, in more fetuses than a woman wants or can carry safely. A woman had been detected to carry as many as 8 live fetuses at one time. With the aid of ultrasonic guidance a doctor can dispatch the excess fetuses and leave the desired number undamaged. This had been done in instances as few as twins, aborting one and permitting the mother to have only a single birth - however it is done most often to terminate a twin proven in utero to be defective. It is to be emphasized that multiple fetuses in a womb are associated with a markedly increased complication rate threatening the mother, and in the present day, the fetuses even more. Each added fetus increases the complication rate proportionately, with increasing threats to the chances for any live births at all[49].

There appears to be a relationship between the number of embryos implanted in the uterus and the chances of the occurrence of multiple pregnancies. On the other hand reducing the number of embryos implanted markedly reduces the chances for pregnancy, which, at best, is 20% or less. It is recommended that no more than three embryos be implanted at any one time, or occasionally four under unusual circumstances. Those doctors involved in this practice assert such a limitation to the number of embryos inserted would seriously compromise the chance of some couples to ever have a child[50].

Many ethicists, who oppose abortion of healthy fetuses, say they can justify the procedure of reducing the number of multiple fetuses in some instances, but nevertheless are saddened by it[48]. One ethicist pontificates: "they are wanted children". He goes on to ask where should the line be drawn - if it is morally acceptable to reduce quadruplets to twins, why is that different from reducing twins to a single fetus, or choosing to abort a single fetus? And should doctors agree to selectively abort fetuses on the basis of sex? Obviously, as late as 1988, there was no hesitancy for some ethicists to resort to the fallaciousness of "slippery slope" reasoning, fallacious because of the assumption that the situations used in their analogies are identical, when in fact they are not.

On occasion the father has intervened in an effort to prevent abortion. In every instance, so far, the courts had eventually upheld the woman's right to make her own decision in this matter. The attorneys for the fathers in these cases had used two grounds for their suits to prevent an abortion: paternal rights alone; or more recently, the unusual approach of basing the paternity action on the rights of the fetus. Most of the parents involved in these cases were unmarried, however even a husband would have no say in the matter, since the U.S. Supreme Court, in 1976, struck down a Missouri law that required the husband's consent for a woman to have an abortion. The Supreme Court in September 1988 denied an emergency petition to intervene in lower court decisions denying an estranged husband the right to prevent his wife from having an abortion. Three previous emergency petitions in similar cases had been denied by individual Justices that year. In November 1988 the Supreme Court, without comment or dissent, refused to hear an appeal of an Indiana Supreme Court decision that a husband had no right to interfere with a wife's decision to have an abortion. The speed and unanimity of this action was taken as clear indication that the Supreme Court had no desire to reopen this part of the abortion debate.

1. Discussion and Conclusions

The majority opinion in the world seems to favor abortion and, in conformity with the purpose of legal systems (see Chapter Two), this is reflected in the laws of the majority of countries. Abortion, at least before fetal viability, is legal throughout almost the entire world despite the vociferous, and even violent, reaction of those opposed to it. It is this minority who, in their righteousness, extend their aggressions to terrorism in order to intimidate legislators and the courts to act in their favor. They attempt to prevent abortion facilities from functioning, and in the U.S. hostile anti-abortion activity is on the increase[51]. The harassments consist of picketing, vandalism, "no-show" appointments to upset scheduling, bombings and arson. Despite these illegal actions, while adding to costs (for increased security), the number of abortions have not decreased. The proportion of patients that obtained abortions from providers under harassment (clinics not in hospitals) was 83% in 1987.

Nevertheless, the aggressions of the anti-abortionists can be effective, at least in the short run. For instance, a French company had developed an anti-progesterone drug (RU 486 or mifepristone) proven to be successful when used, in causing 80% of women to abort, safely and without side-effects. It is taken orally, and must be used within 49 days after the last menstrual period. In France, surgical abortions can be done legally up to 12 weeks after the last menstrual period. Further, if the new drug was supplemented 48 hours after ingestion by an injection or vaginal suppository of prostaglandin E, the combined treatment was found to be 96% effective, and still with no serious side effects. Also, the cost of the pills ($48) was but a small fraction of that of surgical abortion. An important feature of this new abortion-inducing drug is that it privatises the matter of abortion. It permits abortion to be accomplished at home, eliminating the trip to the hospital or clinic, and the surgeon and anesthetist as well. It, therefore, is akin to the "pill" that caused so many Catholic women to desert the directives of the church against contraception. If abortion became a do-it-yourself method in the privacy of the home, a prime target of the anti-abortionists would be dissipated.

The new drug was approved for distribution by the French and Chinese governments in September 1988. All this caused considerable excitement and anticipation among those involved in birth control movements, particularly in Third World countries which lacked medical facilities for surgical abortions. The new drug, however, was removed from distribution a month after it had begun, because the company feared a boycott of its other products and the possible violence threatened by anti-abortionists around the world. This caused an unusually intense response by physicians, family-planning associations and the World Health Organization. It was emphasized that the drug could prevent the annual 200,000 deaths due to botched abortions (mostly, by far, in non-industrialized countries), and that the drug had great potential for the treatment of cancer of the breast and prostate[52].

Within 48 hours after the company stopped distributing RU 486, the French Government, through a decision of its Minister of Health, ordered the company to resume the distribution of the drug. The Minister declared: "From the moment governmental approval of the drug was granted, RU 486 became the moral property of women, not just the property of the drug company." The drug was said to have been used in 15% of abortions in France within less than one month after its introduction for general distribution. The company was happy to resume distribution after being ordered to do so by the government, stating that the government directive had removed them (the companies) from the moral controversy.

There appeared, in 1988, to be little chance that an abortifacient drug would be on the U.S. market for many years to come. It was said this was less due to the fear of boycott (of other products of a company) by anti-abortionists than to the possible costs of product-liability suits in the litigious climate of the U.S., which need to be added to the heavy costs of initial development[53]. This fear of product-liability suits already, in general, had stifled research for contraceptives by American companies[54]. Several small companies and non-profit groups in the U.S. were anxious to obtain a license to produce RU 438, but were unsuccessful because they were regarded as not large enough to distribute it widely. Anyway, it was believed it would take 5 years to get the Food and Drug Administration to approve it.

Six months after the introduction of RU 486 in France (where, already, 100 women a day were using this pill and accounting for one-fourth of the abortions in that country) the company had not yet distributed it in western Europe, despite successful clinical trials having been carried out in over 20 countries. This was because of the vocal opposition of anti-abortion groups and threats of boycott of the company's other products. While China had approved RU 486, it was doubted that it had the technology to mass produce the complex compound.

It is predictable that even if the minority are successful in some of their endeavors opposing abortion, it would only be temporary. Women will do what they view to be in their own best interest, and if the majority favor abortion, they will prevail, and its technology will advance. Democracy is the result of an evolutionary process and, consistent with this point of view, its principles must triumph over the long run, though how long that run might be, is not predictable for many, if not most, issues. According to this view, in a democracy laws are not for creating a behavior pattern, but *flow from* what the majority, and usually a goodly majority, favor in behavior. The law is not viewed in this manner by theists or those inclined to a metaphysical approach to life[9]: "...the delicate question of the legality of abortion cannot be left to 'vast' majorities. It requires extremely careful moral consideration: something certainly more subtle and responsible than the political horsetrading...leading to the present situation in which, whatever the intention of the 'vast majority' in Parliament, we have virtually abortion on demand."

An evolutionary ethical theory offers support for the morality of induced abortion on evidence other than that given or implied above, in the discussion of its judicial history. On the surface it would appear that any interference with the process of reproduction is counter to the evolutionary purpose. However, opposing this perception is the fact that induced abortion had been tolerated in many societies since ancient time and presently it is rampant throughout the world - without apparent deleterious effect to societies or to the species. In some communities, and even nations, it is sponsored as a population control measure with the purpose of improving their overall welfare (see Chapter Nine - "Population Problems"). Secondly, with modern techniques for diagnosis of deformed or diseased fetuses, abortion permits the avoidance of these burdens to society, and also prevents the possibility that such fetuses would survive to propagate their genetic defects. Induced abortion in these instances re-enforces naturally occurring abortion which is said to terminate one third of pregnancies, mostly because of fetal abnormalities. Enhancing the prospects for achieving these goals could count as an evolutionary plus for a group, tribe or nation.

Even infanticide, no matter how abhorrent it is in our civilization, has a history of being practiced by many primitive peoples for the obvious purpose of benefiting the group. It was applied to deformed newborns and used in locales with limited resources of space and/or food, as on some islands. Each of these motives served clear evolutionary purposes. Infanticide is analogous to the elderly committing suicide when no longer useful to their group, as among the Eskimos. Small scale hunter-gatherer societies did (and still do) write off the elderly, the handicapped, or even the severely injured when they no longer can fend for themselves or keep up with group movements[55]. These acts are evidences of favoring the group over certain individuals, under the circumstance of a stressful environment. Similar reasoning is applicable to contraception.

Contraception, which is as appalling to religious fundamentalists as is abortion, in modern times is used widely as a measure of population control. Secondly, it may be viewed as of advantage to individuals in advanced societies: rather than just serving a licentious purpose, it satisfies their physiological need and yet permits them to retain their efficiency. This is especially true for women, who are more and more looked upon as the source for the doubling of the availability of elite minds, to the benefit of modern civilization (see Chapter Two). The use of contraception and abortion permits women to plan their families so as to interfere the least with the other contributions they have to offer society, and thus adding to its enhancement and welfare.

While an evolutionary theory for the origin of ethics does not always permit the prediction of the ultimate resolution of a moral dilemma, as explained in the introduction to this book, the benefits to women from contraception and access to abortion does allow one to hazard a prophesy in this area. Using the reasoning in the preceding paragraph, the contributions to future societies that can be made by liberated women will make it mandatory for a nation to sponsor contraceptive practices and abortion, if it wishes to remain competitive. It is reasonable to assume that the needs of society will determine the resolution of these issues, even though, in 1989, it appeared that the outcome seemed to depend on the judicial interpretation of constitutional rights rather than the formulation of public policy through public discourse.

CHAPTER 9. PROBLEMS OF REPRODUCTION - ARTIFICIAL CONCEPTION

1. Artificial Reproduction

Artificial insemination was introduced in the late 19th century. In 1978 the first child was born in England as the result of *in vitro* fertilization (IVF) and embryo transfer, and shortly thereafter the concept of surrogate motherhood was created. The year 1984 marked both the birth of the first child from a frozen embryo and also a child from a surrogate embryo transfer (the woman carrying the embryo to term not being the one supplying the ovum). All of these techniques have as their objective the providing of children for the one of each six couples estimated to be infertile in the U.S., some 3.5 million couples.

The procedures are expensive and it was estimated that more than $1 billion was expended in 1987 in the U.S. by infertile couples in their quest for conception[1]. In 1988 the average cost per couple was more than $2,500 for diagnostic and medical treatment of infertility. If the treatment included *in vitro* fertilization, the median cost was $5,000 to $6,000 for each of such attempts. Even though more still was spent to prevent pregnancy, that could soon change. A question is: how much society should invest in technology that only a select minority, those who are white and middle class, will use?

An obvious answer is that society as a whole should not be required to invest in artificial reproduction since natural reproduction, if anything, can be too efficient. Over-population is thought by many to be a world-wide problem on a par with the degradation of the environment and the threat of atomic warfare. However, if individuals wish to expend their personal capital to satisfy their personal need to have children to rear, that undoubtedly is perceived by the majority of present day society as an individual right. This is reflected in governmental attitudes in appointing commissions to recommend rules for regulating artificial reproduction, with no hint that it should be proscribed.

There have been efforts at one or another time to have insurance plans pay for these procedures and, up to 1989, with only limited success, and justifiably so. In 1989 a woman member of congress indicated that she would introduce legislation that would require full infertility coverage by the health insurance plans offered to the 3 million government workers. Her support for this position was based on the premise that procedures overcoming infertility of couples were "family building activities".

1.1 Artificial Insemination

It was estimated that 172,000 women underwent artificial insemination each year in the U.S., resulting in about 65,000 births (30,000 of which were from donor sperm)[2]. The technique of artificial insemination has been expanded by the freezing of semen and establishing "banks" that can maintain frozen semen for years. This was viewed[3] as having many advantages: supplying a wide selection of donor semen on demand and in the absence of the donor; time to analyze semen for sex selection or appropriately timed pregnancy; storage, pooling, and concentration of many oligospermic samples of the husband, if the cause of the infertility is only the number of motile spermatozoa; *in vitro* treatment of impaired quality sperm for future use in artificial insemination; preservation of semen before vasectomy, or before surgical, chemical or radiological cancer therapy; and it provides time for testing of semen for genetic and sexually transmitted diseases. The latter advantage over fresh sperm is important in the prevention of the transmission of AIDS, particularly when it was reported that only 44% of doctors tested the fresh donated sperm for HIV, and only 48% screened potential donors for genetic disorders[4].

It was reported that more than 28,000 births had been achieved world-wide by 1986 using cryobanked sperm, with only about 500 husbands being used. Only 1% of children produced from cryobanked sperm had birth defects compared with 6 to 7% of naturally conceived children. It had been pointed out that couples using sperm banks expect the highest quality sperm and should the sperm not be screened for disease and genetic defects, this could be grounds for malpractice. In 1988, because of the AIDS epidemic and some evidence that sperm can carry the virus, the American Fertility Society recommended that fresh sperm no longer be used for artificial insemination. All specimens were to be frozen and quarantined for 180 days. At the end of that period the donor should be retested and confirmed as seronegative.

Anonymity is considered to be a right of sperm donors and a necessity for the collection of specimen and the successful use of the technique. The primary purpose of anonymity is to protect the donor from any claims the resulting child might have on him. On the other hand, couples have been annoyed by donors to see "their" children and in two cases of non-anonymous sperm donations, donors had won visitation rights in court. Still, some physicians believe children produced by donor sperm have a right to know their genetic background, especially for medical reasons. Anonymity of donor sperm produces the possibility of incest, unknowingly, by children of the same donor to different mothers. To reduce the chance of this occurrence the American Fertility Society guidelines originally set a limit of 15 successful pregnancies for any one donor. When it was noted that this could be even too many in a small community, the guidelines were amended to 5 pregnancies within a city and 15 nationally. The Warnock report in Great Britain (*vide infra*) recommended to Parliament that there should be a limit of 10 children that can be fathered by one donor; there should be a gradual move to a system where semen donors should be given only expenses (also mentioned by the American Fertility Society); and that a central semen donors' list be kept against which clinics could check new donors.

Twenty-three states have laws that declare a man who gives sperm anonymously and nonspecifically to a woman not his wife, as through a sperm bank, has no legal right in any resulting child. In Sweden the law provides: that only married women, or those co-habiting as common law wives, should be allowed insemination with donor sperm; and that the written consent of the husband or co-habitee must be obtained (which makes him the legal father).

It has been remarked that children produced by artificial insemination from a sperm bank might suffer all the pangs of adoption: a disquiet over their genetic background and the urge to discover it; a concern that their biological father does not care for them; and the possibility that a parent might not feel responsible for them. Children have demanded that sperm banks open their records so that they may learn who are their natural fathers. Although it is estimated that over 250,000 children have been born in the U.S. by artificial insemination of the mother with sperm not from her husband, only half of the states had laws that recognize the consenting husband as the lawful father[5].

All of these problems cause ethicists to be concerned that the use of donor sperm reduces the begetting of children to a contractual basis placing parental rights and responsibilities of the participants above the best interests of the children. While the usefulness of anonymity is recognized, it is believed that careful record keeping should be enforced to preserve the rights of the children so conceived[5]. This is because not to do so would be a deception agreed to, without participation of the person most involved - the child. Since it may turn out to be an important psychological, medical or genetic issue to the child some time in the future, records of donors must be kept. This same reasoning is applicable to the use of donated embryos, the use of which is discussed below. The law in Sweden states that information about the donor of sperm should be kept for at least 70 years in a special record and be made available to the child "when mature enough". On the other hand, this loss of donor anonymity has severely reduced the number of sperm donors in Sweden and Swedish women have gone to Britain to receive donor insemination[5A].

Other problems arising from sperm donation might well require counseling and are related to the donor, the woman impregnated and her husband (should he not be the donor). It might be discovered that the donor has a medical or genetic defect of which he had been unaware. The donor is usually young (average age is 23) and has not yet started his own family, but when he does, he may be remorseful for a variety of reasons. The woman may feel traumatized to have been impregnated by a stranger and the husband may feel cuckolded or guilty of being infertile. It is considered, therefore, to be unethical by some[3] if provision for counseling is not made by those offering the service of artificial insemination.

The use of sperm banks by unmarried women to satisfy their yearning for a child has raised some controversy. The modern emphasis on women's right to equality of opportunity has led many able women to seek a career at the expense of matrimony. The issue raised is: what constitutes the family?[6] Some sperm banks furnish sperm only to married women, as is the law in Sweden, others are much less restrictive.

A final concern in the use of artificial insemination is that it might provide the means for future efforts in eugenics. There is fear that, little by little, regulations will be enacted to use only certain sperm and women for selection of special attributes. The existence of the "Nobel prize sperm bank" is cited as an example.

1.2 *In Vitro* Fertilization

In vitro fertilization (IVF) consists of a woman being stimulated by hormones to produce egg cells and collecting them by a minor surgical procedure - laparoscopy, or transvaginal or percutaneous aspiration. The egg cells are mixed with sperm in a dish and the now fertilized eggs (embryos) are placed into the uterus. The embryo develops in the uterus and by 7 to 8 weeks it has sufficient characteristics to be labeled a fetus, until delivery. IVF was reported to be successful in 23% of attempts by one Australian clinic, a much better result than any others reported. More usual success rates range from 11.1% to 13.1% of live births (averaged from large numbers of IVF clinics) and are probably more typical of what can be achieved[7].

IVF was expedited by the discovery, by Australians, of how to preserve eggs and embryos (or "pre-embryos": fertilized egg cells not yet divided into the embryonic stage of development) by freezing them. Originally, IVF consisted of stimulating a woman to produce multiple eggs, collecting and fertilizing them and quickly inserting the fertilized ova into the uterus. If more than three embryos were inserted into the womb at once, the chance of multiple births was greatly increased and the extra embryos not inserted, were wasted. Freezing the extra embryos permits their preservation for future attempts, if needed, and for experimentation on embryos, which is believed will improve the success rate of IVF. Freezing of embryos for future use causes death of one in three. Fundamentalists believe this is "killing life" and therefore the procedure is unethical[8]. Incidentally, there has been discussion as to the moment of fertilization, which is of importance in the moral debate, and wherever the matter of embryo research is discussed. The House of Lords of the British Parliament, in their debate, assumed for legal purposes, that an embryo existed when the process of fertilization was completed, and this was heralded by the appearance of a two-cell zygote.

Worldwide, 15,000 IVF babies were estimated to have been born by 1989 (one third of them in the U.S.), and 169 centers in the U.S. were offering IVF, ranging from university hospital programs to clinics that do nothing else. In the U.S. by 1988, 600 babies per year were resulting from IVF. The cost varied between $4,000 and $6,000 per IVF attempt, and most insurance plans covered little or none of it. In 1987 about 7% ($70,000,000) of th $1 billion dollars spent in the effort to overcome infertility was expended on IVF[9]. A conservative estimate of the success rate for each IVF attempt in the U.S. was said to average only 11% during 1987 and 1988.

In Great Britain there were 29 IVF units in 1987 and Australia had 15 units. In France, which boasted of one of the highest IVF success rates, 3,600 babies were born in 1987. French doctors reported that in early 1989 4880 such pregnancies were in progress[10]. Human IVF in China sounds somewhat absurd in view of that country's strenuous efforts to curb its population growth. Nevertheless, an IVF center was established at the Peking Medical School in 1984 and while successful IVF have taken place, no embryo transfers have been done.

There is controversy about the success rate of IVF. In fact, Australia was reported about to discontinue funding IVF clinics because the success rate was only 9% and therefore each baby so conceived cost the government more than $33,000[11]. Another report stated that the crude live-birth rates in both British and Australian clinics remained less than 10%[12]. Among this group there was considerably increased risk of prematurity and developmental abnormalities, reducing the number of completed live births to nearer 5%. Some used the low success rate to condemn the practice, and from the overall public health point of view the procedure, since it was not even close to being cost-efficient, was believed to be unethical to have it so widely available at that time (1989)[6A]. Others used the low success rate as an argument to expand research on IVF.

Still newer methods to overcome infertility, gamete intrafallopian transfer (GIFT: the ovum and sperm both are placed in a woman's fallopian tube), and peritoneal oocyte and sperm transfer (POST), by the end of 1989 had not yet been fully evaluated. They are akin to IVF but the embryo is created artificially in the women, and not in a laboratory plate.

Children conceived by IVF carry no increase in risk for malformations or developmental dysfunctions than conventionally conceived children[13]. Eighty-three IVF children were compared with a group of 93 other children matched for age, sex, race, maternal age, parental education and income. There was no statistically significant difference between the two groups for major congenital abnormalities (2/83 and 1/93, respectively), and the IVF children scored as high or higher on mental and psychomotor indexes. As a matter of fact, by 1990, research on embryos permitted scientists to be able to identify the sex of three-day-old embryos in the test tube[14]. Thus in instances where a male could inherit a serious congenital disease only female embryos would be used for IVF, and abortions avoided for such male fetuses. There are about 200 genetic diseases linked only to males, such as hemophilia, the most severe form of muscular dystrophy and a form of mental retardation. Such embryo analysis could be used for choosing the sex of a child, but the discoverer of the method declared that purpose would be unethical. Medical ethicists usually consulted by the press agreed with this conclusion, but added that embryo analysis would be less emotionally trying than abortion. They also opined that embryo analysis would probably be too cumbersome and costly to make it widely used for choosing a baby's sex without any medical reason.

All the problems, previously mentioned, that could arise with children resulting from artificial insemination by donor sperm are sure to be magnified with IVF. They need to be dealt with, and probably by legislation. That there can be problems of commercialization in the processes of IVF and surrogacy also is apparent; accusations that the buying and selling of children was involved already have been made. This too, will require legislation. Doing research on embryos, made available by IVF (or flushed from a woman's uterus, for that matter) has caused serious moral discussion. Another ethical and legal question is: who owns the frozen embryo? The parents; their estate if they be deceased (this actually came into question as a result of an airplane crash); the laboratory; the state? A judge in Tennessee was faced with this problem in 1989 when he had to decide who "owned" seven frozen embryos of a couple about to be divorced. On the theory that life begins at conception, he awarded "custody" of the frozen embryos to the "mother". How she should dispose of the embryos in her custody was not stated in the judge's decision. The questions remain: must all the embryos be implanted in her uterus at some time? Should she succeed in bearing a child on the first attempt, need she go on to have, say, six more? Could she decide to have some, or all, of the embryos destroyed?

In an attempt to settle these issues, commissions have been established in Australia (the Waller Commission of the state of Victoria) and in England (the Warnock Parliamentary Commission). The state of Victoria had already passed a law in 1984, the Infertility (Medical Procedures) Act, with most provisions to be effective in August 1986. The Act specified that all proposals for research on human embryos be cleared by a government appointed committee, and provided for criminal penalties for researchers conducting unauthorized research. It did legalize cryopreservation of embryos and implicitly acknowledged that they belong to the parents by directing them to make disposition of unused ones, in advance, in case of their death. The law allowed experimentation only on "surplus" or "spare" embryos (ones left over from attempts to implant IVF embryos into a womb), and forbid the creation of embryos specifically for destructive research. It banned payment to surrogate mothers for carrying embryos to term. It forbid the sale of human tissues, including sperm, ova, and embryos; forbid cloning or fertilizing of a human ovum with an animal sperm cell; or using children's gametes (sperm cells or ova).

Australian scientists felt the 1984 law in Victoria was too restrictive of research on IVF[15] and this was particularly onerous because they were in the forefront, world-wide, in this field of investigation. They inveighed against those moralists who believe it is better to let children be born with disease that could have been prevented, because cells of the pre-implantation embryo had been given legal status equal to children and research on them consequently restricted. The Victoria Law, and the one contemplated for all of Australia, did not permit the necessary research that would enable the screening of embryos for genetic defects. Therefore the usefulness of the freezing of ova was eliminated for all practical purposes, since freezing might cause an increase in the incidence of chromosomal abnormalities in embryos derived from them. It was recommended that this be thoroughly investigated before freezing of ova is offered to patients[16].

Since permission to do embryo research was not granted by Australian law, an ethical dilemma was created: to illegally test whether frozen ova produced embryos with increased chromosomal defects, or to offer a procedure to women that might lead to an increased risk of spontaneous abortion in the first trimester, or the need for a therapeutic abortion after amniocentesis in the second trimester revealed a deformed fetus. It was the latter course that seemed unethical to most physicians. The procedure of freezing and storing ova was felt to be important because it would reduce the number of laparoscopies a woman would have to undergo in an effort to utilize *in vitro* fertilization.

The use of frozen ova focuses on female infertility, since it allows for bypassing the tubal lesions that cause two thirds of the infertility of couples in Australian IVF programs. There were 12% of infertile couples in these programs that were the result of sperm abnormalities. The latter can be treated, *in vitro*, by microinjection of a single sperm into an egg[16]. Like the freezing of ova, microinjection of sperm needs testing to assess its safety before being offered to patients as an alternative to the use of donor sperm. The microinjection of sperm might injure the ovum or the sperm used might be defective. The genetic complement of a sperm cannot be determined before its microinjection, so it is important that the chances of using a defective sperm be investigated. The 1984 law prohibited the necessary experiments that would make microinjection of sperm ethically feasible. However, an amendment to the 1984 act was passed in 1987 that specifically allowed a limited fertilization of an ovum (the fertilized ovum was not to be allowed to develop) so that research on microinjection of sperm could proceed.

On the other hand, some scientists are skeptical that research on human embryos is proper[17]. Several embryologists have criticized such experiments and accuse those that do them, of serving their own vested interests, exaggerating its benefits to further their own ends. A leading French investigator withdrew from IVF research because he was concerned that genetic screening and sex determination of the embryo produced by IVF opens the way for eugenics. These remarks were taken from an article by an Australian philosopher of science[17] who also believed there is a tendency to treat human embryos in the laboratory "like rat liver". He stated: "Human embryos are *not* rat liver, and the only reliable mechanism for ensuring that they are not treated as such is through government legislation and licensing." He recognized this did hamper research on embryos but, "on balance, at this stage of our social, political and economic development we have more to gain than to lose by opting for regulation and restriction." Further, he hoped that the restrictive legislation then in force in Victoria, aided by the Vatican's stand against IVF (see below), would become applicable to IVF research wherever it was being done.

Like Australia but unlike the United Kingdom, laws in the U.S. relating to parenthood and reproduction are primarily in the jurisdiction of the various states. There is a federal law requiring approval of the Ethics Advisory Board of the Department of Health and Human Services before any embryo research can be federally funded. However the Ethics Board was abolished in 1980 and for this reason there has been no federal financing for this type of research, at least up to 1989. This, in practical terms, prevented research involving IVF since funds for medical investigation are very limited from sources other than the federal government. The abolition of the Ethics Board principally resulted from the opposition to such research by religious and right-to-life groups, but there was also a series of political "snafus" preventing activation of the Board.

In July 1988, when the Reagan Administration was drawing to an end, it responded to years of pressures from the National Institutes of Health and various professional groups and some members of Congress and announced, through the Department of Health and Human Services, that the Ethical Advisory Board would be revived. It was doubted that the *de facto* ban of the Reagan administration on IVF research could come to an end before it left office. There also had been legislation appointing a Biomedical Ethics Board consisting of 12 congressional members who in turn were to appoint a 14 member expert advisory committee. This committee was to advise on IVF research. However the committee had not yet been activated in late 1987, due to a dispute over the views on abortion of some proposed members. Because of this new development, there was expected to be intensified campaigning against and for IVF research by right-to-life groups and organizations representing the interests of infertile person.

The Warnock Report to the British Parliament (1984) would permit embryos to be fertilized for the sole purpose of research, but under careful regulation by a board set up for this and other reproductive research projects. There was agreement by the Australian and English Commissions that experimentation on embryos should not be done after they had been in existence for 14 days. It is at that time that the "primitive streak" appears - the grouping of cells that will go to make up the embryo itself. Also, it is at 14 days that the *in vivo* embryo embeds itself in the uterine wall, and gestation is reasonably certain to continue. Prior to being embedded, 60% of embryos created by natural reproduction are lost for one or another reason and most of the time these losses are unnoticed by anyone (not even the women). It appears setting 14 days as the time limit for embryo experimentation was a concession by the members of these commissions (most of whom were undoubtedly quite sophisticated) to those fundamentalists who regard this to be the time that life begins.

The Warnock Commission believed that the human embryo should be protected by law, but that the law should permit embryo research under carefully limited and publicly regulated conditions, in licensed centers. It viewed surrogacy (q.v.) as harmful: to society, to easily exploitable persons, and to the family. No legal sanctions against surrogate mothers were recommended, but it was suggested that organized commercialization of surrogacy be made a crime. It went on to recommend licensing of donor services for artificial insemination, capping the number of children from one donor at ten, and biologic children be given access to information as to the ethnic origin and genetic health of the sperm donor. Approval was given for egg donation for IVF, but donors of ova, or of sperm, were not to be paid, other than for their expenses.

Late in November 1987 the British Government published a White Paper on Human Fertilization and Embryo Research. This was intended to allow members of Parliament to decide, hopefully in 1988, whether or not research on human embryos should be permitted to continue. This was an unusual procedure and indicated the government did not wish to assert a position in the controversy between the bio-medical community and the "right-to-life" movement.

The White Paper proposed to create a Statutory Licensing Authority, which, with distinct rules, would issue licenses to institutions and practitioners to carry out IVF treatment or to do IVF research under strict control. It would also be a criminal offense to manipulate the genes of a human embryo, to clone such an embryo, or to create hybrid embryos (i.e., half animal, half man). The Government believed that Parliament would find research in the areas of infertility, prevention of congenital defects, and the improvement of contraception acceptable. The Government would not be able to override the Authority's decisions, but it would retain power to appoint and dismiss its members. The Authority would have at least half lay members, and at least one-third would be doctors and scientists expert in the area. This part of the White Paper, a reiteration of the Warnock Report, was welcomed by the bio-medical community. Doctors were anxious to do research on embryos (up to 14 days old) for purposes of preventing genetic diseases and to improve contraceptive methods.

However, the White Paper went on to offer an alternative course of action, banning all research on human embryos, which would please the faction that believes even an embryo less than 14 days old (the limit for research recommended by the Warnock committee) should be considered a full human being. Apparently the British Government did not believe a meaningful majority Parliamentary opinion could be reached on their White Paper. At least not so by November 1988, since no provision was made for a vote on it in the Parliamentary agenda presented in the Queen's speech for the coming year. Since embryo research was proceeding in the interim, the "pro-life" forces were particularly affronted by the unexpected delay in the debate and vote.

In July 1989 the British Government accepted a report of a committee appointed the previous year (The Polkinghorne Report) which approved research on fetuses and the use of fetal tissue in therapy (as for transplantation). However, the woman must give explicit consent of the use of her fetus for research, after either a spontaneous or induced abortion. If it be an induced abortion, then the consent for use of the fetus for research must be obtained separately from that for the abortion. It reiterated the Warnock Report saying: live fetuses aged more than 14 days should be considered in the same way as children and adults - i.e., any procedure carried out on them should, in general, carry only minimal risk of harm, and any greater risk should be, on balance, for the benefit of the fetus. For further items in the Polkinghorne Report see Chapter Eleven, under use of fetal tissue for transplantation.

Finally, at the end of April 1990 the House of Commons of the British Parliament voted (free of party control) 364 to 193 to allow research on human embryos up to 14 days old under the strict control of a statutory licensing authority. The House of Lords had already voted to support such research by a three to one margin.

The meagerness of the moral pro-life position on embryo research, at least to anyone committed to evolutionary medical ethics, is pointed up by their insistence that experimenting on an embryo, since it is a potential human being, is a desecration of the "sanctity-of-life". Yet, others with a similar feeling for the sanctity-of-life would permit embryo experimentation. The latter that only when the embryo is in utero is it a potential human being. Thus, experimentation *in vitro* can be moral because an embryo out of a womb has no potential for development. Another argument offered against embryo research is that it would be a "slippery slope" to research on more developed embryos and then on fetuses, and then abortions would be encouraged to provide embryos and fetuses.

Despite opposition from scientific groups, in July 1988 all major German political parties were in favor of approval of legislation expected to come before the West German Bundestag that would make it a crime to conduct research on human embryos. This very conservative approach was because of sensitivity to the possibility of linking research on embryos to the abuse of human experimentation by the Nazis in World War II[18]. In February 1989, the Council of Europe's Assembly issued a recommendation on the use of embryos and fetuses in research that was generally more restrictive than that of the Warnock Committee. It was thought that this reflected a Catholic influence, as well as the above mentioned German reaction[19].

In March 1987 the Vatican released a doctrinal statement, "Instructions on Respect for Human Life in its Origin and on the Dignity of Procreation: Replies to Certain Questions of the Day." The statement expressed satisfaction with the progress in the biological sciences insofar as it adds to therapeutic resources, but feared its domination of the procreative process, which would be contrary to nature. The human body is a totality with its soul, forming the person. Therefore the human body cannot be evaluated in the same way as the body of animals. Intervention on the human body affects not only the tissues but also the person. When science comes to the aid of an ill person, it is working to the integral good of human life, but it must not decide on people's origin and destiny. God has determined how procreation is to be done, to alter that process is immoral. God, who is love and life, has inscribed marriage into humans, and, therefore, marriage possesses specific goods in procreation which cannot be likened to those existing in lower forms of life.

The Vatican Statement went on to affirm the inviolability of the right of an innocent human being to life "from the moment of conception to death." The transmission of human life is special and entrusted by nature to a personal and conscious act and is subject to the all-holy laws of God. "For this reason one cannot use means and follow methods which could be licit in the transmission of life of plants and animals." "Man is the only creature on earth that God has wished for himself and the spiritual soul of each man is immediately created by God;...".

On the above bases, the Vatican prohibits contraception, abortion, artificial insemination, *in vitro* fertilization and surrogate motherhood. The fact that homologous gametes (gametes of the two spouses) would be used, would not make any manner of artificial reproduction moral, even if masturbation were not involved. If *in vitro* fertilization be done, despite its condemnation, it is immoral to experiment on the zygote or the embryo, because they already represent the biological identity of a new human individual. In all probability ensoulment takes place at the moment of fertilization. Freezing of embryos or attempts to influence genetic inheritance (even the determination of sex of a zygote) are contrary to the personal dignity of the human being and his or her integrity and identity. Contraception is immoral because: "it deliberately deprives the conjugal act of its openness to procreation and in this way brings about a voluntary dissociation of the ends of marriage."

Treatment of embryos or fetuses in utero with the objective of preserving them is permissible, if there is no disproportionate risk of harm to them. Even prenatal diagnostic procedures are considered morally licit if the purpose is to preserve the embryo or fetus. If the diagnostic purpose comprehends the thought of inducing an abortion, it is perceived that all connected with the act - the doctor, the mother, the spouse and/or relatives - would be participating in an illicit act.

The Catholic Church stated it was sympathetic to the plight of sterile couples and realized the desire for a child often is heightened by this circumstance. It recommended this desire be sublimated with adoption, or by educational work, and/or assistance to other families and to the poor or handicapped children.

There was universal agreement that artificial reproduction requires governmental regulation, although in almost all nations this was still in the discussion stage. The Vatican's Doctrinal Statement recommended to the various public authorities that they recognize what the Church views as inalienable rights of the person. These "human rights" include: "a) every human being's right to life and physical integrity from the moment of conception until death; b) the rights of the family and of marriage as an institution and, in this area, the child's right to be conceived, brought into the world and brought up by his parents."

There was dissent from the Vatican's 1987 statement, even within the Church. Some American Roman Catholic theologians expressed their dissent to parts of the Doctrinal Statement referred to above[20]. U.S. opinion polls revealed there were only 40% of Catholics who agreed with the Church's position advocating a constitutional amendment to ban abortion. About half of Catholic women thought abortion was acceptable for the results of contraceptive failure; more than three-quarters thought it acceptable after rape or incest, when there was a severe abnormality of the fetus, or when the woman's health was threatened; half of all women who felt abortion was morally wrong nevertheless thought it should be legally available; Catholics were, roughly, equally divided between those who thought government funds should or should not be provided for abortion; 68% of Catholics supported the Supreme Court decisions on abortion[21].

Many non-Catholics support the Vatican's position on these dilemmas of reproduction, particularly in regard to abortion. The majority of such non-Catholics can be classified as fundamentalists in their religious beliefs, and often are otherwise bitterly opposed to Catholicism.

1.3 Surrogacy

The use of a woman's uterus to nurture a baby for adopting parents or parent other than herself, is called surrogate motherhood. A woman can be impregnated by artificial insemination with the sperm of the adopting father or donor sperm. The other form of surrogacy is for a woman to have her uterus implanted with an embryo produced by IVF with gametes other than hers, and then she would be a pure surrogate, and not also the biological mother. Preservation by freezing of embryos, sperm and, more recently, ova together with surrogate motherhood permits the possibility of a child having five parents: a donor of an ovum, a donor of a sperm cell, a surrogate mother, and two adopting parents.

Of course any combination of these parents is possible. An interesting permutation of surrogacy occurred in early 1987 in South Africa when a 48 year old grandmother became the surrogate mother for her daughter and son-in-law. The daughter had had a hysterectomy after the birth of her first child and was desirous of a larger family. Her mother was implanted with the embryos resulting from IVF of the daughter's ova with sperm of the son- in-law. On October 1, 1987 the grandmother surrogate gave birth to twins. A London newspaper had contracted with the family for the exclusive rights to the story and films of the birth, for a sum said to be more than $500,000.

Surrogate motherhood has been utilized ever since IVF proved feasible in 1976, but relatively infrequently. The number of surrogate births that have taken place is not certain, but by 1988 it was estimated to have been as many as 2,000 in the U.S. Of these, 238 surrogacies were arranged by the same attorney[22]. It was estimated, in 1988, that 100 babies were being born to surrogate mothers annually in the U.S.[4] Charges in California in 1986 were reported to be $12,000 for the surrogate mother, $2,500 to a psychologist, $6-7,000 to the agent, and the medical fees brought the total to $27-32,000[23]. On only three occasions did the surrogate mother, on delivery of the baby, decide to keep the child; in two of these instances the commissioning couple asked the court to enforce the contract.

Surrogate motherhood escaped public notice, for the most part, until the Baby M case captured international attention in 1986. The issue in that case was whether the natural mother could renege on the commercial contract she had made to be a surrogate for a specific fee and keep the child. The surrogate had been inseminated with the sperm of the intended adopting father, but nevertheless wished to raise the child with her own husband. Another pertinent fact was that the intended adopting mother, age 41, was not infertile as had been purported in the contract. She presumed she had a mild case of disseminated sclerosis and did not wish to run the risk of aggravating the disease by becoming pregnant. Strengthening the claim of those who looked upon the entire matter as the buying and selling of babies was that the adopting couple were of distinctly higher economic and educational status than the surrogate or her husband. This matter of class distinction was troubling to many in society, as was made obvious by numerous letters-to-the-editor in leading newspapers.

The trial court awarded the child to the adopting parents on the grounds that the contract was valid and should be enforced and that, in the best interests of the child, the father would be the better parent. The decision did state that the contract, even if valid, could only be enforced if it were in the best interests of the child. The Judge stated that the surrogate had agreed to bear a child and not sell one, and the adopting father was also the natural one, and therefore he was not buying the child. The Judge authorized the immediate adoption of the child by the biologic father and his wife, the commissioning couple. According to a newspaper poll the Judge's decision was in line with public opinion in the U.S., at that time.

Other items were raised at the trial beside the claim that commercial surrogacy was wrong because it was the buying and selling of babies. They were: testimony of feminists that the rights of the natural mother transcended all other considerations; the opinion of some that the contract between the adopting parents and the surrogate should be legal and binding: commissioning a child is no worse than adopting one - indeed Baby M was better off since she was the natural child of the adopting father.

Feminists believed surrogacy was wrong and should be banned because it created a caste of female "breeders", a unique and tragic form of slavery. They felt it was akin to female prostitution: while a woman has a right to do with her body what she wants, she should not be driven by economic desperation to the choice of allowing herself to be exploited by men. They believed the surrogate mother had the right to keep the child because the "bonding" between mother and child at birth is of such elemental importance to the well-being of mother and child that it must be given priority over any vague claim by the biological father of the right to procreate through artificial insemination. They also cited a study that found most women who gave up children for adoption were troubled for decades by a feeling of emotional loss. The feminists agreed with the brief filed by the New Jersey Catholic Conference which condemned surrogate motherhood as a practice that traffics for profit in human lives.

A spokesman for the National Committee for Adoption, an association of non-profit adoption agencies, expressed an uncompromising stand against surrogate parenthood[24]. He viewed it as a practice being used to break down barriers to selling babies for adoption - a use of "slippery slope" reasoning to support his opinion. Again, this illogical form of reasoning is utilized to bolster personal preference and, possibly, interests.

Natural parenting is not without its problems. One child in five in the U.S. lives with a step-parent, often after a bitter custody battle following divorce. Child abuse and/or neglect by natural parents is increasingly being recognized. Those in favor of adoption claim adopted children are always wanted and for this reason are often better off than natural children. Certainly the same can be said for surrogate children. Indeed, surrogacy might be looked upon as an improvement on adoption since, most often, at least one adopting parent is the biological one. Most surrogate arrangements have yielded great satisfaction to all parties concerned and, on this basis, a utilitarian might well approve the entire situation as offering the greatest benefit for the greatest number.

Emphasizing the ambivalence on the matter of surrogate motherhood was the report of a committee on ethics of the American Fertility Society. The committee, representing a Society consisting of 10,000 doctors, scientists and fertility specialists, said in late 1986 that they had serious ethical reservations about surrogate motherhood. They said much was unknown about the physical and psychological effects of this practice on the people involved. They did not believe it was right to use surrogate motherhood for nonmedical reasons, such as the inconvenience of carrying a fetus to term. It was looked upon as unethical to pay the surrogate anything other than her expenses and for her inconvenience. The committee said it recognized that payment would be necessary in some cases. They went on to say that if surrogacy should prove to be useful, a change in the law would be appropriate for assurance that the couple who contract with a surrogate mother are viewed as the legal parents.

The New Jersey Supreme Court, in February 1988, overturned the lower court decision on the Baby M Case. In a 7 to 0 decision they declared commercial surrogate motherhood contracts were illegal because it conflicted with the state adoption law which forbid the payment of money to obtain a baby for adoption. While the surrogacy arrangement was mitigated by the adopting father also being the biological one, nevertheless the surrogacy contract amounted to the private placement of a child for money and thus, potentially, was a criminal act. Also, it was considered to be degrading to the woman. The Court restored the right of the natural mother, under the adoption laws, to change her mind about the adoption after the birth of the child and when she knows "the strength of her binding to the child". Custody of Baby M was awarded to the natural father, being in the best interests of the child, and the adoption of the child by the wife of the natural father was voided.

The Supreme Court of New Jersey probably was influenced in the custody award by the biological mother having divorced her husband, becoming pregnant and remarrying, all subsequent to the decision of the trial court. Parental rights, however, were restored to the natural mother, including the rights to visitation with the child and to attempt to regain custody, if she so desires. Visitation rights were extended to the biological mother's other children and her parents. This decision treated the problem similar to that of divorce of biological parents, awarding custody of the child to one parent with visitation rights to the other. The decision of this prestigious Court undoubtedly will be the guiding principle for future legal attitudes to surrogacy.

A previous attempt to outlaw the practice of commercial surrogate motherhood on the ground that it involved the illegal sale of babies was denied by the Kentucky Supreme Court. In its decision the Court said: "If there are social and ethical problems in the solution science offers, these are problems of public policy that belong in the legislative domain, not in the judicial, under our constitutional doctrine of separation of powers." Judges in other states, and legal commentators, have expressed similar opinions that the existence and/or regulation of surrogate motherhood was primarily a matter for legislation.

While Baby M was the first case litigated in the U.S. to decide the custody of a surrogate-born child, there had been several previous such cases in England[25]. In one case, the first such case which occurred in 1978, the trial Judge ruled the contract unenforceable on the grounds that the contract was for the purchase and sale of a child, and that was against public policy. This was upheld by a three Justice panel of an appeal court, who were even more outraged at the practice of commercial surrogacy. Both courts awarded the child to the natural mother, the lower court giving visitation rights to the father, but which were denied by the appeal court.

In 1985, with advice from the Warnock Commission, the British Parliament enacted the Surrogacy Arrangements Bill which forbid, under penalty of fine and imprisonment, advertisements to bring together parties to a surrogacy or the making of commercial arrangements for this purpose[26]. The government did not wish to penalize infertile couples nor prevent women from being surrogates if they genuinely believed they were helping other women unable to carry a child. The legislators agreed commercial surrogacy was abhorrent, representing the sale of children, and there was the danger of exploiting low-income women as "rich people's baby farms". These provisions essentially reflected the views of Lady Warnock, the committee's chairwoman[27]: "There is a deep and widely held belief that the relationship of a child to the woman who carries it and gives birth to it is different from the relation of that child to its father. This is the center of the moral objection to surrogacy, whether artificial insemination by a donor or *in vitro*, and indeed there could be, for the committee, no other objection to *in vitro* surrogacy since we found no moral objection to IVF itself.... The surrogate mother is closer to the child, both in space and time.... The moral repugnance stems from the thought of a woman deliberately becoming pregnant for money, knowing she will give up her child."

Lady Warnock did not find surrogacy by a sister or a friend to be repugnant: "The child himself, if he guesses or is told that his aunt is his mother, will in some sense have gained not lost. He was born out of love and charity, not greed". These sentiments, or intuitions, of a woman renowned as a moral philosopher has important bearing on the ethical discussion of artificial reproduction from an evolutionary point of view, to be presented below.

Because of, and despite, the Surrogacy Arrangements Act, two more such cases came before the English Courts at about the same time the Baby M case was being litigated in the U.S.[25] In the first case: "The proposed adopters and the mother and her husband had made a surrogacy agreement. The surrogate mother and the father had intercourse only until the woman conceived: this was no love affair. The father and his wife were a devoted couple, but the wife was unable to conceive a child. They were unable to adopt and regarded surrogacy as a last chance. The surrogate mother had been deeply moved by the plight of childless couples, and, with the support of *her* husband, she had advertised. Other couples had responded to the advertisement and offered large sums, but the mother chose the adopters because she felt rapport with them. A sum of 10,000 pounds was agreed, though the surrogate mother had said she had not entered the agreement for financial reasons, and this was accepted. The payment was regarded as compensation for loss of earnings. She was paid 1,000 pounds and then 4,000 pounds during the pregnancy but refused the remaining 5,000 pounds because she had made money from a book, written under a pseudonym with the identity of the child carefully concealed."

The Judge decided there was nothing commercial in the case, and anyway the contract had been made before The Surrogacy Act had been passed. Therefore the adoption order was made. Not to dispute the legal decision, but the finding of no commercial intent is somewhat difficult for an American to understand from the strange facts of the case, as given above.

The surrogate agreement in the second case also was made in 1985, possibly just before or coincident with the action of Parliament. "The mother was a married woman who lived alone with a small son now aged 7, and she was on social security. In 1985 she entered into a surrogacy agreement with a childless couple and conceived by an artificial insemination donor. A lump sum payment was agreed on delivery of the babies, who proved to be twins.... When the twins were born in September, 1986, she refused to hand them over. The babies were made wards of court, the twins remaining with the mother until the dispute over custody was resolved." The judge awarded custody to the mother six months after the birth of the twins. He reasoned that the welfare of the babies was paramount and "that these babies are bonded with their mother in a state of domestic care by her of a satisfactory nature."

The status of surrogacy legislation was being debated in the legislatures of the majority of the states in the U.S. By May 1988, the laws in four states (Louisiana, Indiana, Nebraska, Kentucky) made surrogacy contracts unenforceable and two states, Arkansas and Nevada, had recognized such contracts as enforceable, subject to judicial review. Bills seeking to ban, regulate,or study surrogacy had been introduced in more than 20 other states. The overwhelming majority of the bills would ban surrogacy or payment to the surrogate. Three bills had been introduced in Congress: one would ban the practice, one would forbid federal enforcement of the contracts, and one would bar the use of federal funds in helping war veterans form families through surrogates. Other provisions of some of the proposed state bills would require that the women seeking a baby be proven infertile; require psychological screening of surrogate mothers; licensing of lawyers and doctors making surrogate arrangement, or else requiring court approval for all such contracts; some provisions were designed to enforce legitimate surrogate contracts; to give the surrogate time to change her mind and keep the child (as in adoption). Adding to the furor were reports of a surrogate dying of heart failure in the eighth month of her pregnancy and the birth of a surrogate child with AIDS whom no one would take[28]. A previous case had been reported of a surrogate mother giving birth to a handicapped child not wanted by any of the parties to the contract.

In September 1988 a Michigan State Court ruled that a Michigan law making surrogacy illegal, and arranging such a contract a felony, was constitutional[29]. The American Civil Liberties Union had contested the law, but dropped its opposition when the state said it would enforce the law only if the contract required the mother to give up the baby. A Detroit based attorney, active in arranging surrogacy contracts, said this limited interpretation of the law would not impair his activities. Instead of making monetary payments contingent on mothers waiving their rights to the baby in advance, the contracts will provide for payment after the mother has agreed to turn the baby over to the adopting parents (most often the father and his wife). The ACLU said its position was that they agreed baby selling should be illegal, but that a woman had the right to "rent her womb" for compensation, while retaining her rights as a parent. The ACLU concluded that under the state's interpretation of the new law couples would be free to enter into agreements with women to bear surrogate babies and be paid for their valuable services. If a surrogate mother wanted to keep custody of the child, the issue then would be decided by a court based on the best interest of the child.

The Ontario (Canada) Law Reform Commission was the only working group that has reacted positively to the concept of commercial surrogate motherhood. A majority of the commission believed that legislation forbidding the practice would merely drive it underground and only aggravate the problems foreseen for it. They recognized their position would be controversial, but the problem, in their opinion, could not be solved to everyone's satisfaction.

These discussions and the decision of the New Jersey Supreme Court in the Baby M case reflected the consensus at that time, at least among ethicists and legislators in the U.S. and England: that commercial surrogacy contracts should be forbidden because they include the buying and selling of children. It was also recognized that there could be a "special bond" between the natural mother and her baby, and therefore she could change her mind about giving it up, even if previously she had agreed to it. On the basis of this special bond that develops between mother and child, an ethicist could conclude that a surrogate has not the ability to give informed consent to a contract to give up a child she has not yet conceived. These were close analogies to all legislation on adoption, and it seemed inevitable the analogy to adoption would dominate, at least legal, attitudes to surrogacy contracts and surrogacy children in the future. Despite all of the above discussion, and legislative action even banning commercial surrogacy in five states, by 1989 there still was no diminution in this activity, not even in New Jersey[30].

Partially avoiding the numerous legal and ethical objections to the usual type of surrogacy (in which the surrogate's ovum is utilized, as well as her uterus) is the implantation in the surrogate's uterus of a fetus created by the IVF of an ovum of a women unable to carry a pregnancy with the sperm of her husband. It would be proper to call such a procedure "true surrogacy", or "gestational surrogacy", to avoid the implications of the, so far, more usual form of surrogacy. This still was viewed by some as "trading in children", but the availability of "true surrogacy" was being advertised in 1989 by several well-known hospitals.

2. Population Problems

The status of the species *Homo sapiens* in terms of its numbers should have some bearing on the discussion of many bio-ethical dilemmas. For instance, repeated reference to the effect of over-population on the environment often creates doubts, or should, in the minds' of physicians as to what ought to be the proper function of medical practice for the best interest of society. This is most obvious in the ethical dilemmas associated with reproduction and dying, and does not seem so pertinent in the ordinary care of individuals - maintaining and restoring their health and relieving their anxieties.

It took thousands of years for humans to reach the population total of one billion, in 1850; it required only another 136 years to reach a total of 5 billion in 1986. The rate of growth of the world (1.7% per year) is slowing and it is possible the population could stabilize at 10.2 billion in 2085. However, updated figures produced in 1989 by the United Nations put the population number at the end of the 21st century at 11.3 billion, because of the slower than expected expansion of family programs. Or, if more vigorous efforts are not made to control growth, the final number could be 14.2 billion. But, according to The Population Crisis Committee, if contraceptive use is extended to 75% of the world's fertile couples by 2000, world population could stabilize at 9.3 billion late in the 21st century[31].

In 1990, in southern Asia about 34% of fertile women were using modern contraceptives, while in Africa the figure was as low as 14%. In the Moslem world the proportion of people having ready access to contraception is as low as 13%, due to religious leaders opposing the limitation of families.

A slowing in population growth is most notable in developed nations, 1% per year; but undeveloped countries, at their 2.1% rate of growth in 1987, will double their populations in 35 years, and by

2085 nine out of ten persons will be living in them. Without China (1.44% growth rate in 1987) the growth rate of undeveloped countries was 2.4%. The birth rate was falling everywhere, but the death rate was falling even faster. The U.N.'s 1988 median projections for Third World countries by 2025 was that Egypt would grow from 51 million to 94 million; Nigeria, from 105 million to 301 million; Mexico, from 85 million to 150 million; India, from 819 million to 1,446 million. In 1989 the developed countries were home to roughly one quarter of the world's population, by 2025 they will have less than one in six persons. By 2025 the combined populations of North America, Europe, Japan, Oceania and the Soviet Union will be less than that of Africa's.

The United Nations Population Fund stated in 1990 that if the population growth by late in the next century is to stabilize at the lowest possible predicted option (7.5 billion), women in developing countries will have to reduce the average number of children they bear from 4.2 to 2.7 in the period 2000-2005 and to 1.9 for 2020-2025. This would require a massive investment in education and the providing of contraceptive hardware and ready access to sterilization.

There are world-wide efforts to improve the health of children and their ability to reach adulthood. This is being led by the Task Force for Child Survival set up in 1984 by the World Health Organization, UNICEF, the World Bank, the United Nations Development Programme and the Rockefeller Foundation. It was the contention of the director of this program that the improvement of the health of children would reduce the world population. Seeing more children surviving into adulthood would reduce the birth rate, provided there were more contraceptives available. This could be wishful thinking to offset an apparent contradiction, and only time and data will provide the answer.

Amidst the plethora of people in the world there are communities whose numbers are falling. In those communities the leaders perceive the need to encourage an increase in the birth-rate up to at least 2.1 children for each woman of childbearing age, the generally accepted level at which a society must reproduce to sustain its population (birth rate per woman is also called the "fertility rate"). This is true of those of Russian extraction in the Soviet Union, as opposed to the Moslem peoples of the Central Asian portion of that nation. Various European nations also feel compelled to encourage their birth-rates, West Germany and Italy have birth rates of only 1.4 children per woman. Japan has a low, and falling, birth rate: 1.66 in 1988 and 1.57 in 1989.

The low Japanese birth rate was ascribed, by a cabinet minister, to the Government's policy of encouraging women to obtain a higher education[32]. The Japanese feel pressed to increase their birth rate because of fears that their quickly aging society will create a health-care and welfare burden that will be borne by a shrinking work force. Surprisingly enough, the Chinese community of Singapore is under a similar compulsion, and Catholic Quebec also with a fertility rate of only 1.4 is giving cash bonuses to parents of a third and each subsequent child. The problem created by such incentives is that affluent (double income), upwardly mobile couples are not tempted by the bonuses, but the poor, with already too great a family burden, will be. Anyway, bonuses for increased number of children have generally been ineffective in resulting in anything but very temporary and meager increases in fertility rates in industrialized countries. The birth rates of the U.S., England and France are similar, about 1.8 per mother.

The low birth rates in developed countries has already led to the aging of their populations and a shrinking supply of young people for their work forces. This puts greater demands on ingenuity to increase their productivity to take care of the needs of the workers as well as those of the large non-working aged population. This, in turn, puts a premium on education so as to increase innovation and the quality of the work force. As an example, the predicted shrinkage of the work force should give greater opportunity to women and thus help the feminist movement overcome male prejudice. Any impairment of the productive potential of one-half of humanity certainly will not be affordable.

In 1986 the National Academy of Science reported that the undue rate of population growth in the Third World, while not the main cause of all their problems, is more likely to impede progress than promote it[33]. Conservatives in their opposition to population control have utilized the argument that if market forces are given free play, they are sufficient to insure development no matter what the rate of growth. Others, probably the majority, adamantly deny this. The discussion is about whether capital dilution from increasing population, anywhere, has a positive or negative effect on development. An undue increase in population increases the drain on energy resources, but this can be, and is being, met with conservation efforts and innovation. If the growth is rapid (high birth rate), the age structure becomes younger and more resources need be placed in education. If the birth rate is low, an increasing population means an older age structure, and more resources go to health and other individual services. Are such activities capital creating or capital depleting processes?

High population densities help agriculture, but only to a point; industry is not benefited at all, because of labor saving technology. An increased population and increased resources to education could mean the creation of more innovators and more progress (see Chapter Two). However excessive populations mean a lower proportion receive education, and education of a poorer quality. Of course, the basic motivation of fundamentalists and conservatives in this discussion is their opposition to contraception and abortion.

It is interesting to note that the 19th Century population boom in the West was accompanied by great economic growth, which presently is not so in the Third World. In the West, as fewer children died young, parents eventually opted to have fewer babies. In the third world, because of religion in Latin America and for cultural reasons elsewhere, this is not happening. In Asia and Africa, parents feel they need help to support their families, and progeny to look after them in their old age. One observer, nevertheless, concludes size and population growth rates of poor countries are seldom crucial to their material prospects. What mattered most, in his opinion, was how well a society and its leaders coped with change[34].

Previous Malthusian predictions that the human population would outgrow its ability to feed itself have been confounded by the facts. Thirty years ago this prediction of Malthus was repeated, and India and China were given as outstanding examples of countries that already had outgrown their ability to feed themselves. Today, both are self-sufficient in food and even, on occasion, net exporters of grain! This has resulted from innovations in crop seed, irrigation, improved fertilizers and pesticides, and the sponsoring of private initiative. It was estimated in 1988 that the world's ability to produce food would outpace population growth for at least 10 years. Many observers believe the world will never outgrow its food supply because of continuing innovation (most recently, it is biotechnology that is offering the greatest promise to increase and improve the food supply). Where food is short (as in Africa), it is the result of poor political leadership and management, and this is agreed upon by all. It is also agreed that African weather and soil are poor, particularly in the Sahel, emphasizing even more the need for good management and use of new methods.

On the other hand, the United Nations Population Fund report, *The State Of World Population 1990*, declared that food production was no longer keeping pace with the increase in numbers: in the late 1980's production per head fell in 25 out of 43 countries in Africa and 17 out of 23 in Latin America. In the 1970's and early 1980's harvests increased virtually every year with innovations in agriculture, but by 1990 that process had stopped. "World food security now depends on the performance of North American farmers and that depends on a global weather system that is increasingly unstable." The report warned that the amount of agricultural land available per person declined at the rate of 2% a year during the 1980's.

The greatest threat of uncontrolled population growth to human health, or even survival, is by its degradation of the environment. By 1990, 15 million acres each year were being added to the deserts by over-grazing, and even greater areas of rain forests were being lost by their being turned into farm land that, because of the poverty of the soil, remained productive for only a short time. Pollution of the environment also is a real threat: in 1989 industrialized nations with only about 11% of the world's population, but still adding to their numbers, were responsible for over 90% of the emission of carbon dioxide into the atmosphere. All of these problems could be overcome by a coordinated political and economic will of the entire world, if that could ever come about. Indeed, the intensifying tensions in the struggles of life created by larger populations makes coordination on many of these problems less likely, and therein lies the severest demographic threat. The Third World needs help, and then uses loans to increase the destruction of rain forests; wealthy industrial countries can afford smog control, newly industrialized nations cannot; communities contest access to water (i.e. Northern and Southern California); farm subsidies in the West, at the behest of their farmers, keep food prices artificially high there (hurting their own people), but low on the world market which discourages Third World farmers in their efforts to produce.

Population growth was a big issue in the early days of the environmental movement, but fear of alienating developing countries and fierce opposition to family planning by right-to-life movements caused activists to back off from the issue. By 1989, the link between human activity and global warming was helping to refocus attention on the threats of population growth[35].

Despite the evidence that the growth of the entire world population was slowing, there were those who believe that this was not a certain trend and that the population explosion in developing nations still could be disastrous. They (The Population Crisis Committee) believed that the decade of the 1990's was the last one in which there would be freedom of choice to control their population growth. They believed all-out efforts to promote the spread of modern contraceptive devices in the third-world must be undertaken. It would not only take the allocation of funds, but also political will and encouragement of the desire of families in developing countries to have fewer children.

There were a goodly number of still others who believed that the focus of present efforts to conserve the environment (reduce energy demands, preserve rain forests, banning CFC's) were doomed to failure. They were of the opinion that a negative population growth, to reduce the world population from 5 billion to perhaps 1.5 to 2 billion, was the only way to preserve the environment. In their view population size is a variable just as is *per capita* consumption of energy, and in an industrial society both factors needed to be addressed if the optimum standard of living was to be preserved.

3. Discussion and Conclusions
(abortion, artificial conception and population problems)

Most people have reached the conclusion that the wealthy nations must use every means to protect the environment while doing as much as possible to promote population control in the Third World. This, from a world-wide view, dictates support for contraception and abortion, and makes promotion of artificial reproduction appear to be incongruous.

It is interesting to recall that in 1974 at the World Population Conference the Third World accused the West of a capitalist (imperialist) ploy to weaken them by sponsoring population control measures, and they were supported by the Soviets and China. At a similar conference held in 1984 in Mexico City this position was abandoned by the Third World and the Soviets and China, but it was supported by ultra-conservatives from the U.S. (such as the religious fundamentalists and some government representatives). This change of approach by the U.S. was followed in 1986 by the conservative Reagan Administration cutting off all funding for the family planning unit of the Agency for International Development. Increased contributions for this purpose by large American philanthropic foundations partially made this up, demonstrating the efforts of elitists to counteract the effects of the strident minority who are fundamentalists[36].

An evolutionary approach to the ethical dilemmas presented by contraception, abortion, artificial conception and surrogacy is partly expressed in the above paragraph. In those areas whose populations are out of control, contraception and abortion are most important, and their value for the welfare of communities is clear. In societies where population control is not pertinent, they serve the purposes of individuals: prevention of the grief or economic strain of an unwanted pregnancy, or alleviating the stress of infertile individuals who cannot respond to the evolutionary drive to reproduce. The serving of such individual purposes, overall, can be viewed as a contribution to the well-being of society. The permitting of satisfaction of sexual urges without undue consequences, in situations which do not represent unreasonable sexual license, also may be discerned as a contribution to the well-being of the community. It relieves individual tensions and provides for the better performance and behavior of individuals. Freeing women to satisfy their sexuality without the consequences of unwanted pregnancies gives them the opportunity to contribute their abilities to the advance of contemporary civilization (doubling the pool from which elite minds can be drawn).

There is an aspect of success in population control measures that could prove to be evolutionarily deleterious. Chinese demographers agree that family planning has helped farm production and the wealth of the average rural worker by increasing the amount of land available to each individual. However, too sharp a reduction in fertility could eventually reduce per capita domestic production. If their present policies succeed, two-fifths of the Chinese population will be over 65 by the year 2050 and depending for support on a depleted work force. This could occur, too, in the advanced industrial nations that have no national policy on population control, but where fertility is declining. Of course it can also be presumed that when the deleterious effects of a declining fertility become evident, factors causing it will be altered, possibly by decree (i.e. in China) or spontaneously in the West.

The justification for medical practitioners to condone artificial reproduction has to be part of their mission to care for the individual: in this instance it is to relieve the anxiety created by the inability of a woman or man (usually a couple) to reproduce. A bio-ethicist emphasizes[37] that a request for IVF is better based on personal need than the right to reproduce, and IVF funding by government or insurance programs should be viewed in terms of it providing a therapy to relieve distress. While preventive medical practices can clearly be identified with preservation of individuals, therapeutic medical practice contributes to the well-being of the human species and its societies through its benefits for individuals.

The problems of surrogacy, with current interest heightened by the Baby M case, fall into the category of individual therapeutic care. The moral issue, biomedically, is not different from that encountered with other techniques of artificial reproduction. Surrogacy has many additional legal and social problems that tend to make the bioethical issues appear more complicated than they really are. The problem of class distinction between adopting couples and surrogates, and analogies to prostitution may be viewed as ethical issues, but they are in the social and not medical category.

Discussions on surrogacy bring out the special relationship between mother and child and because of it, the right of the mother has been established to change her mind about giving up her child, even to its father. The denial of the right of fathers to intervene in preventing abortions is further affirmation of the special relationship of females to their children, even potential ones. Certainly, the emotional circuitry inherited by females that gives them the feelings of attachment to their offsprings must be a biologic evolutionary process. The recognition of this special relationship between mothers and their children would seem to be evidence for the importance of an evolutionary process in ethics, especially when considering the moral dilemmas of reproduction.

Population problems are of different dimensions in various communities: a need for more people to sustain their populations by the industrial nations, and too many people elsewhere. It would seem unreasonable to accept contraception and abortion in one part of the world and forbid it in another, and the same can be said for artificial reproduction. This would appear to be so, particularly, in a world that has been made relatively small by modern means of travel and transmission of information. However, the benefits the human species has derived from increasing individual freedom can justify such a discordant approach to the solution for the ethical problems associated with reproduction.

The success of the principle of freedom for the individual in the advancing of civilization combined with an evolutionary origin for ethical principles establishes what ought to be the outcomes of the present debates on the solutions of the reproductive and population dilemmas. Freedom for individuals to make their own decisions about personal matters, such as reproducing or not, combined with what is best for their community means that the proper solution for one society can be the opposite of the proper solution for another. Moreover, in accord with the Panglossian theme of this book, those are the solutions that will eventuate.

CHAPTER TEN. DYING

1. Introduction

Ethical problems related to dying arise at the beginning and at the end of life. In the post-natal period the issue is whether a deformed or handicapped infant should be preserved. At the end of life it is whether or not it should be prolonged. Of course, it is the scientific advances in medical care that make these issues acute.

Discussion generally begins with the difference between active and passive actions with respect to dying. Ethicists will write pages on what they recognize (at least implicitly) as only a possible moral distinction between a doctor withholding treatment (passive euthanasia) or actively contributing to the ending of life (active euthanasia). The argument considered to be most persuasive against euthanasia is the "slippery slope" one: that justifying it in one circumstance will be used to sanction its broader and broader application until it would be used entirely uncritically. As has been noted before, slippery slope reasoning is really reasoning by analogy and therefore its validity is similarly limited. The circumstances of two situations must be strictly identical, a condition that rarely pertains, for reasoning by analogy to be proper.

Most practicing physicians do not believe there is a moral distinction between active and passive euthanasia. Indeed, how can it be right in some instances not to treat a patient who is hopelessly ill and suffering, and yet look upon active euthanasia as wrong?[1] Nevertheless, there is an intuitive abhorrence of actively participating in the death of an individual. Probably an instinct embedded in the brain of all individuals, and enhanced in physicians by their training to preserve life, can explain such an intuition. Another basis for abhorrence of euthanasia is that all experienced physicians, at one or another time, have erred in their prognosis. A seemingly hopeless situation turned out not to be so, either totally not so, or a period of life of a satisfactory quality intervened before the demise occurred.

The withholding of sustenance (food and/or liquids) to facilitate death would count as an active form of euthanasia to most health care attendants. All too often one receives the impression that undue extension of the discussion on active and passive euthanasia is a maneuver to delay the decision on whether euthanasia in any form is moral. As one ethicist put it[2]: "In all, I hope more to display the issues involved in a difficult question than to advance a particular set of answers to particular dilemmas."

2. Infanticide

Infanticide has been discussed previously under abortion. It was noted that most believe there is no moral difference between a fetus and an infant: neither can be construed as a person; both are living humans and have the same potential. The fundamentalist, who believes life is sacred at any stage after conception, will admit to no distinction between the fetus and the infant, and both most be preserved no matter how severely deformed. Others feel that the infant does give them a different reaction than the fetus *in utero* and they would be more hesitant to concur in its demise.

The rapid advances in genetic screening and *in utero* diagnosis of fetal malformations, if fully implemented and complemented with induced abortion, would reduce markedly the number of deformed infants. At present, it is estimated that there are 200,000 infants born annually in the U.S. (6% of all live births) that are deformed, premature, or so ill as to require intensive neonatal care. The cost of this type of care in 1989 well exceeded the $2 billion spent for it in 1983.

An English Ethical Working Group noted that there were two principles applicable to the ethical problem in the treatment (or withholding it) of infants with spina bifida in particular, but certainly applicable to malformed infants in general[3]. They cited the utilitarian principle of minimizing unhappiness and the deontological one of the sanctity of human life. They recognized that "in certain circumstances these principles were in conflict with each other, and the moral task was to do justice to both.....". They favored "to lay upon the doctor the *prima facie* duty" to preserve life, but at the same time there was no obligation to use extraordinary means to preserve it. It was further stated that if the child was so deformed that its future would be painful and/or unhappy, any special procedures to preserve it would be considered "extraordinary". In elaborating on this guiding principle there was a definite bias to the preservation of life of the deformed infant and used as a reason to convert an extraordinary treatment to being an ordinary one ("He may not be able to contribute anything to society from a utilitarian point of view, but society can contribute something to him"). If the burden on the parents would be too heavy for them to bear, this should not sway the doctor's judgment but other agencies should be sought to ease their burden. In considering factors that would enter into the balance in judging to treat or not to treat infants with myelo-meningocele and paraplegia with incontinence, the committee appeared to be impressed with the report of "social workers' cautious judgment" that the families' experiences in raising these children was "not altogether a negative one", if the IQ was above 90. How the IQ could be predicted in the immediate postnatal period, is not stated.

The committee recognized that an utilitarian would be exasperated by their report. The utilitarian would recommend that it would be better for all concerned if active steps were taken to end the lives of the more handicapped infants (i.e., myelo-meningoceles with paraplegia and incontinence). The committee concluded that the ethical conflict at this point to be irresolvable. The only argument against infanticide that might be persuasive to even an utilitarian is that birth is one of the significant boundary lines in human affairs which, when passed, substantially changes our attitudes. The infant is thus regarded as a member of the human community (but not a fetus) and is perceived to have the same rights as are ascribed to other members of that community. Hence infanticide was believed by the committee to be morally different from feticide. The committee was convinced that "active steps to shorten a baby's life ought not to be taken." It should be added that the committee consisted of ten members, of which four were physicians (one an ophthalmologist), and two were clergymen.

Two philosophers argue that infanticide is morally permissible[4]. They believed that the principle that all human life is of equal value did not apply if quality-of-life was to be a consideration. The value of a life is a function of its quality, its quality a function of its richness, and its richness a function of its capacities or potentialities for enrichment. It is a fact that the potentialities for enrichment are severely limited or absent in some newborns. They also attacked the principle of sanctity-of-life as being of religious origin and therefore not necessarily acceptable to those whose ethical views are not so grounded; also the principle is speciest since it is only applied to human life. Certainly, the capacities of some animals are equal or superior to those of some humans, and the quality of life of some animals exceed that of some humans. If gender and race are not morally relevant to the wrongness of killing, why should species be?

These authors believed what was relevant to the morality of infanticide was that the infant is not a continuing self, it is not able to see itself as existing over time, have desires for the future, nor even the desire to go on living. In other terms, an infant is not a person. Though the majority of infants will become persons, not all will: the irreversibly comatose and severely mentally enfeebled newborns are examples of the latter. The purported problem with this approach is the providing for safeguards against "slippery-slope" reasoning leading to the killing of healthy, but unwanted, new-borns. The answer to the latter was that people are constituted with intuitions and inhibitions against such an act.

The law generally confers full legal rights to an infant and courts, when appealed to, have ruled against infanticide even when the baby was severely handicapped. On the other hand, doctors have seldom been convicted of murder when they have permitted, or even facilitated, the death of a severely handicapped baby; they have escaped punishment by juries and judges because of technicalities and without resolution of moral or legal issues[5]. A further insight into the public's attitude toward handicapped infants (at least in Britain) is the difference in treatment decisions made by parents of babies with Down's syndrome and congenital heart disease[6]. In the experience of a major English pediatric cardiac clinic, parents of normal infants with a serious cardiac abnormality choose operation with a high immediate mortality but if successful, a long adult life without major cardiac disability. Parents of similar infants but also suffering with Down's syndrome (Mongolism and mental retardation) usually refused operation, knowing that their child would have little chance of surviving through a short adulthood, at best.

This problem received wide attention in the U.S., and abroad, because of the famous Baby Doe case and the activity of the conservative U.S. government administration in office at the time. Baby Doe was born in April 1982 with Down's syndrome, and the always fatal malformation of tracheo-esophageal fistula and esophageal atresia (unless repaired). The obstetrician, himself a parent of a child with Down's syndrome, counseled the family against surgical intervention. The family physician and the pediatrician urged that the surgery be done. A consulting pediatrician also recommended surgical intervention to repair the esophageal and tracheal defects. The obstetrician told the family that the baby would be profoundly retarded and would likely have congenital heart disease requiring multiple operations and, in any event, had poor chances for survival. This opinion of the obstetrician was said to be inaccurate, and it contradicted the assessments of the other physicians on the case. The family chose not to correct the esophageal atresia and fistula.

The hospital where the child was born sought to protect itself in the conflict and requested a court to review the case. The County Court Judge, in view of the lack of a medical consensus, allowed the family its own choice. He also judged the family to be a loving one and was doing its best to act in the interest of the child. An appeal was taken to the State Supreme Court and the County Court decision was upheld. Baby Doe died before a U.S. Supreme Court appeal could be heard.

At the end of April 1982 a memorandum was sent by President Reagan to the Attorney General and the Secretary of the Department of Health and Human Services (DHHS) noting the Baby Doe case and citing the federal law that prohibited discrimination against the handicapped. In May 1982 the Secretary of DHHS notified all health care providers that: "It is unlawful for hospitals receiving federal assistance to withhold from handicapped infants nutritional sustenance or medical or surgical treatment if required to treat a life-threatening condition." In March 1983 the DHHS issued an interim final rule requiring all hospitals receiving federal financial aid to display conspicuously in each obstetric, maternity, pediatric and intensive care nursery a notice stating that "discriminatory failure to feed and care for handicapped infants...is prohibited by federal law. Persons having knowledge of such...were to contact the Handicapped Infant Hotline", and anonymity would be given to callers. The signs were to be in place within 15 days after the directive was issued. The DHHS took authority to investigate and, if needed, initiate legal action to save the life of a handicapped infant. DHHS officials were to be given access to hospital facilities and records at any time, day or night.

A Federal Judge issued an injunction against the DHHS directive finding no rational or factual basis for the DHHS order, and the signs were removed. In early July 1983 the DHHS proposed a rule not unlike their previous one, but the signs could be smaller and be displayed only at nursing stations. The proposed rule would not compel medical personnel to attempt to perform impossible or futile treatments; "yet the basic provision for nourishment, fluids and routine nursery care is a fundamental matter of human dignity and not an option for medical judgment." It was stated the evidence supporting the need for this rule was based on the concern that handicapped children were being denied appropriate care because of their handicap. The purpose of the proposed rule was "to acquire timely information concerning violations...and to save the life of the infant." The American Medical Association led a legal challenge to the proposed rule and another Federal Judge, in May 1984, declared the proposed rule of the DHHS to be unlawful and therefore invalid. He declared the Rehabilitation Act of 1973 not to be applicable, and he noted that in the two and a half years of controversy no violations of the Rehabilitation Act had been established by the DHHS.

Later in 1984 the Congress passed legislation establishing treatment requirements for handicapped newborns: an offense would occur when there was a failure to respond to an infant's life-threatening condition with appropriate treatment (nutrition, hydration and medication). Exceptions would be, if in the treating physician's or physicians' reasonable medical judgment, the infant is chronically and irreversibly comatose; treatment would merely prolong dying or not be effective in reversing all of the infant's life-threatening conditions or otherwise be futile in terms of the survival of the infant; finally, if provision of treatment (even nutrition and fluids) would be futile in terms of the survival of the infant, and thus the treatment itself would be inhumane. The law authorized the DHHS to develop regulations and to develop model guidelines for hospital committees for reviewing relevant cases, educating families and offering counsel.

The DHHS version of these new rules (the new Baby Doe, or Baby Doe II rules) were put into effect in April 1985.

These new regulations placed a considerable burden on neonatologists as to when they should, or should not, sustain a premature infant[7]. There were at that time (1988) insufficient data to assess the expected quality of life for each premature newborn in terms of the variables in birth weight, maturity and degree of illness that each presented[8]. Thus decisions could not be based on the expected quality of life as in older children and adults, but only upon whether survivability was possible. "Unfortunately the latter is also difficult to predict for an individual at the time care is initiated, and only becomes clear-cut when the infant can be recognized as dying despite maximal assistance." In the view of these pediatricians, when assessing 'quality of life' most emphasis was given to the medical diagnosis and future of the infant. Less emphasis was given to the resources of the family and its ability to shoulder the burden of the various problems that a particular child might have.

The Baby Doe rules intimated that there was general agreement on when life or death will ensue or how much suffering was likely to result, "when, in fact, there is only ambiguity, equivocation, and disagreement."[7] In the Baby Doe ruling by the DHHS "Definitions which imply precision, are not precise." Nevertheless, paramedical attendants were encouraged to report what they believed were discrepancies from the rules, exposing the hospital and physicians to litigation. The hospitals were encouraged by the Baby Doe Rules to form infant care review committees and were provided guidelines for their functioning. These committees were to have a majority of the laity and non-pediatricians. Nevertheless, in the view of these pediatricians[7] such committees would effectively be making medical decisions by proxy. By 1984 56% of hospitals with neonatal care units had infant care review committees, and they increased to 66% in 1985.

Physicians, of course, resented the invitation of the DHHS to spy upon them and the license given to hospital personnel, so inclined, to exercise their right-to-life passion. This is not to say that hospital attendants did not act emotionally in the other direction, though most often doing so surreptitiously. It cannot be doubted that if hospital attendants are encouraged to act in one direction (to preserve a hopeless life, no matter what) that those inclined to an opposite persuasion (to end what appears to them to be a hopeless life) also are abetted.

The American Roman Catholic Bishops and officials of the American Jewish Congress agreed, in July 1985, on the principle that life is to be sustained almost regardless of quality-of-life considerations. They said that medical treatment only could be withheld when the dying process had begun or where there is no hope of benefit from the treatment[9]. In June 1985, the U.S. Commission on Civil Rights took testimony as to whether treatment of severely handicapped newborns was an issue of civil rights and discrimination (*vide infra*).

A child was born on Long Island, N.Y. in October 1983 with multiple birth defects causing mental and physical impairment and came to be known as Baby Jane Doe. Repair of the myelo-meningocele, it was stated, might prolong her life but would not correct her severe retardation. Her parents, after consultation with doctors, clergy and social workers, chose not to authorize the surgery. At this point a Vermont lawyer, a right-to-life activist and not acquainted with anyone involved, took the parents to court to force an operation[10]. The Court of Appeals denounced the suit as offensive and upheld the parents. The Reagan Administration took up the case and appealed to the U.S. Supreme Court.

On June 9, 1986 the Supreme Court ruled in a 5-3 vote to uphold the Appeal Court's decision. It invalidated DHHS rules requiring hospitals receiving federal money to post notices encouraging staff members (including nurses, aides, orderlies) to report any denials of treatment to handicapped newborns[11]. These were the original Baby Doe rules promulgated in 1984 and based on section 504 of the Rehabilitation Act of 1973. Other of these DHHS rules that expedited access by the federal government to medical records and which ordered action by state child protective services to force compliance also were struck down. The Court explained that where treatment of infants was withheld, it was at the request of the parents and not based on the handicap. Therefore there was no discrimination against the handicapped, and the handicap anti-discrimination law did not apply. Forty-nine cases had been cited by the DHHS where treatment had been withheld, but, admittedly, in all instances it was withheld with parental consent. It should be kept in mind that the new Baby Doe, or Baby Doe II, rules, set forth in 1985 and based on the amendments to the Child Abuse Prevention and Treatment Act passed by Congress in 1984, were still in effect as of 1989.

An important issue that applied was why should a handicapped infant be denied the rights of an adult disabled person? Mentally competent adults have the right to refuse life-sustaining medical treatment if they feel the quality of their lives are intolerable (*vide infra*). Even if such an adult is incompetent, courts recognize the decision to stop treatment can be made through a surrogate. The Baby Doe rules denied this analogy, implying that quality-of-life should not be a consideration in the treatment decisions involving infants. One commentator[12] asked: "Why shouldn't Granny Doe be required to receive the same level of aggressive treatment as Baby Doe?" Furthermore, the penalties for doctor and hospital in the Baby Doe rules were so great that most physicians judged it wise to practice defensively and treat all infants, regardless of the infants' or their families or the communities best interests[13].

Despite the Supreme Court ruling, medical treatment decisions on newborns went on being challenged. The federal Child Abuse Prevention and Treatment Act of 1984 still required states to investigate Baby Doe cases and take appropriate action if the provisions of the Act (see above), the so-called Baby Doe II regulations, were not fulfilled. Generally, hospitals had to report Baby Doe-type cases to a state child protective service agency. Usually the hospitals only reported those cases in which parents wanted treatment stopped, in spite of recommendations to treat. If state officials agreed with the hospital, the case could be taken to court for appointment of a legal guardian to make the child's medical decisions. Pediatricians and hospitals, however, no longer needed to fear the intrusion of Baby Doe squads even though the Baby Doe II regulations remained onerous[14], and probably tipped decisions too far in favor of supporting even the very disabled infants.

The issue of the treatment of severely disabled newborns was exaggerated, undoubtedly, by the support of the Reagan Administration for the ultra-conservative position on the sanctity of human life, no matter what its condition. This was brought out by its aggressiveness in the Baby Doe cases and confirmed in the hearing held by the U.S. Commission on Civil Rights in June 1985 to determine if the treatment of such infants was an issue of civil rights and discrimination[15]. Many doctors, nurses, social workers and parents testified on the extraordinary financial burden caused by these infants and the strain placed upon the families. They testified as to the poor quality of life of the many infants who survived intervention. Government witnesses led by the Surgeon General, a former pediatric surgeon, maintained the right of the government to intervene, charging that decisions against treatment really represented discrimination because of babies' handicaps. The Surgeon General testified that pediatricians and families are sometimes unaware of all the community resources available to such infants and their families. Other witnesses, including social workers and neonatologists, testified such resources are woefully inadequate.

Following the Supreme Court decision in June 1986, and with the waning of the Reagan Administration, public attention to the issue subsided. This was helped along by the Right-To-Life-of-Oregon organization being sued by parents of a severely disabled newborn for which, on the advise of their doctors, they agreed not to request extraordinary treatment. The anti-abortion group had obtained a court order in 1983 requiring the hospital to provide life support treatment to the infant. Seven days and $10,000 later the child died, despite the added care. The Right-to-Life of Oregon settled the suit, in 1987, by paying the parents $217,500 for interfering with their custody[16].

There is little doubt that moving the locale of births from homes to hospitals also removed it from the private to the public sphere. Should a malformed infant be delivered at home, its fate rested on the decision of the parents with the advice of the physician. My father, who died in 1933, told me that it was customary in his general practice for nearly all families to agree to neglect malformed infants; almost all babies were delivered in the home in his era. It was also an era in which, rightly or wrongly, the doctor-patient relationship was far stronger than at present. In hospitals there are in attendance numerous health workers, some of whom would have no hesitancy in forcing their own ethical priorities onto the situation. Hospital administrators, believing the organizations they manage to be at legal risk as well as themselves personally, feel obliged to act on this priority.

The attention given to, and legal activity in, this area makes it understandable that pediatricians and neonatologists in the U.S. bend even further than is their natural inclination to treat vigorously every infant no matter how deformed nor (almost) how small. It is fear of the law being brought down on them, by some bystander or change of heart of a parent, that impels pursuit of treatment that might be against their best medical judgment.

In the U.K., legislation has never been attempted to lay down rules on the maintenance of the lives of deformed infants. In their view it was for judges to apply the right test (the welfare of the individual) and to make decisions on the evidence before them. It also seemed to them that doctors will and should bear the traditional burden for deciding, with the family, when treatment should be withdrawn and for implementing such decisions[17].

In summary, the problem of what to do about deformed infants is more acute today because many very handicapped babies who would have died naturally can now be saved. Is the price for saving all these severely deformed infants indiscriminately so high in emotional and financial terms that it is deleterious to the community? The trend would seem that the majority agree it is, but the aggression of the minority who believe that the sanctity-of-life overrides all other issues, obscures the attitude of the majority. In the U.S., despite repeated assaults by religious fundamentalists (including physicians) of the Reagan Administration to keep *all* infants alive (no matter how deformed), court after court, sensing the mood of the majority, have struck down their attacks.

Infanticide has been used in many societies to rid themselves of the burden of handicapped individuals and, indeed, still is[18,19]. It has been reported by anthropologists to have been used to control population growth in locales with a shortage of food or space, as on some islands. Female infanticide has been a custom, and still is, in various parts of Asia. The evolutionary significance of infanticide previously has been discussed under abortion.

In the absence of a moral dilemma (from an evolutionary point of view), the problem, as in all of medical practice, is the accuracy of prognosis. Admittedly the accuracy of prognosis is of particular concern when irreversible action is involved, as in euthanasia and infanticide. It, therefore, would be appropriate to have a panel convened of as many experts as is deemed feasible and yet able to reach a conclusion. Their recommendation, to treat or not to treat, should then be presented for the final decision to the mother and to the family, since they would be the ones to shoulder the burden and/or emotional strain no matter what would be the conclusion of the experts. Some ethicists believe that it is right for "society to intervene and protect children for whom parents refuse care (including treatment) when such care does not constitute a severe burden and the child can be brought to a good quality of life."[2] This statement is immediately following one recognizing the primary decision in this matter, on the basis of autonomy, rests with the mother and the family. In reality, it cannot be both ways, and those predisposed to the fundamental ethical position of the sanctity-of-life will always interpret the facts in favor of treatment (as illustrated by the Baby Doe Rules).

3. Euthanasia

The advances in medical science and technology have had as some of their most profound effects, the extension of life and the ability to prolong the terminal state. Both effects have added greatly to the cost of medical care, but it is the cost of the latter that is resented, because, to most people, it seems pointless. The quality of the life in the prolonged terminal state usually ranges from barely tolerable to absolutely miserable. Until the last fifty years nothing more than rudimentary supportive care could be offered to terminal patients and,therefore, no ethical dilemmas were created. The new ethical dilemmas, other than created by increased financial cost, are how decisions are to be made in the use of the present array of treatments which can prolong survival.

Compounding the problem are changes in customary medical practice and in the definition of death. Up until the modern era the vast majority of people died at home. With the change in the financing of medical care, by far the majority of people die in hospitals (80%). Not only does this increase the cost of dying, but it makes dying a much more public event than it had been previously. In addition to the patient and the doctor and the family, there are now on the scene the variety of health workers that staff all hospitals. Also the administrative staffs of the hospitals are involved, in at least their legal capacity as managers for the hospital. All of these people have their personal view on the value of life under differing circumstances, and many, even if not a family member, have little hesitancy to impose their view on the situation. Some may act on what they believe is their legal responsibility, or from fear that they will expose themselves, or the institution, to a legal assault. Another possible motivation is that the training of para-medical personnel in life-preserving techniques supplies them with a *raison d'etre*, resulting in their need to use their specialized knowledge as often as possible, regardless of the consequences; in fact, the life-saving techniques in such a circumstance pursue "lives of their own".

As an example, an elderly relative (age 84) suffered a severe heart attack and in all probability had a severe cerebral ischemia at the time. A rescue squad revived him on the scene and transported him to the cardiac intensive care unit of a medical school hospital. It was obvious to those that knew him that he had suffered serious brain damage. It was the desire of his wife and entire family and his attending physician that no heroic measures be used to prolong his life, and it was so stated on his chart. The specially trained intensive care personnel was of another mind, and he was revived on several more occasions only to die after seven weeks and still in the hospital. The total hospital bill was in excess of $38,000, in 1980.

The cost of treating aged people in their terminal illness is not known precisely. It has been said that the U.S. spends 1% of its gross national product on the health care of elderly persons in their last year of life - a matter of $38 billion in 1984[20]. Other pertinent statistics from that year are that 3% of all individuals who received Medicare reimbursements (some 24,000 decedents) were those who incurred charges greater than $20,000 in the last year of life (total = >$600,000,000), or 6% (56,000 decedents) had benefits of more than $15,000 given them in their last year of life (total = >$900,000,000). While these costs for terminal care appear exorbitant, it should be understood that physicians are only able to judge the effects of their care of the elderly retrospectively, not prospectively. Many more Medicare beneficiaries who are hospitalized during any year are discharged, survive and function than die within the succeeding 12 months: the ratio of those who survived to those who died within 12 months was 4 to 1[21].

Ethicists recognized that, as a result of the effect of economics on decisions concerning life-sustaining treatments, there was a two-tier health system in this area. Some patients had to forego beneficial treatments on grounds of cost while others, who could afford it, had the right to request all possible treatment with little regard to considerations of benefit, and none at all to overall health costs[22]. Nevertheless, doctors were advised not to be involved in cutting costs or rationing resources at the bedside for the benefit of society. Yet, it was stated, doctors had the duty to advise patients with limited resources about the cost-worthiness (cost versus benefits) of any proposed treatment.

Until the modern era death was determined to have occurred only when the heart permanently stopped beating, and it is still an accurate criterion. However, it now is agreed that the brain too is a necessary component of the life process, and should it permanently cease to function, the person can be declared dead. In order to certify that a person is brain-dead the brain stem must have ceased to function, proven by absence of reflexes depending upon it (corneal, pupillary, vestibular and, especially, respiratory). It is also necessary to prove the cerebral cortex is not functioning, by determining the patient is unresponsive and irreversibly comatose and that there is no activity in the electroencephalogram. One significance of using the brain as the criteria for death is that heart and circulatory functions can be maintained by mechanically ventilating the lungs and providing fluid and nutrition intravenously or by a tube inserted into the stomach. This creates an ethical dilemma for those people who are still convinced that the ceasing of cardiac function is the only criterion of death. Another factor with ethical significance is that the bodily organs can be kept viable in a brain-dead individual until it is convenient to "harvest" them for use in transplantation operations. The dilemmas this creates are discussed in the chapter on transplantation.

The President's Commission for the Study of Ethics in Medicine and Biomedical and Behavioral Research proposed, in 1981, a Uniform Declaration of Death Act to include the criteria for brain-death. Thirty-eight state legislatures adopted this recommendation by 1984, and even in those states which only authorized the traditional definition of death (permanent cessation of heart and lung function) the use of brain-death became standard medical practice: meaning that when brain-death had been established, removal of life support systems was countenanced by the courts. There is general agreement that heart and lung functions need not be maintained when brain-death has been confirmed.

The first dilemma concerns the resuscitation of a suddenly unconscious patients as a result of the failure of circulation. It is obvious that when a person whose status is unknown is come upon in a sudden state of unconsciousness, all measures for supporting life should be undertaken. The dilemma arises (usually in a hospital or nursing home) when a patient whose prognosis is known to be hopeless, suddenly has a failure of the circulation. Should he, or she, be resuscitated? Ethicists contend that the patient's desires in the matter are paramount, and it is necessary to obtain their permission not to resuscitate beforehand. It is a matter of observing their autonomy.

Some physicians have suggested that discussing do-not-resuscitate (DNR) instructions with some patients would provoke unnecessary anxiety[23], and this would not be a beneficent action. It is suggested also that, since one cannot predict who will suddenly have a heart arrest, resuscitation would have to be broached with virtually everyone on hospital admission. My own experience confirms these suggestions, and in addition there are many patients, even in their most healthy and competent moments, that never could be rational about this subject; at least not with a specialist they have known for only a short while. Ethicists, and those with a legal temperament, deny this to be true and believe such discussions "gently" done could be "settling" to patients. Again, they produce no empirical evidence for this opinion, which ought not be too difficult to gather.

New York State, enacted in August 1987, the first law in the U.S. requiring hospitals, nursing homes and mental institutions to establish clear rules for do-not-resuscitate orders and for the state health department to draft guidelines for them. This Act was the result of at least four years of public discussion and pursuant to the recommendations of a special panel appointed by the Governor in December 1984. The law required that patients be permitted to decide in advance to forego resuscitation, even if they are not terminally ill, and to appoint a proxy for themselves should they become incompetent. If this above provision was not taken advantage of, the law affirmed the presumption that all patients consent to be resuscitated if they suffer cardiopulmonary arrest. If a patient was incompetent, doctors were to solicit consent from family members for a do-not-resuscitate order only if the patient's illness is terminal. The law granted civil and criminal immunity to doctors and nurses who carry out lawful do-not-resuscitate orders. It also required that do-not-resuscitate orders be reviewed every three days in hospitals and every 60 days in nursing homes. Physicians were to establish whether a patient was competent or not, and if they disagreed the issue was to be mediated.

Prior to the above law, it was believed do-not-resuscitate orders were carried out secretly by many institutions or that they used a slow response (slow code) for some patients, to effect the same result[24]. Many others were concerned that some patients were resuscitated against their will. Several undesirable consequences of this New York law were reported in 1990[25]. Firstly, if the complex document is not completed in its entirety, every patient must by law undergo cardiopulmonary resuscitation (CPR). Secondly, a terminally ill patient, say with metastatic cancer or end-stage heart disease, who presents at an emergency room must undergo CPR before being permitted to die. Finally, Many spouses or children find it difficult to sign the papers that they feel, symbolically, seals their beloved's fate. Therefore, the unconscious, hopelessly ill, terminal patient has to be subjected, by law, to the indignity of futile CPR. This observer goes on to say: "Cardiopulmonary resuscitation has been, and continues to be, performed and withheld by physicians in an entirely appropriate manner in the vast majority of instances where the choice applies. Caught up in the tide of 'patient rights' and physician 'paternalism', New York State legislators have made the monumental error of mandating patient or surrogate involvement in every instance of CPR. The bitter fruits of their deliberation are being reaped throughout the hospitals of New York State."

The Committee on Ethics of the Stanford University Medical Center[26] showed some confusion on the matter of cardio-pulmonary resuscitation. They rightfully pointed out that it was cruel to resuscitate debilitated, terminally ill patients. This could be avoided by having obtained prior permission from the patient or the legal surrogate to withhold resuscitation. It then was pointed out that "only 14%" of those who received cardiopulmonary resuscitation survived to leave the hospital and these patients were always admitted to an intensive care unit (ICU), which in itself was a very unpleasant experience. The conclusion drawn was that these facts should be used to persuade patients to give do-not-resuscitate permission in advance.

Confusion arises from interpretation of the data: a practicing doctor would read "*as many* as 14%" instead of "*only* 14%" survive to leave the hospital. Also the issue of the unpleasantness of an intensive care unit would apply principally to those who might achieve leaving-the-hospital status, and they probably would regard the ICU experience as worthwhile. As a physician, these reasons offered by the committee to obtain permission not-to-resuscitate, are not convincing. It should suffice to point out that when patients who are hopelessly ill, and life no longer of value to them, come under a doctor's care, that it is ethical to ask for permission not-to-resuscitate. Physicians need no persuasion in this direction, neither on technical nor on ethical grounds. It is rather that patients and families are, too often, not as understanding as ethicists in their writings would have us believe - so that, for either humane or legal reasons (arousing suspicions about their proposed care), it is uncomfortable to discuss, in advance, do-not-resuscitate orders with many patients or families.

When attitudes of 200 hospitalized patients toward life-support decisions were ascertained via a questionnaire submitted to them, only 16% reported that they had discussed life-support with their physicians. "However, an additional 47% desired such discussion."[27] The authors could have stressed that at least 37%, and as likely as many as 45%, did not which to discuss it, and that the information was gathered impersonally by questionnaire.

An investigation added age as a criteria for the situations in which cardiopulmonary resuscitation (CPR) is a hopeless gesture[28]. In the first part of this study it was confirmed that patients suffering with cancer or sepsis did not leave the hospital, even if revived after a cardiac arrest. These observers then added another category to the list of those not leaving the hospital after CPR: patients over the age of 70. This was so despite the same percentage initially being revived as that in younger patients.

It seemed just as futile to an attending physician in a long-term-care institution (nursing homes or chronic-care hospitals) to use CPR on most, if not all, of his patients[29]. It was observed that even the percentage of revivals was far lower than in an acute facility, but it was the uselessness of prolonging the lives of patients who suddenly arrested in these facilities that was his principal point. He argued for physicians to make the decision not-to-resuscitate in these instances, unilaterally. In his view, physicians are not required to provide or discuss useless therapy with patients: patients or guardians have no right to expect useless therapy. It is unfair to place the burden of decision on the patient at the end of life, or a possible burden of guilt on a surrogate. It was suggested, in passing, that to discuss DNR (do-not-resuscitate) with all patients and/or their surrogates is a waste of time better spent on other problems, even in a long-term-facility. (Ethicists, in general, have no sympathy for the latter point, even for the staff of an acute hospital.) He proposed to evaluate patients in long-term-facilities over a period of months and to give DNR orders on those who are severely demented or chronically ill and for whom CPR is clearly futile.

An ethicist related, fairly, the technical arguments offered by the above physician in favor of a unilateral decision on DNR orders[30]. Yet his rebuttals, based on interpretation of the meaning of "futile", appear to be sophistries. For instance, he questioned: can treatment efforts that postpone death by even 24 hours be called futile? He ended this portion of his rebuttal with the statement that the physician gave opinions disguised as data. In regard to the question of needing to conserve public resources by rationing, the advice given to physicians was that they continue to separate concerns about patient welfare from broader social and economic policy issues. "As professionals, we are there to serve our patients. As citizens we can vote or lobby for policies that limit individual choice in the interests of a broader social good." This sounds good, but for the problems of the rationing of medical care, it is far off the mark (see Chapters Three and Eleven). Finally, patient autonomy in preference to doctor beneficence, referred to as paternalism, is revealed as the real basis of this ethicist's thesis.

Another physician-ethicist disagreed that age alone should ever be used as a criterion for a DNR order[31]. He cited another review of this question which concluded that age was not a good predictor for the long term outcome of CPR, even though, as a group, the aged did less well. It was, rightfully, suggested that extending the data offered above[28] well could reveal that perhaps 2% of patients over 70 would make it out of the hospital, and then the conclusion would be against using age as the only criteria for a DNR order. He supported discussion of a DNR order with all patients, and recommends that the new data on the poor outcome of CPR in the aged be used in persuading appropriate older people to forego CPR voluntarily. Actually, in ten other series, the reported percentage of patients over 70 given CPR and that survived to leave the hospital, varied from 3.8% to 17.1%; clear appraisals of the quality of the lives of those leaving the hospital were not offered, though the inference was that it was generally poor.

Still two other ethicists, writing on do-not-resuscitate orders[32], believed when they were based on a rationale that the life preserved would be of a quality that neither the patient nor family should find of value, the physician could write a DNR order without actually determining the patient's values in the matter. "The decision that cardiopulmonary resuscitation is unjustified because it is futile is a judgment that falls entirely within the physician's technical expertise." It was pointed out that this recommendation differs from that of the Presidential Commission's[33], which was: in all resuscitation decisions attending physicians had a duty to ascertain patients' preferences.

While logical reasoning supports the recommendation that the patient's attitude to the value of life was irrelevant when the physician had determined there cannot be "any meaningful prolongation of life" after resuscitation, it is a departure from reality. In practice, if a physician in the U.S. wishes to stay clear of legal entanglements, he best comply completely with the terms that comprehend "informed consent" before penning a DNR order. To resuscitate or not-to-resuscitate must be decided by physicians in a pragmatic manner, or they will surely suffer undesirable consequences. Resuscitative measures in an acute-care hospital must be instituted unless there is documentation in hand or on the chart (a living will that has been updated and suitably witnessed, consent of an acknowledged proxy and/or an unanimous agreement of personal family members). In addition, when a do-not-resuscitate order is placed on the chart it is wise to notify the hospital administrative authorities and obtain their written agreement.

A second dilemma arises when a patient appears irreversibly comatose and the criteria for brain-death are not met - how long should the support systems be maintained? An important issue, then, is to establish an accurate means of prognosis for patients in the comatose state.

For this purpose, 210 patients in coma due to cerebral anoxia or ischemia for at least six hours, but not brain-dead, were surveyed[34]. Fifty-seven per cent went on to die without consciousness ever being restored, 20% attained only the vegetative state (eyes-open wakefulness without evidence of cognitive awareness) and 13% recovered independent function. If at the initial examination brain stem function were impaired (pupillary light reflexes absent), and/or evidence of widespread brain dysfunction persisted for at least 24 hours, the prognosis was grave - only one of 94 such patients regained independent function. More importantly, no patient remaining in coma for more than 7 days ever became independent, and no patient still in the vegetative state at one month ever regained consciousness.

It is necessary before treatment can be withheld in patients not yet brain-dead that there be precise guidelines for predicting when unconsciousness is certain of being irreversible. The data in the previous paragraph is thought not to provide such criteria[35,36]. It cannot be denied, except if all the required signs for brain-death are present, very early neurological examination leaves a small, but significant, margin for error in predicting a hopelessness of outcome for hypoxic-ischemic coma. However, the data does indicate that if the focus would be on what length of coma, together with what persistent neurological signs, are necessary to predict with certainty a hopeless state of unconsciousness, such guidelines are possible.

Presently, coma is defined as a sleeplike state of unarousability, and when unconsciousness (loss of self-awareness; total cognitive loss) is permanent it is called the persistent vegetative state (or cognitive death). The vegetative state can come on abruptly as a result of injury or it can come on more slowly as the result of progressive disease, both conditions causing widespread loss of cerebral cortical function. Decreasing numbers of patients recover from the vegetative state with the passage of time and the longer the vegetative state persists the less complete is the recovery; there is virtually no recovery after six months. The older the vegetative patient is, the less is the chance for recovery.

The dilemma of when to prolong life can be divided into two problems that have a difference, albeit perhaps only a subtle one.

They are: one, when patients are hopelessly comatose and are being kept alive by life-support techniques; and two, when patients are well known to be suffering with hopeless diseases and deteriorate but could be kept alive with continued treatment. When is it proper to withdraw life support (machines that breath for, and/or maintain the circulation of, the patient), or in the latter instances, withhold treatment? A distinguished group of physicians addressed themselves to these questions in 1982[37].

Their first conclusions were that the patient's role in decision making was paramount, and that a decrease in aggressive treatment of the hopelessly ill patient is advisable when such treatment only would prolong a difficult and uncomfortable process of dying. They expressed no reservation in discussing with mentally competent patients their impending demises. "If the terminally ill patient's ability to make decisions becomes progressively reduced, the physician must rely increasingly on the presumed or prestated wishes of the patient." In instances where the patient is incompetent from the outset, the physician must rely on a proxy designated in advance by the patient. This should be part of a "living will", now widely recommended be made by individuals when in good health and mentally competent, to designate how they wish to be treated in their terminal illness.

A living will is a written statement prepared in advance which tells the attending physicians that life-prolonging medical procedures are not wanted when the patient's condition becomes hopeless and there is no chance of regaining a meaningful life. The idea of a living will was first proposed in 1967 at a meeting of the Euthanasia Society of America. By 1988, three quarters of the states had passed natural death acts recognizing the rights of dying patients and their living wills, if in existence. It was said as many as ten million Americans have living wills, but they are the better educated class, and those with access to lawyers.

Other reasons for living wills not being more widely utilized are that close relationships between doctors and patients are required for the former to broach the subject when the latter is sick or elderly, and such close relationships now seldom exist in the U.S. (see Chapter Three); doctors fear that raising the subject for discussion will cause patients to feel abandoned; and lastly, when patients are young and healthy there is a complacency that prevents discussions on living wills being completed, even if raised. Actually, in a study of patients in two intensive care units from whom life-support systems were withdrawn (93) or withheld (22), over a period of one year (1988- 89), only 9.2% were reported to have had living-wills or were reported to have had discussed the issue previously with family or friends[38]. While the total of 115 cases from whom life-support systems were withdrawn or withheld represented only 6.7% of the 1719 patients admitted to the two intensive care units monitored, they did represent 45% of all the deaths there.

There can be no serious objection to living wills, but they, and designated proxies, may not always be helpful. Living wills, of necessity, must be vague since not every contingency can be foreseen and, in practice, the actual circumstances that occur, most often cannot be anticipated. The designated proxy may not be available, or so distraught, or conflicted by multiple interests as not to be helpful in taking responsibility for the patient. Many believe that a better answer than a living will is to encourage the appointing of an agent to make medical decisions under the authority of durable power of attorney acts. All 50 states recognize durable powers of attorney and nine recognize that agents may make medical decisions on the principal's behalf[39]. Problems have been encountered with this procedure also: large numbers of people (particularly those in long term care) have no one to appoint as an agent or proxy; and it was thought that even when there was someone to appoint, it was too great, if not an impossible, burden to impose. Then again, there may be uncertainty, if not an error, on the part of the physician as to the exact prognosis in the terminal state.

In England in 1989 living wills still had no legal status, but it was thought it might be desirable to provide for them in a climate where "the duty to respect a patient's autonomy increasingly makes medical paternalism uncomfortable,"[39]. The same observer made several other pertinent comments: "But in pragmatic Britain, probably justifiably priding itself in a trusting relationship between doctors and patients, the question to be considered is whether documents such as living wills are needed...and whether they would help or hinder the search for solutions to individual clinical dilemmas.", and: "Certainly the best results are likely to arise from continuous care by a practitioner who 'knew the patient's mind'." This also was the judgment of F. Rouse, the reviewer of this subject for the Institute of

Medical Ethics (in England)[40]: he said that living wills and appointment of agents are second best to patients being fortunate enough to have the same doctor over a long period of time, who knows them well, and to whom they have repeatedly spoken on the matter. In the U.S., late in the twentieth century, the latter is an unlikely circumstance.

That such was unlikely to be the situation in the U.S. was noted by previously quoted observers of this scene[37]. They said that people who died in hospitals were attended by physicians who were relatively strangers, and that there was a dearth of family doctors whom patients and families had come to know over many years, and to whom they could turn for trusted advice. Reasons for this differing circumstance in the U.S. are, firstly, that there are more than twice as many specialists as general practitioners, the reverse of the situation which existed several generations ago, and abroad at present. Secondly, the adverse legal climate, recently contributed to by the emphasis on patients' autonomy as opposed to doctors' beneficence, makes physicians hesitate to make decisions that could be medically sound and conserving of the public wealth. An example of how far the balance is being tipped against the position of the doctor is the appeal by an ethicist to eliminate the word "order" from a doctor's not-to-resuscitate order[41]. He believes such a word distracts from the concept of respect for patients and their autonomy, and that they are to be cooperated with, not ordered.

The usual handling of decisions to be made in the terminal illness of an incompetent patient (in the author's last experiences) was to involve the closest family members available, carefully documenting their discussion and proceeding on an unanimous decision. If no family was available and the patient was incompetent the hospital "risk manager" was notified who consulted with hospital counsel, presumably with the intention of obtaining a court order. If there was a family dispute and the hospital wished to curtail treatment or have a do-not-resuscitate order followed, it could ask for a judicial review. Judges have said the existence of a living-will eases their burden of making a decision.

Other factors complicating the decision-making of physicians and leading to a greater effort to preserve life, no-matter-what, are that society has become more secular, and has a misunderstanding of scientific advances. The conviction that there is life after death, and probably a better one, is less strong, and patients and their families are far more interested in this life than eternity. Rapid advances in modern medicine lead much of the public to assume that, since they hear and read about new treatments for many diseases, that all phases of all illnesses are now treatable. Moreover, a litigious society tends to believe that good outcomes are always possible and that bad outcomes are inevitably someone's fault.

The objectives of living-wills or other legal instruments with similar purpose, to prevent the dehumanizing of dying and cost containment, are often confused by a misunderstanding of certain facts. The first is that patients need to be categorized as to whether they are young or old, and how this categorization relates to the "dehumanizing" of dying. The persistent chronic-vegetative-state with essentially only the brain stem functioning is almost exclusively confined to the young and is not to be confused with mental incompetency in the elderly. The true persistent vegetative state in the elderly is seldom, if ever, prolonged and therefore does not pose the problem as in the young, either from the emotional impact on families (certainly there is none to such patients) or cost-containment. In the situations where elderly patients are judged to be incompetent due to dementia or loss of brain function (as due to strokes or Alzheimer's disease) there is almost always a greater or lesser degree of cognition remaining or other mitigating circumstance present that makes relatives or proxies seldom inclined to abandon them, no matter what the cost. The impression is that there are only a minimal number of these elderly patients who approximate the fully decerebrate state, without any cognition at all, that is called the persistent vegetative state. It would be most helpful if sufficient data were accumulated to confirm, or disaffirm, these firm clinical impressions that living wills in the elderly seldom become operative. One study by a physician-lawyer did lead him to conclude that directives had little effect on medical decision making and the care of patients[42]. "In reality, most physicians in California and Vermont knew little about directives, had little experience with them, and rarely, if ever, changed the care a patient received because of them."

The second generally unrecognized fact is that containing the costs of medical care in the terminal state is a matter of rationing, and living wills are not a means of rationing. To ration in any manner, other than by the market-place, requires that it be done by physicians against a background of a firm doctor-patient relationship (as explained below, and clearly expressed above by Rouse). To begin with, cost containment in the mentally incompetent aged cannot be affected by a living will since too often no one would agree they are truly terminal and without, at least some, cognition. In the care of the truly terminal elderly it is a matter of limiting tests, consultations and expensive treatments (that will have no real effect on the eventual outcome). Living wills do not pertain to these situations since these are not dehumanizing procedures. In the present climate of the U.S. to legislate or to regulate against doing these tests or procedures is impractical, even should there be a living will. It is impractical because of the deterioration in the doctor-patient relationship and the lack of incentive for doctors to behave otherwise. It should be clear to all, that incentive is necessary to change the behavior of any large body of people, or rather in this instance, removal of the incentives for doctors to do excessive procedures or treatments in the terminal state.

In summary, it does not appear that living wills are the answer to their stated objectives. The young, in their usual state of well-being, are unlikely to be sufficiently provident to have them, and the elderly, if they do have them, will seldom find them applicable, or always accomplish the purposes intended: to provide every death with dignity (or ease the dying process) or contain costs. It would seem the facts offered above would explain the relative lack of interest in these documents abroad. An added down-side effect in the U.S. is the emphasis active, contemporary doctors believe they must put on unnecessarily emphasizing a fatal prognosis. As an illustration, a prominent, teaching oncologist insisted on repeating to a patient with a terminal cancer: "We have agreed no unusual measures will be taken at the end." When remonstrated with, he stated: "We modern doctors don't practice as you did." The only practical result was causing the patient to have a severe depression in the last six weeks of her life. Yet, all measures to prolong her life were taken, and no expense was spared.

Indeed, with there often being uncertainty in the exact prognosis of a terminal state, and even the possibility of error being made, it would be understandable if one used a living-will in order to say that no possible treatment be overlooked in his or her care. This attitude might well be re-enforced by the recent campaign of a well-known bio-ethicist to limit the care of the elderly at a certain given age, no matter what the circumstance. This cut-off in the care of the elderly was proposed as a form of rationing to contain the overall costs of medical care[20,43].

The dilemma related to the initiating of, or the withdrawal from, life support systems of those irreversibly comatose, has been referred to the courts on several occasions, more so to decide when life need no longer be supported. It is estimated that there are at least 10,000 Americans (mostly young) irreversibly comatose at any one time, and keeping them alive causes extended periods of anguish to their families and costs the families and society large sums of money[44]. The widespread publicity attendant upon these court cases, in addition, cause much unnecessary anguish among the elderly, who are already concerned with their own impending demises. The elderly mis-identify themselves with these mostly young, chronically decerebrated or persistently vegetative patients, and then are encouraged to agonize over the terms of their living wills or other similar legal documents. Despite all this, no clear legal guidelines have been enunciated that could help physicians with this problem. Therefore, essentially the same pragmatic approach as previously recommended above is in order. That pragmatic approach, in fact, generally is adopted, whether there is or is not a living will, because physicians and hospitals fear that they will be exposed to malpractice suits based on the perceived neglecting of the rights of patients or of some family member, and/or on accusations that not everything that could have been done, was in fact done.

Then there is always the chilling case in 1983 of the two California physicians who were arrested for murder, by direction of the county prosecutor when, with the consent of the spouse and children, they ordered the cessation of intravenous nourishment and hydration of an irreversibly comatose man. They eventually were cleared of the charge, but only after a protracted period of time, which included their being convicted, and then its reversal on an appeal to a higher court.

One difference between a decision on continuing treatment of a terminal state from that of a problem in CPR is that there is available more time in the former for doctors to consult with each other and with ethics committees. Consultation permits, first, the confirming that the medical prognosis is indeed hopeless and then, that all concerned with the cessation of life support are legally protected. Contrary to the situation in abortion and the fate of disabled children there is relatively little moral debate on withdrawing life-support treatment from hopelessly ill patients who are comatose.

The most recent exposition on this subject was by the Stanford University Medical Center Committee on Ethics[26]. They re-emphasized that patients, or their legal surrogates, were the sources of authority for what happened to them. "It is one of physicians most vital skills to be able to communicate with patients, or their proxies, and overcome their stresses, fears, and from being overwhelmed by unfamiliarity with the setting." The committee stressed the lengthy amount of time necessary to accomplish this objective and suggested a "proven facilitator" be used, if necessary. The inference is that if properly handled practically all patients, or their legal surrogates, can be fully apprised of the situation and sufficiently at ease to render an ethically and legally informed consent. Physicians to behave ethically: "must ascertain, whenever possible, the views of each patient or representative on the balance between quality and mere prolongation of life - the concept of proportionality.... Thus, at a minimum, every important change in a patient's condition demands that decisions about proportionality be re-evaluated. Such reassessment requires carefully exploring the ambiguous feelings of families as they make decisions or attempt to influence those of the patient." At this point (and after their discussion of the do-not-resuscitate problem, cited above) it should be obvious, at least to an experienced doctor, that at a minimum, 34 of the 48 committee members were not practicing physicians.

Another recommendation of this ethics committee was that the American Hospital Association's Code of Patients' Rights was an appropriate basis for decision making about life support. The Code includes: the patients' right to receive considerate and respectful care; to receive information on all aspects of their illness in terms they can understand; to receive as much information about a proposed treatment or procedure as necessary for them to be able to give an informed consent; to participate actively in decisions regarding their medical care; to have all the patients' rights extend to the person who may have legal responsibility to make decisions on their medical care.

The Stanford Ethics Committee next admonished physicians to provide against the normal human instinct to give sustenance (as food and water and supplementary oxygen) reflexively, when it well might *not* be a caring act. Similarly, doctors should take care *not* to treat a complication that can be overcome in a dying patient, just from frustration with inability to treat the underlying fatal illness - as using antibiotics for infection or steroids for cerebral edema. Also, physicians should be careful, in dying patients, not to proceed in a manner that made it difficult to forgo initiating treatments that would only prolong the patient's agony. The placing of intravenous lines for hydration and nutrition might make it difficult "to refrain from treating the infections and chemical imbalances that might provide a humane release."

The Vatican had not expressed itself on these matters but a growing number of the Catholic clergy and theologians were taking the position that artificial feeding and hydration were analogous to artificial respiration and were "extraordinary" medical treatments. Extraordinary care was not required to be maintained if life was burdensome, as contrasted with "ordinary" care which would be immoral to withdraw[45]. The Roman Catholic Archbishop of Chicago (head of the Bishop's Committee on Pro-Life Activities), in May 1988, called for a national consensus opposing euthanasia or assisted suicide for individuals who were sick, infirm, comatose or in pain. He confirmed, nevertheless, that the withdrawal of artificially provided food and water from certain patients for whom these measures were useless or excessively costly or painful was allowed[46]. He spoke against any broad policy on this latter point, but decisions were to be made on a case by case basis.

Medical ethicists seriously debate whether stopping nutrition and hydration is comparable to stopping other life-sustaining treatment. Daniel Callahan, an ethicist, despite later recommending the use of age as a criterion for the withholding of medical care (see below), argued that the giving of food and water is a fundamental of human relationships and, therefore, it is morally repugnant to cause death by withholding nutrition and fluids[47]. Others contend that it is ethically permissible to withhold fluids and nutrition if by sustaining them the prognosis, nevertheless, would be hopeless[48].

The first case coming before a court, on whether it was justified to withhold life-sustaining care from a patient not terminally ill, was that of Karen Ann Quinlan in the State of New Jersey in 1976. This 22 year old woman suddenly suffered a cerebral anoxia for reasons that never became entirely clear. In any event, she remained in a vegetative state and on a mechanical respirator for several months. Her adopting father sought permission from the court to have her removed from the respirator insofar as he had been informed by the attending doctors that there was no hope of her ever regaining cognitive function. The doctors testified she was not brain-dead, but that there was no form of treatment could make her cognitive or functional. They also said that she would not survive without the respirator; how long she would live without it was unknown. The medical consensus was that removal of the respirator would neither conform to medical practices, standards, nor traditions.

The Supreme Court of New Jersey felt that the patient's right to privacy, as expressed through her guardian due to her incompetency, was more pressing than the State's interest in the preservation and sanctity of human life and defense of the right of the physician to administer medical treatment according to his best judgment. The court authorized the discontinuation of the life-support apparatus and proclaimed that there should be no civil or criminal liability of any participant in the act. Mechanical respiration was discontinued on the court order, but the patient lived on for 10 more years, without regaining consciousness.

The Court then turned to the question of what limits should be placed on the power of the family and the guardian to decide to withdraw the respirator. Firstly, they said, the guardian must be appointed by the court and then the family and treating physician must concur with the decision of the guardian. If the treating physician did not agree, then the agreement of a consulting physician would be acceptable. Finally, a hospital ethics committee, or like body, must agree that there was no reasonable probability of the patient (in this case, Karen Quinlan) ever emerging from the comatose state to a cognitive, sapient state.

After the decision in the Quinlan case there was by 1988 some legislative enactments and over 50 judicial decisions concerning termination of treatment in similar circumstances[49]. It became well established in the U.S. that competent patients have a legal right to refuse treatment or care. This right had been extended to incompetent patients in some instances, as when there was a valid living-will available and created when the patient was competent. Also, some state legislatures and many courts had granted power to an incompetent patient's family to make the decision to withhold or discontinue treatment when there was no indication of what the patient, when competent, would want or would not want. Lastly, it became well recognized, legally, that patients can refuse, and thus their physicians can withhold, any type of treatment including artificial nutrition and hydration.

However, controversy remained as to whether care can be withheld only from patients who are terminally ill, or also from those not so, but whose condition was a burden to them and they were still competent to request they not be treated. In other words, can hopelessly ill, competent patients but not yet terminal be assisted legally and ethically to commit suicide by withholding vital treatment?

In mid-1988 a bill was close to enactment in the state of Victoria in Australia that would make medical trespass (as treating a patient against his or her will or the decision of his or her legal proxy) a criminal offense. If passed, as seemed likely, it would be the first such criminal law in the English-speaking world.

Controversy also surrounded the criteria for deciding whether, or not, care can be withheld from incompetent patients. The New Jersey Supreme Court had made three rulings involving all the issues related to the termination of care. Apparently in legal and legislative circles the decisions of this court have particular prestige in these matters, as well as in other bioethical dilemmas. In general, the New Jersey Supreme Court believed the right-to-die decisions rest primarily with the patients, their families and doctors, not the courts.

The first such case was Kathleen Farrell, a 37 year old woman with advanced amyotrophic lateral sclerosis and dependent on a respirator. While living at home she requested the right to discontinue the respiratory assistance. The Court strongly affirmed the right of a competent patient to make such a request, but outlined some procedural safeguards for a patient at home: there should be two non-attending physicians to certify the patient's competence and clear understanding of the prognosis and the available treatments; and secondly, it should be made certain that the patient had made a choice without coercion. The Court insulated physicians and others who follow this procedure, both from criminal as well as civil proceedings. It was also stated that judicial review was unnecessary in future cases, unless a conflict arose between physicians, family or any involved parties.

The second case was Hilda Peters, a 65 year old woman said to be in a permanent vegetative state and maintained in a nursing home by nasogastric tube feedings. Before becoming incompetent she had executed a power of attorney authorizing a male friend, with whom she had been living, to manage all medical care for her if she became incompetent. However, in the document she did not specify the termination of life-sustaining treatments. Nevertheless, the friend requested that naso-gastric feeding be withheld. He said he had discussed the issue with the patient before she became incompetent. The nursing home opposed the removal of the feeding tube, and it was also denied by the ombudsman (see below). The New Jersey Supreme Court approved the removal of the nasogastric tube, saying that the patient had left clear and convincing evidence of a desire not to be sustained by a life-support system. This was the first higher court in the U.S. to rule that a power-of-attorney law not specifically permitting the proxy to make a decision on ending health care, could, nevertheless, terminate medical treatment. Also the decision reaffirmed that feeding by nasogastric tube, or other means of artificial nourishment, constituted medical treatment that could be terminated. More important, the Court made clear the illness need not be a terminal one: "all patients, competent or incompetent... terminally ill or not terminally ill, are entitled to choose whether or not they want life-sustaining treatment." The judges believed that such decisions were private matters for the individual.

These decisions joined other state court rulings on similar matters. In California, the court recognized that a 28 year old competent woman (Elizabeth Bouvia), with such paralyzing cerebral palsy that she had to be spoon-fed by others, could starve herself to death even though her illness was not terminal. In Massachusetts, in a 4 to 3 decision the Supreme Court permitted the nasogastric tube to be withdrawn from a man (Paul Brophy) in a permanent vegetative state but not terminally ill who had clearly stated, before becoming incompetent, that he did not want life-saving treatment. The reasoning used in the latter case was that the life-expectancy duration is not of consequence in the permanently vegetative state since there are no benefits from continuing physical existence. Also, the Massachusetts Supreme Court said that in the Brophy case continued nasogastric feeding was artificial and, therefore, an extraordinary rather than ordinary care. They also said that to discontinue nasogastric feedings was not murder nor aiding suicide nor subjecting Brophy to a painful death. It was merely allowing the underlying disease to take its natural course. However, one dissenting judge said the removal of the feeding tube was aiding suicide; another said the state's interest in the preservation of life had not been given appropriate weight; the third dissenter felt the majority decision degraded human life "in favor of death and against life".

Despite the above rulings, the New Jersey Supreme Court made clear that the termination of care for incompetent patients suffering with organic brain syndrome, Alzheimer's disease, or other severe mental impairments should be restricted. They had ruled that life-sustaining treatment could be removed from non-vegetative patients with severe and permanent mental impairments only if they had a life expectancy of less than one year (in the case of Claire Conroy, a case similar to the "second important case" they had decided on and quoted above, insofar as both states of which they were examples, made the patients incompetent). The Justices explained this latter position by stating such patients, even though incompetent, have some consciousness and some interaction with their environment, making life expectancy a key criteria for decisions in their cases.

This latter decision was criticized[49] on the technical medical ground that there was no distinction in Conroy's mental status and the chronic vegetative state. It is true that some patients with advanced organic brain syndrome and some with Alzheimer's disease do not differ, in any important way, from the chronic vegetative state in regard to their meaningful awareness of their environment. This critical attorney stated: "By medically sustaining rudimentary reactions of patients with advanced Alzheimer's disease or organic brain syndrome if they are not terminally ill, no human benefits, save existence, are being realized, at least by the court's own reasoning." (Lawyers and courts clearly use consequentialist reasoning in matters that deal with euthanasia). Criticism was also directed at the legal inconsistency in the distinction, made by the Justices, between patients in the chronic vegetative state and patients with severe mental deficit syndromes who are not terminally ill. They prevent the latter patients from choosing, through proxies, whether or not they want life-sustaining care, thereby violating their right to refuse medical treatments.

The New Jersey Justices gave recognition (in their 1985 Claire Conroy decision) to the ombudsman system as an acceptable one for nursing home oversight[50]. The use of an ombudsman in nursing homes was to complement the presence of ethics committees in hospitals which, particularly since the Quinlan case, had assumed the task of verifying the status of, and prognosis for, patients recommended for cessation of treatment.

The ombudsman system had been established several years before to investigate physical and mental abuse of elderly patients in nursing homes. The Court, in its Conroy decision, called upon the ombudsman now to examine all cases in nursing homes in which life support, including feeding and hydration, was proposed to be withdrawn at the request of a guardian, family, friends, attending physician or the nursing home itself. The ombudsman was to investigate immediately and report within 24 hours to the Commissioner of Human Services and other appropriate authorities. The ombudsman would appoint two physicians not associated with the patient or nursing home to examine the patient and to provide an opinion on the patient's condition and prognosis. If these two doctors agreed and the guardian or family or next of kin too, and the ombudsman agreed that the standards of the court were met (as detailed below) then life support, feeding and hydration could be withheld. The authorization by the ombudsman would remove any civil or criminal liability from any of the participants.

Objection was expressed to a political appointee, the ombudsman, being involved in such a technical and sensitive situation as determining when maintenance of life should be abandoned[51]. It was believed by this author that it would be better to have voluntary institutional ethics committees composed of doctors, nurses, and public representatives to supervise such decisions. The use of such in-house committees would help maintain privacy in the making of such determinations and assure their being arrived at expeditiously by keeping them out of the legal system.

Another important decision by the New Jersey Supreme Court was in the case of Nancy Jobes, handed down in June 1987. The problem was similar to that of Hilda Peters (detailed above), but the patient was younger and the vegetative state was the result of an accident, not a natural process. Nancy Jobes was a 32-year-old woman who, six years before, had been pregnant and was involved in a car accident. The fetus was killed and at the operation to remove the dead fetus she suffered a severe cerebral anoxia which left her in a permanently vegetative state. She did not require respiratory assistance but was fed through a nasogastric tube. The husband and her parents, after she had remained in this condition for five years, requested that the feeding tube be removed and she be allowed to die. The nursing home, to which she had been confined, refused and they were supported by a number of right-to-life activists. The Court decided that the feeding tube could be removed, and a little over a month later she was declared dead. The nursing home had appealed to the federal courts but the appeal was refused. The family expressed great relief that the ordeal was over and stated that "it's nobody's business but our own". The nursing home lawyer proclaimed: "I think we've seen the death of a good part of civilization," and the head of the New Jersey Right-To-Life Committee commented: "The final solution to a burdensome medical problem is now to starve and dehydrate the individuals to death."[52]

In 1985 the New Jersey Supreme Court had set three standards for patients with severe and permanent mental impairment, the presence of any one of which would suffice to withhold artificial nutrition and hydration. First was a subjective standard: the patient when competent had provided clear indication (as a living-will) that he or she would have refused such treatment. Second was a pure objective standard: when the burden of life outweighs its benefits, as when sustaining life would only perpetuate severe pain. This must be evaluated by the patient's proxy. The third, the limited objective standard is a combination of the first two: there being some evidence that the patient had previously expressed opposition to such treatment (as in a conversation) and if the burden of life outweighed its benefits. The Court believed that none of these standards had been met in the Nancy Jobes case: there was no good evidence on her attitude when competent, and being in a vegetative state she could feel no pain. They therefore used another, the substituted judgment standard - that the incompetent person's surrogate (the family in the Jobes case) should try to ascertain the patient's actual interests and preferences.

This last standard is at variance with the opinion of the President's Commission which had stated in 1983 that such a conception (imagining what the patient would want) is impossible. All the surrogate could do is offer an unverifiable guess. This opinion had been explained by the President's Commission in convincing detail[33]. Therefore, in the opinion of an attorney and ethicist[53], while the Court's decision in the Jobes case was correct, a *good* reason for it was not offered. He observed that the Justices recognized this by stating the courts should not resolve these agonizing decisions, but the legislature should give guidelines for the withdrawal of life-sustaining treatment. This ethicist believed this issue has not been resolved because society is devoted to individual self-determination and governmental moral neutrality. Since incompetent patients cannot be self-determining, and the substitute judgment standard was invalid, and a government can't be morally neutral in making such guidelines - local communities will have to debate their own values in the issue of terminating care for incompetent patients. Despite this admonition, by 1989 this was not yet being done.

The highest court of New York (the Court of Appeals), in October 1988, ruled that an elderly woman who had suffered a series of strokes and could utter only a few words and whose life could only be sustained by artificial feedings, must be kept alive even though her daughters insisted that she would prefer to die. The 5-2 decision stated that the majority was unconvinced that the patient "had made a firm and settled commitment, while competent, to decline this type of medical assistance."[54] The New York court held that the patient had to have stronger evidence of their desire, such as a living-will rather than the hear-say evidence of relatives.

The Missouri Supreme Court, in November 1988 and in a 4 to 3 decision, barred the family of a hopelessly comatose woman (Nancy Cruzan) from depriving her of food and water. This reversed a decision of a lower state court. Missouri's Living-Will-Statute permits the withdrawal of artificial life-support systems from hopelessly ill or injured persons, but it specifically forbids the withholding of food and water. In addition, the majority of Justices said they choose to err on the side of supporting a policy in favor of life and respect the right of incompetent persons to live, on the possibility they may choose to do so despite a severely diminished quality of life and the opinions of their surrogates.

Thus, the N.Y. and Missouri state courts favored more judicial intervention, as opposed to the New Jersey's Supreme Court's position of leaving these matters primarily with the families and doctors of the patient. Earlier decisions in a number of state appellate courts (California, Florida, Massachusetts) and numerous trial courts in other states also affirmed the position of the New Jersey Supreme Court. By 1989, the courts of nine states had authorized cessation of feeding hopelessly comatose patients.

At about the time of the above New York and Missouri court decrees, in the first U.S. Federal Court decision on this matter it was ruled that a Rhode Island State Hospital must remove the feeding tube from a woman hopelessly comatose for two years. The judge stated this was in support of the principle of individual self-determination: the patient in question having expressed the desire to her family, when competent, not to have her life artificially maintained.

Finally, the U.S. Supreme Court in June 1990 upheld, 5 to 4, the above cited Missouri Supreme Court decision barring removal of a gastric feeding tube from a young woman (Nancy Cruzan) who had been in a vegetative state for seven years following injury in an auto accident. The majority agreed that her family had not shown by "clear and convincing evidence" that she would have wanted the treatment stopped. However, 8 of the 9 Justices did endorse the view that there is a constitutional right, as part of the "liberty" guaranteed by the 14th Amendment to avoid unwanted medical treatment when clearly and convincingly expressed, as in a valid living-will. The 14th Amendment's due process clause prohibits the Government from depriving any person of "life, liberty, or property without due process of law."

Some legal observers linked the problem of the right-to-die to that of abortion, the question in both being that of a constitutional right to privacy[55]. State courts had sought to balance the state's interest in preserving life against the individual's interest in being free of intrusion of unwanted medical treatment. The New Jersey Supreme Court had held in the Quinlan case that an individual's right to privacy grows as the "degree of bodily invasion increases and the prognosis dims." This position reflected the approach in the Roe v.

Wade decision on abortion: that as pregnancy advances the right of privacy of the woman to make her decision on abortion wanes as the state's interest in the life of the fetus grows and, after viability of the fetus is reached, the former is overshadowed by the latter. Anti-abortion groups appreciated the connection and had been active in the Missouri right-to-die case arguing in the state courts to keep the young woman alive. The Missouri Supreme Court majority opinion stated that there was grave doubt that the constitutional right to privacy even applied to a right-to-die case. Anyway, it went on to declare, as long as the medical treatment was not so oppressively burdensome, a patient had no legal interest that could outweigh the policy strongly favoring life, regardless of its quality, that had been adopted by the State Legislature. The Supreme Court in discussing the right-to-die issue in the case of Nancy Cruzan (cited above) said, without further explanation, that the Court did not analyze the issue as a privacy question in that particular case. "We believe this issue is more properly analyzed in terms of a 14th Amendment liberty interest,". The majority opinion traced the "liberty interest" in being free of unwanted medical attention to English common law when "even the touching of one person by another without consent and legal justification was a battery."

Active euthanasia is illegal in all nations but its practice is widespread and publicly acknowledged in The Netherlands. Active euthanasia was said to have extensive support elsewhere[56]. In the U.S., "mercy killings" had come to the attention of the courts from time to time and had been dealt with leniently[57]. In fact, an effort was made in California to place on the ballot a voter initiated referendum to give terminally ill patients the right to choose the time of their own death[58]. It would have allowed doctors to accede to a terminally ill patient's request to administer a lethal dose of drugs, after two physicians had certified death was likely to ensue within six months. The initiative could obtain little more than half of the 372,000 signatures required to place it on the ballot and, given the amount of publicity it received, this indicated the people of that state were really not in favor of euthanasia.

This proposal was firmly opposed by the California Medical Association as being "contrary to the entire medical ethic." The California initiative was supported by several active groups: The

Society for Concern for the Dying, The Society for the Right to Die
and The Hemlock Society. The object of these organizations is to
secure the right of patients to "death with dignity". They recognized
there was little controversy with this position, but they pointed out
the legal and monetary concerns of doctors and hospitals are apt to
result in terrifying experiences for some patients and their families at
the end of life. They did recognize that emotional relatives, or even
just one of a group of relatives, may be the prime cause of the
prolongation of a "terminal terrifying state". They, therefore,vigorously
support legalization of living-wills and such movements as the
California initiative.

It was said that an active debate on legalizing voluntary
euthanasia was going on in China[59]. A survey in Britain in 1985,
sponsored by the British Voluntary Euthanasia Society, reported that
75% of the public agreed that "the law should allow adults to receive
medical help to an immediate peaceful death if they suffer from an
incurable physical illness that is intolerable to them."[60] Only 15% of
doctors agreed!

A working party of the British Medical Association in 1988
issued a report against any form of active euthanasia, and stated that
a patient has no right to request it of a doctor. It agreed that it is
not unethical not to prolong life in the persistent vegetative state
"when the relatives and care team can concur with the conclusion
that the patient is, in a very important sense, no longer there."

The U.K. Institute of Medical Ethics criticized the above
doctors' report as "essentially backward looking and defensive, rather
than progressive and enlightening and, consequently, does not deal
satisfactorily with the new problems and questions which are
arising."[61] They rather more agree with the 1987 report of the N.Y.
State Task Force on Life and the Law, which concluded that: "All
policies about life-sustaining treatment must affirm the value of life
and the presumption in favor of continued treatment. However, when
that presumption conflicts with the individual's decision, the
individual's right to control his or her own treatment must be
respected."

Between 6,000 and 10,000 of Holland's 120,000 yearly deaths
are estimated to be the result of doctor assisted euthanasia despite
it remaining illegal under the Dutch criminal code[61]. Court decisions
had condoned this practice and the government has issued guidelines

for it that soon may allow the procedure to become legal. However this will not occur, at least for several more years, because of the opposition of the Christian Democratic (religious) Party which had the largest representation in the coalition government, as of 1988. Its partner in government, the Liberal Party and the opposition party, the Socialists, favored legalizing euthanasia. A majority of Catholics were in favor even though the church hierarchy was among the principal opponents of euthanasia.

The guidelines issued in 1985 by the Dutch Royal Commission on Euthanasia called for patients, and they must be competent, to put in writing or otherwise verify repeatedly their determination to die. Secondly, euthanasia must be done by a doctor who has consulted at least one colleague. Third, the patient must be enduring a lasting case of "unbearable suffering". Fourth, the symptoms must be physical; depression is not sufficient reason. Fifth, the doctor must make a full report to authorities. Incompetent patients, such as those with Alzheimer's disease, are not subjects for euthanasia in Holland because they cannot request it, and it is not to be done by doctors on only the request of families.

Some Dutch doctors and lawyers were beginning to believe that the subject may be too difficult for legislation[62]. They said: the more you talk about it and the more you try to regulate it the more problems you create. They suspected it might be best to leave it to medical practice, the criminal justice system and the courts. It was said that euthanasia is not really more common in Holland, just that it is more openly discussed. This is probably untrue in the U.S., but it might be so abroad. Apparently, involuntary euthanasia, also, is widely practiced in the Netherlands, and has broad public support according to a Dutch physician[63]. This practice, however, can only add to the adverse effects that widely practiced active euthanasia can have on the morale of aged persons. A survey in the Netherlands did conclude that "the majority of residents of homes for the aged are afraid of involuntary euthanasia"[64]. This fear of the aged was found to be present despite the wide publicity emphasizing that euthanasia was to be carried only at the voluntary request of a competent patient.

In contrast to the active euthanasia practiced in the Netherlands was the legal wrangle over stopping the artificial feeding of a Dutch woman who had been in irreversible coma following a caesarean section 15 years previously. Two Dutch courts had ruled against the husband's petition to have the artificial feeding discontinued because in the courts' opinions the decision to abandon artificial feeding was a medical one that must be left to the doctor. While most doctors (as well as Dutch lawyers and courts) would accept that it was medically pointless to continue feeding such a patient, the nasogastric tube remained in place because the nursing and medical staff at the home were not prepared to oversee the process of dehydration and starvation that would eventually cause her death[65]. Obviously the Dutch courts' belief, that decisions regarding life-support were medical ones and belonged to doctors, is similar to that of courts in the U.K. and opposed to the interventionist stance of U.S. courts in such matters.

A secretary-general of the World Medical Association took note of the increasing calls for euthanasia for our sick elderly population as a need for dealing with the ever rising cost of medical care[66]. At an international assemblage of this organization, meeting in Dallas in early 1985, all agreed some form of rationing for medical care was inevitable because of its rising costs, and this would be a first step to euthanasia.

Others expressed concern that age was used, informally, as a criterion for rationing, as in treatment of breast cancer[67]. It was noted that chronological age does not describe the value of the individual, and the effect of the age factor is indeed remarkably variable. It may be true that populations of elderly are more likely on average to have cognitive impairment, more physical problems and shorter life expectancy than younger age groups. But there is such individual variations that chronological age, by itself, should not be a factor in rationing medical care. This author[67] went on to question whether quality-of-life estimates should be used to decide on treatment, or it being withheld. He explained that this was a subjective assessment of another person's values, and anyway it was a judgment that was highly inconsistent and too often based merely on the patient's age. Another claim for withholding efficacious treatment in the aged is that they do not tolerate aggressive treatment. He rebutted that there was evidence, for both hemodialysis and chemotherapy, that older patients tolerate treatment as well or better than younger patients.

A recent book[20] by a medical ethicist, Daniel Callahan, took as its theme that age, indeed, is a legitimate factor for withholding, even efficacious, treatment and to serve as a criterion for the rationing of medical care. He suggested there ought to be a generally agreed on age - probably between 75 and 80 for most people - that would serve as a cutoff for aggressive, life-extending treatment, even for antibiotics. He believed the rising costs will require rationing of medical care and the use of age as a criterion is the fairest approach. Some others in the coterie of medical ethicists agreed with him, but physicians generally opposed his thesis, bitterly[68,69]. They pointed out that it would be more humane to save money by making the system more efficient. This is especially true in the U.S. where the structuring of the payment system for medical care over the last 45 years has been the greatest cause for its run-away costs[70].

Certainly from a physician's point of view the use of age as the benchmark to ration medical care would present severe, if not insurmountable, procedural difficulties. In the first place, people "age" at different rates: it is well recognized that at the same chronological age there are physical and mental groupings - from the young-young and the old-young through the young-old to the old-old. Then, using contributions to their community as being the implicit factor in the use of age for the rationing of medical care, it should be also the old-young and only the old-old that be denied care, if justice is to be served. Secondly, the distinction between therapeutic measures and treatment to relieve pain and suffering is very often indistinguishable. Not even Callahan recommended that the aged be denied the latter.

A most cogent criticism of Callahan's thesis was that it confounded the very essence of his colleagues' original foray into bioethics - the rights of the individual, their rights to autonomy and informed consent[71]. To legislate rationing based on age and thus make passive euthanasia compulsory, certainly would be repulsive. There are numerous other ways of solving the economic costs of medical care, certainly with greater moral imperative than the suggestion of Callahan. If society could be so "rational" as to decide on a specific physiological age limit to cut off treatment, then one would expect it to be sufficiently rational to cut-off support and/or subsidies for alcohol, tobacco and sugar.

In the U.K., while age is never mentioned overtly as a criterion, the more expensive health care procedures, such as dialysis and coronary by-pass surgery, are rationed by age. This does not remove the doctor and families from the decision making process, as Callahan would do. His recommendation is another example of the basic distrust that medical ethicists have for physicians. One previously quoted English physician, commenting on Callahan's recommendation that all medical treatment cease at a given age as a form of rationing was exasperated sufficiently to remark that much of current medical ethics seems to be "an adventure playground for unemployed philosophers"[72].

4. Discussion and Conclusions

The problem of euthanasia to most physicians is a legal one and not a moral dilemma. The care of the increasingly numerous patients with Alzheimer's disease makes this obvious[73,74]. Doctors need not be told that they need to differentiate, in their treatment of demented or terminal patients, between palliative measures to ease their patient's lot and the withholding of life-sustaining maneuvers. Certainly, as an example, the treatment of pain in terminal patients has accumulated an extensive medical (particularly neurosurgical) literature over the last 75 years.

That life-sustaining treatment should be withheld from patients hopelessly unconscious is obvious to most doctors. The Missouri Medical Society, coincident with the right-to-die problem before their courts (the Nancy Cruzan case), called for legislation to permit withdrawal of life support in such circumstances. As a matter of fact the published guidelines of the AMA and the American Association of Neurological Surgeons recommend withdrawal of feeding tubes and other supporting treatments of patients in the chronic vegetative state. The only problem is that the legalities should not be onerous, and that they be in order at the time when the decision to withhold treatment is made. It appeared imminent in 1989 that the necessary guidelines on the withholding of treatment in such situations would be provided by the courts and the legislatures. Such guidelines are necessary because the dictum that courts had resorted to: to rest on what attitude the patient might have expressed when competent - seldom can be relied on, especially when the victims are young. It is unlikely that normal young people would think to contemplate and to express what they would desire in their care should they become permanently unconscious. Yet relief for the families, and society (since there are 10,000 to 15,000 such cases yearly), is necessary in such situations.

The last observation seemed to be particularly attainable because, as has been previously mentioned, there does not seem to be any large, or too meaningful, constituency for the prolongation of life by continuing treatment of those in a permanently vegetative state, or the terminally-ill aged or demented individuals. Such activity as does exist is a spill-over from those who believe in the right-to-life of fetuses and severely deformed babies. The antiabortionists and pro-life-for-infants groups reflexively apply their sanctity-of-life principle to hopelessly ill patients, but with less enthusiasm, and less so for the aged than the young and, for the most part, only because they believe it reflects on the abortion issue.

A poll taken in 1988[75] confirms the attachment of people to the young in contrast to the aged. The purpose of the poll was to discover the public's opinion as to what treatments should be covered by insurers, if they were unable to reimburse for all. 81% believed it was more important to cover a treatment that would cure 50 very sick children than one that would save the lives of 1,000 people 75 years old and giving each of them three years more of life. Twenty-seven per cent said it was "absolutely essential" and 48% "very important" to cover neonatal intensive care for very small premature babies, at a cost of $150,000 each, in circumstances in which one baby in every three survives to be a healthy child. Another interesting result was that 62% of all who answered thought the law should allow active euthanasia for those who wished it, and were dying and in severe pain; however, only 43% of doctors polled agreed. Other polls have shown 70% to 90% of Americans favor withdrawing life support systems, including food and water, from hopelessly ill or irreversibly comatose patients if they or their families requested it.

Even if moral objections continued to be raised by some, rationally there cannot be any firm basis to oppose euthanasia for hopelessly ill patients for whom, it can be agreed, life is a burden. The falsity of the sanctity-of-life argument is succinctly presented by Sidney Hook[76]. He spells out the depravity of life-for-life's-sake by citing that it can be interpreted as life at any cost and then it means: "there is no value, no cause or faith, no person however close or near, he will not betray to stay alive, no indignity or dishonor he will not swallow, no dictator before whom he will not grovel." On the other hand, some societies under the stress of an extremely hostile environment (as the Eskimos) consider it honorable or necessary to voluntarily terminate life when the individual becomes a burden to the community. This is certainly an evolutionary ethical principle.

A discussion of whether an utilitarian or deontologic ethic should dominate the decision to withhold treatment of irreversible coma or a terminal illness is resolved by the usual reconciliation of these systems[35,37]. It is suggested by the deontologist that "a minimal level of cognitive self-awareness is a necessary condition for being a subject of rights and duties." Since self-awareness is irreversibly lost in hopelessly unconscious individuals, there is no moral obligation to maintain their lives. The inference is, though not stated as such, eliminating "the person" from the unconscious patient frees one to pursue an utilitarian (or consequentialist) course in their disposition.

Physicians are fully aware of the uselessness of life to many aged and terminally ill people and their cost in terms of distress to their families and to the economy of society. Yet, it is obvious from a survey of their writings that the vast majority of them are opposed to euthanasia in any active form. They well may be willing to cooperate with the withholding of the treatment of obviously hopelessly ill patients, especially if they are suffering and the doctors feel legally immune. However, partly because of the natural instinct of all humans and their training as physicians (to preserve life), but also because of their distrust of the situation, they are opposed to active euthanasia, even if it is voluntary on the part of the patient. Their distrust comes from their familiarity with errors in diagnosis and prognosis, and administrative failures and errors in the carrying out of "guidelines", as well as sporadic evidence of false self-assurance in some of their colleagues. All this makes physicians loath to risk such an irreparable error as active euthanasia could be, no matter how infrequent the error would be.

A recent poll of general practitioners in Britain as to whether they would participate in voluntary euthanasia, if it were legalized, showed that 55% would not consider it under any circumstance[77]. Ten per cent might consider it, and 35% would consider it only on patients they knew well, patients who suffered from an incurable physical illness that was intolerable to them, and if the patient made a written request that their life be ended. The Council of the World Medical Association, in May 1987, declared: "Euthanasia, that is the act of deliberately ending the life of a patient, either at his own request or at the request of his close relatives, is unethical. This does not prevent the physician from respecting the will of a patient to allow the natural process of death to follow its course in the terminal phase of sickness."[78] This statement was ratified by the entire Association in October 1987.

It is clear the medical profession remains firmly against active euthanasia, or even assisted suicide, despite the recent emphasis on personal autonomy that in these instances challenge such a tradition. This conclusion has been upheld recently (1988) in discussions on euthanasia provoked by the editor of the Journal of the American Medical Association[79,,80]. Also, a report on active euthanasia issued in 1988 by a working party of the British Medical Association stated it was intuitively wrong. And anyway, they stated, it was infrequently requested by patients. If it should be, it was intimated that the patient's autonomy must be limited; the wish of a patient to have his or her life terminated should lead the doctor to question whether the patient is competent.

To repeat, the problems for physicians that relate to the end of life are procedural and not moral dilemmas, at least in the U.S. Any attempt to set rules for the right to die would be directed at the most obvious cases, which undoubtedly are in the majority. But possible medical or procedural errors cause most physicians to be against legislation for either active or passive euthanasia. In the present climate, certainly in the U.S., it is unlikely that the matter of dying would be allowed to rest on the beneficence of the medical profession towards patients they knew well. Euthanasia resting on the principle of patient's autonomy (often through surrogates) probably would cause few changes from the present, and certainly would not become more widely practiced in the English speaking countries.

There is no dispute on the fact that too much of our resources are expended on those whose death is inevitable in the very short term. This does not prevent politicians and medical ethicists from orating or pontificating on the subject, without offering a solution. It is clear that the free-enterprise system for the delivery of medical care does not lend itself to a suitable rationing mechanism. It logically can do so only through the market-place, and that is not acceptable in a modern liberal society with its emphasis on the rights of the individual, if done openly. The modifications of the medical care system in the U.S. to make it more equitable, so far, have only served to make it more expensive, and reduce what rationing of it could be achieved by the market-place. In a sense, the mixed U.S. system of delivering medical care has given us the worst of both worlds, the free- enterprise and the socialist systems.

Where rationing of medical care does occur more efficiently and equitably than in the U.S. (in Great Britain) the system is much nearer a socialist one (the NHS) - and even there it has to rely on the doctors and the ethics of the medical profession, chiefly their beneficence, to accomplish rationing of medical care[81]. The view of lawyers and judges in the U.K. with regard to treatment for the dying is that doctors will and should continue to bear their traditional responsibility for deciding, with the patient and family, when treatment should be withdrawn and for implementing the terminal decisions. "The UK courts respect the medical profession as the arbiter of clinical competence in negligence claims and will be wise to leave doctors in charge of terminal decisions. By contrast the courts in the United States have taken a much more interventionist stance...and has produced some distressing and depressing decisions following prolonged US court actions."[19]

The futility of ethicists in the U.S. to call upon doctors to obtain from their patients, while still competent, permission to forego terminal life-sustaining treatment as the method to curtail the excessive costs of dying which maintains the principle of autonomy, has been discussed above. The only way to make the dying process less wasteful (and provide for rationing) in the U.S. is through a change in the system of the delivery of medical care[70], and not to expect (or demand) that doctors, under prevailing circumstances, change their performance.

A health care planner suggests the way to ration medical care is to decrease the power of the doctor and increase the activity and power of "Health-plan managers, hospital administrators, insurance-company executives, and government officials [who] will...make difficult decisions about the allocation of scarce resources."[82] In his view physicians are needed only to aid the medical economists to determine the cost effectiveness of their treatments. This planner obviously believes rationing is entirely an economic problem and not an ethical one, and that neither the beneficence of doctors nor autonomy of the individual need play a role. Others maintain justice and equity at the level of the individual will always demand that the final rationing decision rest with the doctor[83], and anyway, no one else wants the job of withholding treatment of the individual patient[84].

For rationing to rest on the decision of doctors, in the U.S., the strength of the doctor-patient relationship would have to be restored. When the cost of medical care, including that of dying, becomes so exorbitant as to undermine the entire economy, perhaps then medical care systems from abroad, where the doctor-patient relationship remained strong and costs are contained (as in the U.K.), will be used as a paradigm for change.

CHAPTER ELEVEN. TRANSPLANTATION
(with additional notes on the rationing of medical care)

1. Transplantations

Transplantation of organs or other body tissues from one individual to another has become an established technique over the last 30 years. The transfusion of blood, actually the first method of transplantation from one person to another, has been going on for even a longer period of time. The progress in transplantations has been constant, and there is every reason to believe it will continue.

The original concerns were, in the first place, whether it was feasible and worthwhile to transplant an organ. Secondly, whether it was justifiable to permit donors to give up an organ (a kidney) for this purpose, even though they had to be close relatives so that the organ would "match" the recipient immunogenetically and not be "rejected". The latter concern has been alleviated by the discovery of drugs that suppress immune reactions in recipients, permitting the use of organs from unrelated cadavers. Also helpful was the redefinition of death to be the cessation of brain function (q.v. Chapter Ten), enabling cadaver organs to be kept fresh and usable by continuing heart and lung function until they could be "harvested" for transplantation. Improvement in transplantation techniques has all but eliminated the relative risk to recipients (as compared with that of their disease), and, for instance, the five-year survival rate for cadaver kidneys exceeds 60%, and for hearts it is better than 50%. The original moral questions raised by organ transplants were answered by these advances, but they have been replaced by new concerns.

The principal newer moral problems are related to rationing: the first of which is occasioned by the existence of a far larger number of recipients than the supply of available organs or tissues; the second is the allocation of the high cost of transplantation;

thirdly, even the appropriateness of its use at all, in view of the ongoing difficulty with the cost of medical care. The difficulties of ethicists in being helpful in solving the problem of rationing in the U.S. is nowhere better illustrated than in their discussion of transplantation[1].

Other moral problems of transplantation originate from variations in views on what are the proprieties in the obtaining of donor organs and tissues. Lastly is an obvious irony that most transplantations require that the donor be a healthy individual who has met with an unfortunate accident. Of course, those most involved in the practice of transplantation are not interested in this incongruity, and their press releases even could be said to help divert the public's attention from it. Efforts to prevent accidents (such as to reduce drunk driving, lower speed limits, etc.) very well could remarkably lower the supply of donor organs and yet, from an utilitarian approach, yield a greater community benefit.

Despite the remarkable progress in organ transplantations, serious problems are still encountered in the quality-of-life of the recipients, particularly if they be children[2]. They must take drugs daily to prevent rejection, and be under constant medical supervision and testing. The anti-rejection drugs are good, but there is room for improvement. Many recipients report a persisting emotional upset from fear that their graft will fail. The families of children with renal transplants are said to be "a gloomy group". It is suggested[2] that indeed there are children whose quality-of-life are so poor that they should be allowed to die. Even in adults, the complications, often as mental side-effects of sustaining drugs (steroids in particular)[3], can cause one to question the worthwhileness of an organ transplant.

The great visibility of transplantation has been irresistible to hospitals and the surgeons involved, particularly with the encouragement it offers, particularly for U.S. medical care providers, to cultivate their entrepreneurial spirit. This has led to failure to emphasize the downside of transplantation such as that liver transplantation is only successful one third of the time, and often it can be a bad experience for the child and the family. Then again, once started, transplant surgeons won't stop treatment even in relatively hopeless situations such as doing a second and even a third transplant in desperately ill children. They say: "She is not brain dead. (but) We can't do anything about it. Nobody believes that in medicine anymore.... If people get to know we don't do everything possible and don't keep going under all circumstances, then they won't send us patients anymore!"[4] The further response of transplant surgeons is that they have made a commitment to a patient once they have done a transplant, and their Hippocratic Oath and the bonding between patient and doctor won't permit them to think of anything - such as half the chance of success of retransplantation in their patient as compared with giving the organ to another child for primary transplantation - but the extension of *their* patients' lives.

The above observations were offered from a conference (grand rounds) on liver transplantation that included anecdotes illustrating that no one, not even a group of doctors, could predict when a transplant patient was hopeless[4]. The anecdotes were offered in support for the all-out efforts once a patient has been transplanted, even for a second or third organ. Hopefully, the functioning of the national organ procurement program will settle the issue more sensibly - even in the muddled (with regard to rationing) medical care system of the U.S. A bio-ethicist, oft-quoted in the media, was in attendance with the transplant surgeons, but was not cited as offering any constructive comment.

Kidney transplants cost $30,000, and heart, liver or other organ transplants can cost more than $200,000 each. Immunosuppressive drugs, which have to be taken by recipients for the rest of their lives, cost from $5,000 to $7,000 per year. By 1989 the average total cost for one year's care for the 1,673 hearts transplanted was $162,000, for the 2,160 liver transplants $216,000, and $52,000 on average for the 8,886 kidneys transplanted. Most agree in the U.S. that it is whether Medicare will or will not pay for a transplant that sets the standard for other insurance agencies and most state Medicaid programs. Congress in 1973 had extended the Medicare law to cover all patients with end-stage renal disease, regardless of their age, and this included the costs of kidney transplantations. Medicare and private insurance companies paid for about 80% of other organ transplants in 1987; but Medicaid reimbursement was erratic among the various states. The most common transplant procedure in the U.S. is of the cornea (keratoplasty), and in 1985 more than 30,000 were done at an average total cost of from $4,000 to $7,000 each[5]. The Total transplant cost in 1986 was estimated to have been $1 billion.

The cost of the Medicare end-stage renal program (dialysis and transplants), which on its inception in 1972 was projected to eventually cost $1 billion, by 1984 was approaching $2 billion, and the new projection was that it would be $3 billion by 1989. By the end of 1985, kidney transplant patients accounted for 18% of all end-stage renal Medicare beneficiaries and 32% of all beneficiaries less than 55 years of age[6]. Because the costs of maintaining patients with functioning grafts is only one third of those for patients on dialysis, and because the quality of life is so much better, renal transplantation is a convergence of the best clinical and economic results for patients with end-stage renal disease. Indeed, such is the stress of dialysis treatment that 22% of people on this treatment voluntarily give it up, knowing they will die shortly thereafter. In Britain it is estimated that every successful kidney transplant saves the National Health Service 30,000 pounds ($46,000).

It is ironic, and a serious condemnation of the U.S. health care system, that new medical technologies and procedures do not become less expensive after widespread use after their initial introduction as do other (industrial) innovations. Indeed, they tend to become even more expensive[7].

Thirty-two per cent of renal transplants in the U.S. are still donated by relatives (12% in the U.K.). Families of children with kidney failure are often placed under severe emotional pressure to donate a kidney for them, especially since it has now been shown that an adult kidney can be safely placed intra-abdominally in small children[8]. The risk of death to the donor is reported to be about one in 5,000. Although recipients of kidneys donated by close relatives still require immunosuppressive drug therapy, results are much better - there being a lower rejection rate than if the donated kidney is from a stranger. Living kidney donors should avoid high-protein diets, and it is recommended that they be observed by a physician at regular intervals after donation.

In addition to the obvious altruism for relatives to donate kidneys (or tissues such as marrow or fetal cells), it is said that often there is a financial consideration for such offerings[9].

Efforts have been made by state legislatures to increase the number of organs available for transplantation. Uniform Anatomical Gift Acts have been adopted by all 50 states providing for mentally competent persons to will their bodily organs for transplantation.

These laws also permit family members to consent to the removal of organs from their deceased relative for this purpose; and most acts include brain-death criteria as determining when death has occurred.

The problem was said to be not so much that families refused to donate organs of a deceased person, but rather that they were not being asked to do so by doctors or nurses who were reluctant to intrude into the grief of relatives, understandably greatest for those most suitable as donors - young accident victims. Thus several states, starting with Oregon in 1985 and followed by New York and California and 38 other states by early 1988, had passed laws making it mandatory for hospital representatives to request families to permit the organs of deceased relatives be made available for transplantation[10]. The U.S. Congress passed a similar law (in 1986) for all hospitals receiving Medicare or Medicaid funds. Under this latter, national law, hospitals also must inform transplant units about all potential donors, and citizens are to indicate their willingness to act as a donor when filling in tax forms and driving license applications.

Many hospitals were found not to be complying with these laws, and even in those that were, there had not been an increase in organ donations[11]. Further, an empirical study published in Britain late in 1989 suggested that required requests would not considerably increase the supply of donor organs[12]. The principal reasons for failure to increase the supply of organs from accident victims in this study were poor condition of the donor body at the time of brain death, lack of compatible donors, and failure of coroners to release bodies. Also, some physicians believe it is unethical to continue to ventilate someone for the sole purpose of organ donation[13].

Since accident victims are the largest source of healthy organs for transplantation, several states had placed on the reverse of drivers' licenses a form to be signed for permission to donate organs in case of death. Only 20% of drivers had signed such a form where offered, and each year fewer than 3,000 of the 25,000 people who died with organs suitable for transplant actually had their organs used. Relatives of 30% of potential donors refuse consent, unless their is indication of prior consent on the part of the victim. Understandably, in light of the malpractice climate, doctors generally will not honor a signed donor's card without first obtaining permission of the family. Despite these efforts, donor organs remained in short supply. There were still 3,500 to 5,000 patients for whom no corneas were available. In 1986, 8,960 kidneys were transplanted (with >10,000 still on the waiting list); also transplanted were 1,368 hearts (with >450 waiting), 924 livers (>300 waiting), and 45 hearts together with lungs (91 waiting)[14]. It was said that half of those awaiting liver or heart and lung transplants, and a third waiting for a heart alone, would die before organs could be found for them.

The National Health Service in Britain transplanted 1,160 kidneys, hearts and lungs from the recently dead in the first six months of 1988, an increase of 39% on the same period of 1987. Nevertheless, the waiting list for kidneys in the U.K. had grown from 2,500 to 3,500 in five years, and the waiting list for heart and liver transplants increased by 60% from 1986 to 1987. Altogether in the U.K., in the first 10 months of 1988 1398 kidneys were transplanted, 338 hearts, lungs, and lung-hearts transplanted (408 waiting) and 203 livers transplanted (33 waiting).

It had been suggested that laws be passed presuming consent to donating organs on the part of all recently deceased persons. The law was recommended to read that people would have the right to object to organ donation, but in the absence of documented objection every one would be a potential donor at their death. Such laws were in existence in France, Scandinavia, Israel, Austria and Switzerland. Critics said the majority objected to presumed-consent laws as being high-handed, and it would only turn people away from voluntarily donating their organs. It was feared efforts to pass such laws only would reduce the supply of available organs.

Under French law, a person's organs may be used on death unless specific instructions had been given to the contrary - or the patient's relatives dissented. In Britain the law was the reverse. The British Human Tissues Act of 1961 specified that would-be donors indicate their desire ahead of time, and doctors must assume that people who do not carry donor cards were unwilling to donate their organs. Despite the French law appearing to be more favorable for donations than the British law, in practice France has fewer donors than Britain, because French relatives are more reluctant to give consent.

Another suggested solution to the shortage of donors was to permit the marketing of organs in anticipation that the commercialization of the process would increase the supply. The permitted sale of one's blood and sperm were cited as precedent, and, anyway, permitting the sale of organs is a legitimate exercise of individual freedom. The sentiment most everywhere has been against commercialization of organ donation. It was perceived as another way to exploit the poor since they would have the greatest incentive to sell parts of their body to the more privileged in our society. This would apply especially to the sale of one of their kidneys by poor people while still alive. It is also visualized by ethicists as reducing the respect for the human body, and by reducing voluntary donations it would diminish these altruistic acts - to the detriment of society.

Actually, it was reported in 1989 that two Turkish men were transported to England and each given 2,000 pounds to donate one of their kidneys to non-related recipients[15]. These transplantations were done in a private hospital and, as a consequence, it was predicted that it soon would be legislated that private hospitals must report all transplant procedures, as the National Health Service Hospitals had been required to do for years.

Condoning the above sale of organs in Britain were reports on this practice in other countries. In India almost all renal transplants, said to be 1,000 annually, were done with paid, unrelated donors. There were myriads of poor people in India willing to give up a kidney for as much as 10,000 pounds. China, too, was reported to be carrying on a thriving business in transplanting organs from paid donors or executed criminals[9]. It was not mentioned in the above cited business magazine article that the increase in the supply of donor organs that could result from its commercialization, would favor the affluent and exclude most all others.

In 1984, the U.S. Congress passed the National Organ Procurement Act providing for a nation-wide organ procurement and distribution network to bring order to the situation. The Act also provided support for local or regional organ procurement programs; establishment of a task force to advise on the implementation of the law, to review medical, ethical, legal and economic issues related to organ transplants, and to evaluate and review the extent of insurance coverage for immunosuppressive drugs; and establishment of a national scientific registry of transplant procedures to evaluate their effectiveness, and to monitor the clinical status of patients. The legislation prohibited purchase of human organs for use in transplantation procedures, with a penalty of $50,000 or 5 years in prison or both for violation of this provision. A principal theoretical basis for prohibiting the payment for a donor organ was that it would harm the inherently fragile system of recruiting voluntary donations.

The task force was appointed and awarded a contract to create the National Organ Procurement and Transplantation Network by October 1, 1987. The country had been divided geographically and one organ procurement agency was to be designated for each area (about 2.5 million people) by the Secretary of Health and Human Services. Implementation of this new network had been delayed and the new deadline was to be March 31, 1988. Contests for overlapping territories in some states (Texas, New Jersey, New York. and Illinois) continued in January 1988. Although the agencies were non-profit organizations, the competition between them was bitter and it was feared the "turf wars" would have an adverse effect on the public in regard to organ donations. Failure of an agency to receive government designation precluded reimbursement for their expenses, and they would have to cease operations. The criteria for settling the matter was to have been that the agency with the most transplants and the lowest costs would receive federal designation. However, local and state health departments made rulings that, legally, clouded the issue.

A problem was encountered in accrediting transplant centers. An early decision was that it be done on a basis of the quality of personnel and environment, rather than on the number of grafts done, or on survival numbers[16]. The latter "are commonly influenced by patient selection, and might lead centers to avoid treating the most seriously ill patients." Along with this, it was not intended that the number of centers approved be limited. Nonetheless, the Task Force on Organ Transplantation in May 1986 finally recommended to Congress that to qualify as a designated center eligible to receive federal reimbursement (from Medicare), a hospital must have performed 25 kidney, or 12 heart, or 15 liver transplants annually. Many private insurers adopted a similar guideline for reimbursement.

A research planner and a member of the task force was quoted as stating that the volume of surgical procedures was positively associated with patient outcomes. He also hopes that the proposed yardsticks for activity would slow the burgeoning of the numbers of transplant centers that had been occurring[17]. There were,by 1985, 71 heart, 36 liver and 178 kidney transplant centers in the U.S. It was not explained how a center could obtain designation if not so chosen initially. Congressional attitudes on this question varied: a liberal Democratic approach was that the rapid growth threatened the entire program; a more conservative Republican Senator questioned why the Federal Government should give centers antitrust immunities by granting them franchises. There was serious competition between hospitals for approval and this added to the procurement process snag, referred to above, by the influence hospitals had on state departments of health. As usual, the demand of health planners and health economists to limit the number of hospitals permitted to do transplants was joined by the entrenched interests already doing these procedures.

Limiting the utilization of any particular innovation in an otherwise completely unplanned medical care delivery system previously had been shown to be difficult, and even counterproductive. This was illustrated in the U.S. by the attempt to limit the number of designated open-heart surgery centers, and to limit the deployment of computerized axial tomography[7]. To the contrary, restriction of the number of transplantation centers in the planned environment of the National Health System of Great Britain is quite rational. Wisely, the U.S. Task Force did not pursue the licensing of transplant centers, leaving the matter up to the states. In many states certifying transplant centers devolved onto the Health Service Agencies whose funding by the Federal Government stopped in 1986, returning the issue to the state health departments.

A system of priorities for distribution of organs has been established (so far by 1988, applied only to kidneys) which included the degree of match between the donor organ and the recipient, the proximity of the organ to the patient, the length of time the patient has been on the waiting list, and the severity of the patient's illness. A final criteria for priority rating was the degree of sensitization of the recipient, meaning how many previous exposures the patient had had to antigen-producing conditions such as pregnancies, blood transfusions and/or, very importantly, previous transplants. If an equal match was obtained between an organ and several patients, the patient with the greater sensitivity would be given the organ.

The theory for the latter rule was that the sensitized person was harder to match and, therefore, had less chance of obtaining an organ. The ethical problem this introduced was that the transplant to a more sensitized person had less chance of succeeding, even if the match was good, than it did in the less sensitive patient. Another aspect of this problem was that persons who had had one kidney donated to them that failed, often had a better priority (because of their increased sensitivity resulting from their failed transplant operation) and were more likely to get a second kidney, even before other, less sensitive individuals got their first donated kidney. The irony was that the latter patients, because of their lower sensitivity, were more likely to have good results. A frequently cited injustice of this nature was the child which received a fourth liver after three previous failures, only to reject the fourth one and go on to die. It was pointed out that three other children on the waiting list might have been saved, if the child in question had been regarded as having had its chance with the first liver.

Perfect matches between a recipient and a kidney will occur about 5% of the time, and such matched kidneys were be distributed on a national basis. No other organs were mandated for national distribution, and centers were free to make regional and national arrangements for sharing excess organs as they desired. A formal policy with regard to foreign nationals receiving organs from the Network was to be announced. An ethicist had commented that it was wrong to give a sizable number of kidneys to wealthy foreigners (as alleged was the practice of one university medical center) since it would increase the distrust of the medical profession and thereby decrease donation of organs[18]. He advocated a quota system for non-resident aliens, but stated that charity dictated that at least some outsiders have access to American organs.

The dilemma with regard to transplanting aliens brought into focus the often encountered question as to how far the beneficence of a physician should extend. Some physicians believed, when interviewed, that they were under obligation to do their utmost for any patient that consulted them, regardless of citizenship. In one center it was reported that 25 to 28% of kidneys were transplanted to non-resident aliens[19]. This center acknowledged, implicitly, that it was not just a question of the surgeon's beneficence that was involved, but that the donor organs could be looked upon as a national resource, since they promptly agreed to keep transplants to aliens at 5% of hearts and kidneys and 10% of livers that became available to them (regardless of how often they were consulted by aliens).

Complicating the problem was that the foreigners given transplants were uniformly wealthy and were charged greater than usual rates. Of course, there were strong expressions of xenophobia to exclude all foreigners, or at least give to citizens first priority, and the strongest outcries were from patients and their families on the long waiting lists (a total of 27,515 on the nationwide computer listing, in August 1987). The consensus opinion of the physician transplant societies was that aliens should be limited to 10% of renal transplants in any one hospital. The probable reasoning was that this gives transplant surgeons leeway in their practices to accommodate to situations in which their duty to a deserving patient cannot, and should not, be compromised by complete exclusion of all but firmly established, legal citizens of the U.S.

The obverse of the problem of transplanting organs in the U.S. to aliens is the situation in Third World countries. In those countries, there are wealthy patients requiring organs and surgeons competent to do the transplantation and desperately needy people who, for a price will give up a kidney. The surgeons complain if they stick by the guidelines of the international Transplantation Society, to which they belong, and not participate in the purchase of organs they will lose their clientele to surgeons abroad. Their countries are not interested in setting up programs for the securing of donor organs, or sponsoring transplantations, or even for treatment for end-stage renal disease, when they do not have funds sufficient for basic medical care. This situation was criticized, in essence, by some who ask (without providing answers, but implying incorrect or impossible ones): should not a patient in Africa receive the same care as a patient in London? "Can we continue to produce miracles for the few that are off-limits to the many?"[20]

Shortly after the alien transplant question was aired the Federal Task Force on Organ Transplantation, in the summer of 1986, called for all people who were in need of heart and liver transplants to receive them "regardless of their ability to pay", and the necessary postoperative lifetime drug costs, also, were to be supplied. At the same time they said the access of foreigners coming to the U.S. for purposes of transplantation should be limited to 10% of kidney transplants at any one hospital. They estimated that heart transplants would cost $55.9 million per year and liver ones, $93 million. They estimated that the costs would be $37.5 million for Medicare, $4.2 million for Medicaid and $14.2 million for private insurers. Medicare was already paying for more than 90% of renal transplants but not the postoperative drugs (an amount averaging about $5,000 per patient per year). The Reagan Administration opposed the recommendation of open financial access to heart and liver transplantation on the ground that it would markedly increase the number of procedures, as it had for renal transplants since 1973, and then it would be too expensive for the national budget.

Despite the progress in the allocation of organs, it was still possible, in 1988, to "jump the queue". Most organ procurement agencies were associated with transplant centers and as a result those on the list of that center received priority for the organs from that particular procurement agency. Moreover, those that could afford several consultations were able to get themselves on the waiting lists of several transplant centers, multiplying their chances to receive an organ. One state, N.Y., was taking steps to consolidate the multiple lists in their jurisdiction, as well as the procurement agencies, to make the distribution of available organs more equitable.

Ethicists cast doubt on the ability of physicians to select patients fairly, and suggest that selection on the basis of "medical suitability" can easily degenerate into "obfuscation"[21]. A common suggestion was that once a pool of acceptable recipients were identified medically, the final selection should be by lottery. It was sobering that in this published symposium on transplantation, which denigrates the ability of practicing physicians to judge the medical status of patients and act in a fair manner, 25 of the 28 contributors were not, and had not ever, engaged in caring for transplant patients.

A study in 1988 revealed even in kidney transplantations, the financing of which for all persons in the U.S. has been by the government since 1972, there still was a 30% more likely chance for a member of a family earning $35,000 annually to have a transplant than a member of a family earning $20,000[22]. This discrepancy, in the principle of equal access to medical care, extended to race and sex. White men in the U.S. were twice as likely to receive a new kidney as blacks of either sex, and a third more likely than a white woman. Twice as many whites donated organs after brain death as did blacks; among living donors, six times as many whites donated a kidney to a close relative than did blacks. About 20% of blacks carry antigens against tissues from white persons that make them less suitable for organs of white origin. Despite these facts on donors, an oft-quoted ethicist believed the recipient discrepancy was the result of one of "medicine's dirty little secrets". He believed doctors have an unconscious bias in their referral of patients to transplant centers[23]. It was not suggested that the U.S. medical care system deprived the poor of personal attention, and that this was the basis of the poor receiving fewer organs, which is in line with other evidences of their poorer health care in general.

A scandal in London came to light in 1988 that had been going on since 1985 (previously mentioned, p. 411. A private hospital had been buying kidneys from Turkish peasants brought to the city for the purpose, to transplant them into wealthy Londoners. The outrage aroused caused a Human Organ Transplant Bill to be immediately introduced into Parliament forbidding any payment being made for the supply of a transplant organ. The Bill also would restrict live donations to close genetic relatives, unless permission was given by an authority that was to be set up. Undoubtedly there would be additions to, and modifications of, the Bill as it traversed through the various parliamentary committees. Some, including ethicists, asked what was wrong in people of their own free will selling an organ? They got some extra cash and the recipients had their lives spared and were relieved of suffering[24].

As mentioned above, the final allocation of an organ to an identified group of suitable recipients is thought by many to be most just if done by lottery. Others say there must be a better way. Many side with the suggestion of Dr. George Lundberg, Editor of the Journal of the American Medical Association, that the most deserving recipient among those available should receive the organ[25]. He said in an editorial: "If I had one liver to transplant and 50,000 possible recipients, I wouldn't let the fact that a great creative genius might drink deter me from giving him or her a needed new liver to allow another 30 years of creativity." Isn't that an evolutionary view: to override justice to individuals by doing what is perceived as the best for the species?

Cardiac transplantation, 20 years after the first one done in 1968, could be viewed as an established valid treatment for end-stage heart disease. By 1988 the hospital survival rate of cardiac transplant recipients was approaching 95%, and the two year survival rate was up to 91% (80% reported the previous year)[26]. Trials with artificial hearts were continuing: they still were feasible only to preserve the recipient's life until a donor's heart was available.

4,992 patients had undergone cardiac transplantation worldwide by the end of 1987 (4,016 since 1980) and there were 94 institutions with active programs in the U.S. alone (up from 71 in 1985)[27]. It was estimated 1,600 to 1,800 Americans received heart transplants in 1987[28]. In the leading cardiac transplant center (Stanford University), 448 patients had received new hearts and 206 were still alive in 1987, the longest survival being almost 18 years and that patient was leading a normal life. The longest survivor in the world had been a Frenchman dying 18 and one half years after his heart was transplanted. The majority of third-party payers (insurance carriers) were accepting cardiac transplant as a valid therapeutic procedure and had made coverage available as was Medicare, and Medicaid to a limited degree.

The success of cardiac transplantation and the continuing shortage of donors raised the ethical problem as to who should receive the available donor hearts. Should the sickest candidate or the one most likely to have the best result (most functional and longest lasting) get preference? Most transplant surgeons believed they should try to save the sickest and least stable patient by giving him or her the first available heart[28]. On the other hand, serious systemic disease likely to limit the functional capacity of the patient, no matter how well the heart worked, might well be a contraindication for transplantation in such a patient[27]. Another probable contraindication was the judgment that a patient was unlikely to be able to follow the rigorous and complex postoperative regime to which transplant patients must submit for the rest of their lives. Addiction to tobacco, alcohol or drugs, or a history of medical non-compliance would be unfavorable factors in such a judgment. These ethical decisions, for the moment, were being left to doctors and their beneficence.

Experimentation in an effort to create an artificial heart had been underway for over 30 years and grant money in excess of $200 million had been expended on it[14]. Attempts at permanent implantation had been made in five patients and although one survived 20 months the experiences were considered unsuccessful because the severe complications (thrombo-emboli and infection) precluded an adequate quality of life. It seemed unlikely that the means to prevent these complications would be available in the foreseeable future. Implantations of temporary artificial hearts had prolonged the lives of 35 patients until a donor heart could be located and transplanted into them. The shorter time the artificial heart was in place the better was the outcome after transplantation.

Some believed the entire effort to create artificial hearts was unrewarding and that large sums of money should not be spent on their development. In regard to permanent artificial hearts it was believed the inadequate results so far and the poor prospects of avoiding the serious complications in the future spoke for themselves. Opposition to temporary artificial hearts rested on the fact that their implantation was so dangerous that it automatically propelled their recipients to the top of the priority list for a donor heart[30]. This was not only frequently patently unfair but also actually aggravated the shortage of donor hearts.

This ethicist added he "thinks it's terrible" and called for a ban on all artificial heart implants. He was particularly incensed because authorized surgeons could implant a temporary artificial heart into a patient without informed consent. The reason given for this circumstance was that the patient's condition could be (and usually was) so poor that informed consent for implant was impossible, but then with improvement on the artificial heart, informed consent for transplantation could be obtained. It was further noted that donor hearts were in such short supply that temporary artificial hearts, for all practical purposes, could become permanent and doom the patient to severe suffering before their certain death; and all this could happen without informed consent. A final point was to be considered: experimental use of artificial hearts was an all or nothing treatment. Unlike a clinical trial with a new drug, withdrawing from an artificial heart experiment - a provision that informed consent allows for in any other clinical trial - means certain death. To most practicing physicians the majority of these comments would seem to be sophistries.

Another ethicist (not an economist) decried research on the development of an artificial heart on the basis that it might be successful[31]. If so, perhaps 17,000 to 35,000 people a year could benefit, but both their length and quality of life after operation could be problematical. His point was that such a success would result in its use becoming a required part of any health care program, and would emerge in an estimated $5 billion (in 1983 dollars) being added annually to the already excessive cost of health care. The result would be that supporters for a good national health insurance program would be further frightened off.

Organs for transplantation into infants, babies and very young children were noted to be in very short supply, and many said they were practically nil. It was estimated there were 400 to 500 infants requiring new kidneys, the same number needed donor hearts and 500 to 1,000 required livers[32]. Transplantation of hearts into infants, mostly for congenital cardiac defects that do not permit survival, raised several additional moral issues. This was because the required donor hearts were so small that non-viable babies (such as anencephalics) and animals (such as a baboon) could be considered as donors. An anencephalic infant is one born only with a brain stem, and the cerebral hemispheres missing or reduced to mere stumps. They can be identified *in utero* and usually die shortly after birth. There are 0.3 per thousand births in the U.S. each year, and although about two thirds are stillborn the estimated remaining 375 anencephalic infants could potentially supply almost all the infant donor organs needed.

The problems with using an anencephalic infant as an organ donor are many fold. In the first place, if such an infant be alive at birth - should one wait until it dies before "harvesting" its organs? If the child appears to be dying after birth is it right to maintain life with machines until its organs are needed? It is illegal to harvest the organs unless brain-death has been established and since the brain stems of anencephalics do function they can not be said to be brain-dead. If the death of the brain stem is awaited, vital organs fail *parri-passu* and by the time the anencephalic infant is legally dead its organs are useless for donation. Adults after a fatal accident, to the contrary, are immediately supported with machines permitting the diagnosis of brain-death and simultaneous preservation of organs in good condition for transplantation.

Doctors said that anencephaly was an easy and certain diagnosis and the infant was sure to die in hours or days. Therefore a law should be enacted equating anencephaly to brain-death so that such a deformed infant's organs could be harvested as soon as the diagnosis was made (as in brain-death). Some ethicists opposed this, fearing a "slippery slope" will be created to justify the use of other damaged or deformed infants for this purpose[32]. They ignore that most always in life it is necessary to draw a line between justified and non-justified actions. It was stated at another time: "if society wants to adopt a policy of sacrificing living patients for their organs, it seems very strange - and a very bad precedent - to start with the most vulnerable patients".[33] These last sentiments were not claimed to reflect any omniscient ethical principle, and their *a priori* logic is not convincing.

In October 1987 a Canadian anencephalic infant was put on a respirator and kept on it until the brain stem failed 48 hours later, diagnosed by the infant failing to breath on its own after being off the respirator for 3 minutes, having been tested for this every 6 hours, and then pronounced brain-dead. The infant, returned to the respirator, was flown to the U.S. and its heart transplanted to another infant, said to have been the youngest heart recipient at that time. This case was met with considerable criticism by the bioethical community[34]. One stated: "calling [anencephalics] dead wouldn't make them stop breathing...[and] we don't usually bury breathing people." The same ethicist in another interview[35] worried that an anencephalic child on a respirator could be shipped from center to center seeking a viable recipient if the intended one died: "Are we going to ship this little body around to 10 states? or 20 states? You might transform a human being...into nothing more than a portable organ farm." Such were an academic ethicist's contribution to the problem, in the public press.

Ethicists feared that widening the definition of brain-death to include all anencephalic babies might be applied to children and adults who are brain damaged, suggesting the specter of human organ farms[36]. "Even suggesting such a change...would cause the public to lose confidence in the transplant system and envision instead a network of greedy doctors seeking a ready supply of organs." These pontifications in the public press sound more like their own prejudices than rational analyses, and are other examples of excessive "slippery slope" reasoning. More often parents of anencephalic infants have stated they received surcease from their grief with the knowledge that their deformed infant would be of benefit to others.

A program to solve the problem was initiated at a center that had specialized in infant heart transplant (Loma Linda Hospital) and consisted of placing the anencephalic infant on a respirator at birth, administering analgesics to prevent pain (on the far-fetched suggestion that the anencephalic infant could be sentient), as well as antibiotics and sustenance. The respirator then was removed every six hours and if the child fails to breath on its own for three minutes, it would be declared brain-dead. The anencephalic baby was to be maintained for seven days and if not brain-dead in this period, life-support was discontinued and the anencephalic abandoned as a donor and allowed to die naturally. This seven-day limit was to dampen the criticism of those who objected to this program in any form. This program was suspended after 12 anencephalic babies were maintained according to the guidelines with only one of them meeting the brain-dead criteria - but no recipient could be found for even this one donor-anencephalic's heart, liver or lungs[37].

Some bioethicists contended that this program was on shaky ethical ground by "keeping one patient alive solely for the benefit of another" [38]. Program officials maintained that the shortage of small organs was severe enough to merit confronting the ethical challenge. It is a fact that most anencephalic infants born alive ceased to respire in the first 24 hours and very few survived for up to seven days. As for the determination of death in anencephalics, doctors generally agreed that death is signified by the absence of spontaneous respiration[39].

A discussion on the effect of the suspension of the Loma Linda program for preserving anencephalics for organ transplant had medical ethicists opposed in their views[40]. Some hoped the moratorium would be permanent, while others feared it would lead to the removal of protection of anencephalics as a source for organ transplant. One oft-quoted medical ethicist's contribution was that the episode (failure of the Loma Linda program) demonstrated the need for systematic discussion of bioethical issues.

A final issue was that there was still insufficient data, by 1988, as to the value of organ transplants to infants and very young children or the long term value of organs from anencephalic infants. There had been only nine heart transplants and four kidney transplants in this very young age group and all were relatively recent, so the long term prognosis was not yet established. A German team reported[41] three cases of transplanted kidneys from anencephalic infants (harvested immediately upon birth) to two children (4 and 11 years of age) and one 25 year old adult. The four year old child had normal kidney function and was doing well at one year and 10 months after transplant. The 11 and 25 year old patients had several bouts of rejection which were overcome, and both were doing well on reduced kidney function at one year and 10 months and two and a half years, respectively. The German doctors believed that important considerations should be that parents make up their minds freely and under no duress as to the donation of the organs of their anencephalic infants, and no remuneration be offered, or given.

From an utilitarian point of view there is every justification to use organs from hopeless anencephalic infants to preserve the lives of many other viable infants. The ethical objections to this practice can only be sophistries resulting from fundamentalist convictions of one or another derivation.

In 1984 a 15 day old infant (Baby Fae) with a cardiac deformity that was sure to prove fatal had the heart of a baboon transplanted into her. The age of the baboon was somewhere between 4 and 12 months old and was used because a compatible human heart was not available. Baby Fae died 20 days after operation but the cause of death was not entirely clear. The heart was not rejected in the usual sense, but there was evidence of abnormal collections of red blood cells throughout the heart, and the blood vessels of the liver, lungs and kidneys of the infant also were "clogged" with clumps of red cells.

The previous four efforts to replace failing human hearts with that of apes all failed. Doctor Christian Barnard, the first surgeon ever to do a human heart transplant, was reported to have said in 1977[42] after abandoning the effort to use primate hearts as transplants in humans: "not because I'm so convinced I'm on the wrong track, but I got emotionally involved with the chimp." Was this not an important insight into this surgeon's mind, and his potential for beneficence? It also was testimony to how close chimpanzees are to humans but, of course, all pet animals can arouse compassion (see Chapter Seven, animal-rights).

One year after the use of a baboon heart for transplant into Baby Fae, the Journal of the American Medical Association published two editorials on it[43,44]. The gist of the editorials was that the surgeon of Baby Fae underestimated the immunological difficulties with xenografts, and that it was unwarranted to continue the effort to use animal hearts for transplantation at that time. Baboons were too far from humans genetically to hope that the immunological rejection of their hearts could be overcome. Chimpanzees and gorillas, being genetically closer to humans, would be better candidates for this purpose but they cannot be bred in large numbers. It was suggested also that the surgeon had not pursued a human heart with sufficient diligence before proceeding to using the baboon's heart, and that the prospects of success with the xenograft were overstated in the consent form.

A bioethicist, stimulated by the Baby Fae case, reviewed the problem of xenografts and concluded that the need for donor organs was such that "it was ethically defensible to allow research in xenografting to proceed"[45]. He observed that many could object to the increase in the killing of animals entailed in xenografting, but he justified it because there was no good alternative. He did concede, for xenografting to remain ethical, all possible other alternatives must be pursued diligently. He emphasized that the vulnerability of human subjects who might be asked to serve in the future for xenograft trials was so high, that unusual efforts of researchers and review boards to respect their autonomy, rights, and dignity were required. Despite the sanctioning of xenografting by a non-physician ethicist, animal-rightists, nevertheless, asserted it was an expression of speciesism.

The Baby Fae case created such publicity for the medical center where she had been treated that, despite the moratorium on any further animal to human organ transplants, a small but significant number of infant hearts became available to it for transplantation. In a two year period, 11 human heart transplants were done in infants and 8 survived, four for more than a year at the time of the report[46]. Nevertheless 13 infants with defective hearts died at that center in that period of time before a human donor heart could be found for them. Consequently the surgeon was hopeful he would receive permission to continue his efforts to establish xenografts as an acceptable alternate to human donors. He was not asking his institutional review board for permission to do so as yet, because the procedure would be "just too visible". He was continuing research in the field using monkeys and baboons. Xenograft research also was being pursued at Columbia University, in Germany and in South Africa.

A still later report from the Loma Linda Hospital, in January 1990, stated that they had done 62 heart transplants in infants, averaging one every two weeks and almost all within the first month of life. Forty-eight of these babies survived and were still alive at 3 to 4 years of age. The cost of the procedures averaged $120,000 each, the postoperative care required was rigorous and the quality of life of these babies still needed definition at the time of the report. Apparently, most of the donors were anencephalic infants, but how this was arranged was not spelled out[47].

Transplantation of the heart together with both lungs were being increasingly performed for almost a decade, despite the severe limitation of donors. By June of 1987 one transplant center in the U.S. had performed 52 heart-lung transplants and an English center in Cambridge had done 27[48]. Transplantation had been successful for pulmonary vascular and other chronic lung diseases, and, in Cambridge, in prolonging the life of patients with cystic fibrosis. A newer procedure, single or double lung transplant without the heart, had been done successfully in Canada. By early 1988 11 patients had single lung transplants by the Canadian surgeons who then did the first successful double lung transplant in 1987.

Liver transplantation had been carried out for over 20 years, and in the institution which pioneered the procedure 300 such operations were being done each year by 1986[49]. By 1988 there were 45 centers in the U.S. doing liver transplants and they had done a total of 924 transplants by 1986. In the year 1989 alone, 2,000 people got new livers in the U.S., but, because of the shortage of livers for donation, there were still 8,000 remaining on the waiting list. In Europe there were 32 centers for liver transplantation, and they had done 1,218 transplants by 1987, most since 1983 and 450 in 1986 (130 in Britain that year)[50]. In this total European group the survival rate at one year was 44% and at two years 41%, and was improving as their experience grew. In the leading American center the immediate survival rate was said to be 80% and this included several patients over 60 years of age, the oldest being 76. These latter patients had caused considerable comment as to whether it was ethical to deprive younger patients of donor livers in view of the length of the waiting list at all times.

Following the lead of Canada, the U.S. Government in March 1990 said that it would pay for liver transplants for people 18 years and older who were beneficiaries of the Federal Medicare and Medicaid programs. The HHS Secretary believed this would save money by lowering the costs of treating patients with advanced liver disease. This Federal decision was thought likely to influence private insurance plans.

Another issue was whether alcoholic patients with failing livers due to cirrhosis should be considered for transplantation[51]. Most national and international medical organizations regarded alcoholism as a disease, and on this basis alcoholics should receive equal access to donor organs. Many people, for puritanical reasons, view alcoholism as a vice and not a disease and object to the concept of spending public funds to give new livers to alcoholics. Alcoholism, moreover, is an indication that most such patients would be poor candidates for transplantation because of not being able to comply with the rigorous post-operative regime. It was suggested that alcoholic patients be abstemious for at least six months before being considered for transplantation; but this requirement would result in many alcoholics, with failing livers, dying while proving themselves.

In June 1983 the National Institutes of Health convened a "consensus development panel" consisting of thirteen transplant experts. They concluded that liver transplantation may be considered for alcoholic patients in whom evidence of progressive liver failure develops despite medical treatment and abstinence from alcohol. It was suggested that treatment for alcoholism itself might be effective in the post-transplant period to improve the abstemiousness and compliance of alcoholics. Like so many other moral dilemmas, and in accord with evolutionary (and consequentialist) ethics, the solution has to await the accumulation of sufficient data. In fact, already late in 1988, a report of the largest series of transplantations in patients with failed livers because of alcoholism supported their being treated no differently than patients with failed livers from any other cause[52]. Their prognosis after transplantation was as good, and only 2 of 35 patients (5.7%) surviving at least six months resumed drinking. In 1988, alcoholic cirrhosis accounted for 138 of the 1,680 liver transplants done in that year, and the figures could be slightly higher because the diagnosis sometimes could be disguised by calling it cryptogenic cirrhosis or cirrhosis of unknown origin.

Pancreatic transplantation for insulin dependent young diabetics had been carried out since 1966, and three-quarters of the more than 1,000 operations since then had been done in the 4 years from 1983 to 1987[53]. The survival rates were steadily rising and by 1988 the graft was functioning at one year in 42% of cases, and the patient survival was 79% at one year. If transplants were done before uremia was present in the diabetic patient, at one year the graft survival was greater than 50% and patients were alive 92% of the time. Technically, it still had to be determined if the trade-off of the insulin treatment of diabetes for life-long immunosupression was worth it. A proper randomized trial was necessary to settle this issue, comparing pancreas transplantation with conventional medical treatment. It was not yet clear in 1988 that pancreas transplantation for treatment of diabetes was justified[54]. A report in 1990 on the effect of pancreatic transplantation upon the neuropathies of 61 patients with insulin dependent (type 1) diabetes did show it was favorable, and the good effect persisted throughout the follow-up period of as long as 42 months[55].

Many insulin-dependent diabetics developed kidney failure, and in the short term they did nearly as well after renal transplantation as did non-diabetic patients with end-stage kidney disease. Nevertheless, there was good reason for concern that accelerated diabetic glomerulosclerosis might develop in the kidney graft. Many surgeons saw combining pancreatic with kidney transplantation as a logical way to protect the renal graft. The results of such combined operations were constantly improving: of 714 operations done from 1982 up to 1989, the patient survival rate was 77%, and 54% were freed from dependence on insulin at one year[56].

Despite these impressive statistics an expert observer commented that since insulin-dependent diabetes was becoming more common, especially in children who have the worst prognosis, the future for pancreatic transplantations was questionable[57]. Not only would insulin-dependent diabetes become a very expensive disease, but there would be a severe lack of donor organs. He recommended added research efforts to find the cause of the disease so as to prevent it; and to learn to grow pancreatic islet cells and thus

overcome the lack of donors. In his view, even learning
cells would be an unsatisfactory solution unless the im
of such cells could be reduced so as to avoid the nee
anti-rejection treatment.

Transplantation of bone marrow does not present the ethical
problems of organ or fetal tissue transplantation. The donors are
alive and only a portion of their marrow need be taken (3 to 5%),
which is regenerated in several weeks. Moreover, still in 1989, the
donor was most often a close relative (usually a sibling) of the
recipient. Even with a sibling the problem of immunologic sensitivity
to the donor marrow remains. Therefore, many local registries, and
a National Bone Marrow Donor Registry, have been established for
those recipients in need of an immunogenetically compatible stranger
to donate marrow to them[58]. Marrow transplantations are helpful in
treating patients with leukemia and those with aplastic anemia.

On average, it is necessary to check 15,000 to 20,000 people to
find one whose tissue type matches that of a patient needing a bone
marrow transplant. It is a fact that matches are more easily obtained
between a patient and members of their own population group - that
is by race or ethnic origin. Unfortunately, as of 1989, the funding of
the National Registry was not sufficient to diversify the listings in that
manner, or to increase the donors registered to adequate levels, so
as to reduce sufficiently the odds against minority patients needing a
marrow transplant matching with donors, to make the Registry really
useful for them.

It was estimated that there were about 11,000 patients who
would benefit from bone marrow transplantation and only 3,000 were
done in 1987. The National Registry hoped to find 100,000
volunteers, but by early 1988 they had found only 15,000 potential
donors. It was projected that at least 500,000 volunteers were
necessary to supply the number of patients in 1988 that were in need
of compatible marrow. The number of responders volunteering to
donate their marrow were labeled as disappointing, but an alternative
view could be that the number willing was evidence for the innateness
of altruism. This was true especially because the volunteers were
being asked to participate in a strange procedure that was invasive
of their bodies, and the solicitation efforts had been relatively modest.
The National Marrow Donor Registry was established by a $3.5

million grant from the Navy. Each bone marrow transplant was estimated to cost $100,000, mostly for the prolonged post-transplant care in a special antiseptic isolation facility necessary for each recipient.

The transplantation of bone was gathering momentum 1989. Donors (from cadavers) were necessary to replace the large quantities of bone that are removed, as in the effort to cure patients with single, primary bone tumors. Bone transplants are most spectacular, of course, when a joint is included in the bone removal. In the transplantation of bone and ligaments, rejection is not a problem, but the donor and recipient must be closely matched for size. It was estimated that 25,000 patients per year in the U.S. receive donor bone tissue, although transplantation of bone including a joint had been rarely done and still was considered experimental.

By 1989, reports of efforts to replace multiple abdominal organs were appearing. This entailed replacement of the liver, pancreas, stomach and intestines and the first cases were those of small children who had their viscera compromised, either accidentally or by disease[59,60]. Multiple visceral organ transplants subsequently were reported in 13 adults near death from hepatic, pancreatic, or duodenal cancer with 11 survivals[61].

While the surgical skill and fortitude of the surgeons were admired, the carrying out of these procedures was criticized as being premature[62]. Resort to the principle of "desperate remedies for desperate situations" without suitable research preparation (specifically, to try the procedure first on animals) or without consideration of the enormous sums of money involved were presented as the objections. The latter objection probably was valid in a period of national economic stress and the failure to deliver even ordinary medical care to a large segment of the population. However, the early reports on multiple visceral transplants can be regarded as research efforts, ethically more defensible by being done on terminally ill humans (with the informed consent of the patients and/or their families) than on healthy animals.

The use of fetal tissue for transplants had been experimented with for decades but recent events promised to bring it to the forefront of public, as well as medical, discussion. Fetal brain tissue possibly can produce transmitter amines and/or induce production of such materials by a host brain, offering the promise of treatment for neurological diseases, and Parkinsonism in particular.

Several patients with Parkinsonism - in Mexico, Cuba, Sweden and England - by early 1988 had had fetal brain tissue (substantia nigra) transplanted to them. Some were reported to have promising results shortly after operation. The results in the two Swedish patients, the best observed ones, were disappointing and the general mood of specialists in the field was one of caution, if not outright skepticism[63]. Nevertheless, the careful, but unrewarding, initial Swedish clinical experiments on fetal neural transplants in Parkinsonian patients did suggest technical improvements that offered hope for success[64]. In fact, by early 1990, distinct success in obtaining a viable graft and an unquestionably clinically improved patient was reported[65].

Experiments with fetal tissue for transplantation in the treatment of diabetes, to induce bone marrow production (as in the treatment of radiation induced anemia) and to repair damaged nerves were also under way. Fetal liver transplantations had been tried in the treatment in a small number with patients of other metabolic and genetic disorders (thalassemia, Gaucher's disease and Fabry's disease) with some beneficial results.

Fetal tissue has the advantage of inducing less immunological response than adult tissues, and there is promise of fetal tissue being cultured in the laboratory. The latter would make large amounts of various kinds of cells from one fetus available to multiple recipients. Culturing cells creates the possibility of genetically engineering them so they would not be rejected.

Human fetal tissue, also, was being used in AIDS research. Late in 1988 transplants of such tissue were being done only to immune-deficient mice, who then were susceptible to, and could be infected with, HIV. Such animal models were more available and less expensive than chimpanzees to study drugs to treat, and create vaccines for, HIV infected people. Also, mice for such experimental purposes were presumably less objectionable than chimpanzees to animal rightists (if not to anti-abortionists, who objected to any use of human fetal tissue). Previously, the chimpanzee was the only "animal" susceptible to infection with HIV.

The human tissue was obtained from aborted fetuses (8 to 12 weeks of age) and this fact alone was sufficient to produce the opposition of pro-life, anti-abortion groups. Others said that abortion was a distressing and negative event under any circumstance, and the chance for it to have a positive aspect should be welcomed. It was this positive aspect that the anti-abortionists disliked the most. They, and others, feared that women will become pregnant for the purpose of aborting and supplying fetal tissue for a beloved relative, or for profit.

Another objection was that the fetuses may not be dead, by some definitions, when their tissues were taken for transplantation. It was agreed that the neural tissue used for transplantation needed to be "living" cells and not dead ones, but some, especially anti-abortionists, were not satisfied that pre-viable fetuses were equivalent to dead ones. That pre-viable fetuses were not technically dead had aroused the opposition of an "activist" who previously had gained attention by his most visible antagonism to genetic engineering[66]. He found the transplant of these tissues distasteful anyway, because it "...is an aging population that entertains the prospect of living off the life-blood of the next generation." He wanted the death of even pre-viable fetuses to be established by electrocardiography, electroencephalography or the confirmation of the cessation of circulatory and respiratory systems by two independent physicians. It should be clear the tissue used in transplantation had been from miscarriages, and abortions done long before the time of viability. The participation of professional activists, and the above quoted one in particular, in these scientific debates added poignancy to the previously discussed role of "fundamentalists" in moral dilemmas.

An oft-quoted ethicist was afraid of commercialization of fetal tissues: "although we've banned the sale of human organs, there are markets in renewable body tissues, like blood, bone marrow and sperm.... I think the commercialization - or commodification - of the body is a bad idea in a society that has a hard time keeping the commercial aspects of life in check in other areas."[67] In a later interview he is quoted as saying that only a few major medical centers should conduct brain-cell transplants because: "Brain transplants is an environment in which charlatans, quacks and rip-off artists can flourish,"[68] Nonetheless, one commercial company reported it was culturing fetal tissue to grow pancreas and neural cells in the expectation of selling the cells, after a few years of investigating their potential. They expected to create enough cells from the tissue of one fetus to treat many people, a prospect the company believed would prevent women ever conceiving just for the purpose of getting fetal tissue.

Other ethicists asked questions without providing answers, satisfied with only the raising of issues[69]. Some questions appear muddled (or foolish) to a neurosurgeon: "Is brain tissue uniquely identified with a particular individual? Do we violate an important interpersonal barrier if we transplant brain tissue from one individual to another, even for a laudable goal as treating Parkinson's disease?" - the answers being very obvious "no's". They implied slippery-slope reasoning was fallacious, but, nevertheless, used it: "This argument is valid and relevant, but neither more nor less compelling here than is the slippery-slope reasoning with regard to issues such as permissibility of abortion (leading to infanticide) or withdrawal of life- sustaining treatment (leading to euthanasia)." Finally, the question is raised as to whether the mother need give consent for the use of the tissue from her pre-viable aborted fetus as a transplant. Or should such tissue be regarded as discarded and used as seen fit by doctors? It is concluded by one ethicist that the mother's consent should be obtained out of respect for her feelings, not because it is necessary[70]. In March 1988 an Assistant Secretary for Health barred the National Institutes of Health from doing experiments in transplanting fetal tissue from elective abortions until the ethical issues were further studied[71]. The directive asked the director of N.I.H. to appoint an advisory committee to study the use of fetal tissue not only from elective abortions but also from miscarriages and stillbirths as well. While scientists supported by government funds were barred from research on living fetuses, research on untransplanted fetal tissues (from spontaneous abortions or stillbirths) that had been funded (federally and privately) for years was unaffected. Ethicists were divided on the issue. One ethicist whose remarks cited above could be construed as obstructionist, on this particular matter was quoted as pointing out how many patients could be helped by the transplantation of fetal tissues.

In September 1988 the above advisory committee concluded (in a 18 to 0 vote, with 3 abstentions) that it was acceptable to use human fetal tissue obtained from legal abortions for research and therapy. The committee made clear they were taking no position on the morality of abortion in making its recommendation. It was their opinion that tissue from aborted fetuses, when it was available, was like other cadaver tissue that would be disposed of and could be used for research and possible treatment (that is transplantation). The testimony against the conclusion of this committee had been presented by Roman Catholic and anti-abortion organizations.

A final report in December 1988 stated, after weighing concerns over abortion against concerns for medical research that could improve the lot of thousands of Americans, that research, including transplantation of fetal tissue, must go forward[72]. The safeguards advocated for the research were: a flat prohibition on the sale of fetuses from abortions; procedures for isolating a woman's decision to have an abortion from any subsequent consent to allow the use of her fetus' tissue in transplantation research; and policies for continuous oversight of federally funded fetal research to insure that these ethical considerations were being observed. Despite the latter statements, of the 21 panel members four, who deeply believe abortion to be immoral, voted against the report. One professor of theology believes abortion to be so abhorrent that he likened fetal researchers to Nazi doctors who experimented on live humans! A professor of medical ethics countered the position of the anti-abortion panelists by citing what ethicists know as the universal moral code. "The universal moral code is based on rationality.... When there is no agreement, we reach decisions by consensus."

This final report was sent to the office of the Assistant Secretary of Health early in 1989, but eight months later there still was no indication that its recommendations would be accepted. The journal Science reported that health officials were pessimistic that the White House climate would be receptive to supporting research that was opposed by the anti-abortion movement. This prediction was confirmed when the Bush Administration announced on November 1, 1989, through the Assistant Secretary for Health in the Department of Health and Human Services, who himself was an anti-abortionist, that the ban on federal financing of research using transplanted fetal tissue would be extended indefinitely. The Assistant Secretary said his decision to extend the ban was a "matter of heart and of mind as well". He said the research pits the rights of fetuses against those of patients who would be helped by it, so he felt obliged to come down on the side of the fetuses[73].

Anti-abortionists, encouraged by the Administration's position against research on fetal tissue for transplantation, hoped to have the ban extended against the federal financing for all fetal research. They were aided in this effort by statements of some doctors and some ethicists who favored the use of fetal tissues in research, but who said they were uneasy about the way some groups obtained and distributed the tissue[74]. These critics were concerned that many abortion clinics did not obtain the permission of the women to have their fetal tissue used for research. Also they feared that some doctors altered the abortion procedure, prolonging it at increased risk to the women, in order to get better fetal tissue samples. While it was alleged some clinics and individuals were profiting from the sale of fetal tissue, it was not denied that many, including the largest suppliers of fetal tissues, distributed the tissues without profit. Nevertheless, one ethicist, frequently quoted by the New York Times and purportedly in favor of fetal research, stated: "This sleazy, scummy world of fetal tissue procurement cries out for Federal regulation." He went on to opine that the only ethically acceptable way to get informed consent from women is to ask for it after the abortion, not before. "The basic premise is that you should keep out of it until the abortion is over. You want to be sure there is no cutting of corners, no risk to the mother, no encouragement to have an abortion."

To the contrary, the Thatcher Government accepted a report of a special review committee (The Polkinghorne Report), issued on July 26, 1989, that the use of fetal tissue for research could be separated from the issue of abortion and that investigation on the uses of fetal tissue could proceed. The Committee, nevertheless, said that consent should be given by the mother separately to the abortion and then subsequently for the use of the tissue from the aborted fetus, with no direct contact permitted between abortion clinics and the institutions using the tissue for research. To avoid the possibility of "personality transfer" between fetus and the recipient of brain tissue, the report recommended that, in the case of nervous tissue: "only isolated neurones or fragments of tissue should be used for transplantation." A government-backed organization was to be set up to collect the fetal tissue and distribute it to research teams. This would create a buffer between those supplying the tissue and those using it so that researchers would be prevented from pressuring women to abort for the purposes of science. They recommended that all proposals for the use of fetal tissue should continue to be approved by local ethics committees and all guidance on the use of fetuses, and fetal tissue, should be based on ethical principles embodied in a code of practice rather than legislation[75].

It was not thought this action of the conservative government of Margaret Thatcher, favoring the interests of the scientific community over the moral views of the right-to-lifers, would influence the Bush Administration to allow fetal transplantation research to be federally funded.

Transplantation is done in most countries of the world, the practice varying, roughly, according to the economic resources of a nation. Japan, whose gross national product in 1989 was the second greatest in the world and whose innovative abilities no longer could be doubted, was an anomaly in not utilizing organ transplantation at all. The one organ transplanted, a heart in 1968, resulted in the surgeon being subjected to six years of litigation before the prosecution dropped it. Apparently there was a national aversion to the practice based on several considerations. The heart was considered as the repository of the soul by many, and therefore the concept of brain-death was not acceptable to them. Secondly, there was an aversion among many of the Japanese to any mutilation of the body after death even though cremation was widely accepted. Lastly, it was said that the notion of the patient as a medical consumer was poorly developed and it was feared that over-zealous and imperious transplant physicians would abuse the rights of patients[76].

Corneas and kidneys, which do not require cadaver donors to have a maintained intact circulation, have been transplanted in Japan for years. Kidneys are still viable grafts from cadavers for 90 minutes after the heart has stopped. However, in Japan only about 600 kidney transplants have been done yearly (81,000 patients on dialysis) and in 1988 456 kidneys came from live donors (usually a parent), the rest from indubitable corpses. In the U.S., brain-dead donors whose hearts were still beating accounted for 80% of the kidneys transplanted. The Japan Medical Association decided to accept brain-death as a valid definition of death in early 1988. Since no legislation is required to permit transplantation and the majority of the public supports it, it is anticipated that gradually it will become acceptable medical practice.

2. Discussion

A review of the literature and a survey of media reports up to 1989 gave the general impression that the ethical dilemmas associated with transplantation of organs and tissues were not very troublesome. This conclusion, undoubtedly, was due to this technique prolonging life and improving its quality for so many (particularly, for instance, the recipients of corneal transplants). The chief problems that were being encountered were associated with a shortage of donor organs and the rationing of those that were available.

The solutions to these problems were not aided by off-the-cuff pronouncements in the news media by presumed experts. For instance, in California late in April 1988 a 19 year old unidentified man was pronounced brain-dead and his heart transplanted after a 24-hour police attempt to identify the victim failed[77]. This was in conformance with the guidelines set up by state's Uniform Anatomical Gift Act, which require a 24-hour police search for identification and relatives, and questioning of visitors to the donor. Several oft-quoted medical ethicists viewed this case with consternation: "To take vital organs out of someone who is not identified is really incredible." Another ethicist stated: "It seems to me this does not sit well with the way we are doing things. It seems to me that this is a variation from practice in this country where someone generally has to agree to the donation." Still another ethicist, a member of the National Task Force on Organ Transplantation, did support the procedure though, perhaps, with some hesitation: "I'm not sure there's any serious abuse if they're complying with applicable law. First of all we're dealing with someone who is dead, it's not like they're harming the person. Those bodies are either going to get cremated or buried."

As another example, the use of anencephalic babies as organ donors does receive opposition from pro-life activists, but this opposition can be interpreted as relatively muted. The very wide discussion by contemporary bioethicists, not opposed perhaps - but emphasizing the "moral" problems - is frightening to present day investigators (certainly as compared with 20 years ago). Those ethicists actually opposed to the use of anencephalic babies for organ donation use fallacious "slippery-slope" reasoning: that if it is condoned, other infants with malformations and eventually adults in a permanently vegetative state will be used as organ donors[78]. The actual bases for their opposition are that vital organs should not be taken from the living for the benefit of others, and they are not satisfied with the proposed criterion for brain-death in anencephalics. Indeed one of these ethicists is dissatisfied with brain-death as the criterion for death of an individual. Similarly, the promising applications of fetal tissues for transplantation are hindered by the expression of premature fears of commercialization in their use and the recommendation that research in this field be restricted "to only a few major centers". This would preclude the advantage that our free enterprise medical system does have to offer and the very real contributions that could come from sources not included in "major medical centers", and/or from the entrepreneurial firms in this field. There are many problems, other than ethical ones, that need to be solved, such as the long term usefulness of infant transplantation and the actual value of fetal tissues and anencephalic organs. As mentioned above, the use of fetal tissues for transplantation is presently "on hold" in the U.S., therefore, it would seem the answers to many of these questions will come from abroad.

It is believed by many, if not a majority of observers, that it may be necessary to presume organs are donated upon the death of a suitable donor, unless specifically denied by the patient when alive, or by the family after death. Presently, some bioethicists assert this is a breach of autonomy and therefore would be resented by the public. An evolutionary ethical approach would be to await the public response and not presuppose it. Evolutionary ethicists, if there are any in the medical field, would assume that if the general perception would be that the presumption-of-donation is in the best interests of the community, it will be made legal and, moreover, that it will come about. Therefore, for persons who have become authoritative figures in bio-ethics to reject presumption-of-donation on an *a priori* basis only delay a decision which will be come upon in a naturally evolved manner.

3. Rationing

The suggestion that transplantation should be abandoned because of its costs and that such moneys would be better invested elsewhere in the medical care system is not a valid one. In a *laissez-faire* medical care system, such as exists for the most part in the U.S., it hardly is appropriate to arbitrarily restrict one segment of it in favor of another. Other, possibly more rational, systems of medical care find the costs of transplantations not to be exorbitant, and the question of who pays for it not to be a problem.

Transplantation of organs and tissues is the technical advance beyond all others that raises the question of the rationing of medical care. In the first place the limited availability of donors immediately raises the question of how to ration those organs that do become available. Secondly, new techniques in medical care, because of their expensiveness, have already been widely discussed in terms of need to ration their availability. Transplantations are, relatively, more recent medical techniques and very expensive, therefore it is normal for them to stimulate discussion on their cost-effectiveness.

As an example, in 1987 the legislature of the state of Oregon, by an overwhelming majority, approved a budget that discontinued the payment for transplantations by Medicaid (which pays for health care of the poor). Their reasoning was that the anticipated 34 poor patients needing heart, liver, bone marrow or pancreas transplants would cost $2.2 million, and this amount would be better spent extending health care to 1,500 indigent patients not covered previously[79]. They particularly had in mind destitute pregnant women and children not covered by Medicaid.

Shortly thereafter a severe public reaction was provoked when a child was denied a marrow transplant to treat his acute lymphatic leukemia, and he subsequently died. Concern grew that transplants were being denied to poor persons whose lives could be saved, even though no such reaction had occurred when two indigent adults had been refused transplants. Others complained that no such visibility was being extended to those denied basic medical care. The self-serving purpose of the transplant surgeons was pointed out, when such surgeons argued that the state should pay for transplants required by the indigent.

Commentators[79] asked: why were transplants chosen to be eliminated when there are so many health-care programs competing for state support? They then cited several reasons as answers: transplants are easily identifiable large scale expenses; relatively few people are benefited; and they are new, therefore easier to displace than older, more established treatments. These observers believed the action of the Oregon legislature was an attempt to allocate limited resources in a deliberate and rational manner. The public did not support their legislature's decision because acute care is always more visible than the need for preventive care (the transplant money in large measure went to preventive care for mothers and children). Finally. it was suggested that, if organ transplantation is an important therapy, it was up to physicians to suggest what treatments are less useful and could be eliminated to make room for it.

The physician-legislator who had sponsored the above Oregon rationing plan for the poor subsequently consulted The Bioethics Consulting Group which, previously, primarily had been helping medical institutions to set-up ethics committees[80]. The head of this group, a Jesuit priest-ethicist, and the physician-state senator, together with interested others, formed "The Oregon Medicaid Priority-Setting Project". It was based on an utilitarian perspective, as explained by the ethicist, of advancing the health of the population as a whole as opposed to the then current practice of doing everything for each individual patient until the money ran out, with everybody thereafter getting nothing. They formed four focus groups of volunteers, each representing a Medicaid population segment (obstetrics and gynecology, pediatric, adult, geriatric). The focus groups consisted of physicians, nurses, social workers, and health and social service program administrators. Priorities were set for all therapies and each group elected a representative to meet with a lawyer, a physician and an ethicist as representatives of Medicaid recipients. The latter committee melded "the four age-specific lists into one master priority list".

When the master list was publicized, it caused "a furor" and the ethicist said this was because the media, especially television, got the story wrong and gave the wrong impression as to what treatment an Oregonian would or would not receive. Actually the items on the master list were each "costed" by an actuarial firm and the legislature was to decide on packages of services that then could be managed in various ways: traditional fee-for-service (costing most); through a preferred-provider organization (costing less); a regular health maintenance organization (HMO); or "an aggressively managed" HMO. The legislature was to choose what benefits were to have what priority and how they were to be managed, when the entire health program was to be funded. Also, the approval of the U.S. Congress would be necessary before the new program could go into effect, since state Medicaid funds are matching ones to those from the National Government. It should be clear this plan was only to ration care for the poor, and those poor whose medical treatment was to be paid for by the Medicaid program. The affluent and well-insured Oregonians would continue to have as much care as they desired.

Subsequently, a similar plan for the rationing of medical services for the poor was proposed for Alameda County of California. It was being sponsored by the county health director and the same Jesuit medical ethicist mentioned above. The local health-care workers were reported to have organized to resist this rationing plan since it only applied to the indigent. Their Vote-Health-Coalition stated the plan would make official the (market-place) rationing that currently was depriving the poor of the quality of medical care available to the affluent.

It will be of interest to see if these rationing plans for only the poor do become legislated. If they are, it is unlikely that they will be tolerated for long by a society that purports to believe in egalitarianism, even if it does not always behave in that manner. Moreover, the plan attempts to categorize and reduce the over 10,000 diagnoses in a standard coding book of disease states into 1,600 entities. The application of the results to the operation of the rationing plan is sure to produce intolerable inequities. If, indeed, this effort to ration medical care in Oregon fails, then the conclusion of most experienced observers, discussed below, would be reaffirmed: that successful priority rationing in such societies can only be accepted if done for all, and then by physicians who are guided by their professional ethics; moreover, rationing of medical care only can be accomplished if done quietly in the privacy of a well- functioning doctor-patient relationship - not by legislative fiat.

Nevertheless, *it is true, and must be recognized, that governments that finance access to medical care for their citizens can never afford all that could be consumed, and so rationing becomes inevitable.* All feasible methods of rationing are done either by the market-place - that is by denying access to medical care for a portion of its population as in the U.S. (the poor and uninsured, said to be 37,000,000 in 1989) - or where there is universal access to medical care, as in England and Canada, by restriction of public funding and leaving to the medical profession, and its ethics, the responsibility that justice be done at the level of individuals[81]. An additional requirement for justice to be observed in rationing is that the autonomy of the physicians be preserved, and not compromised by their being employed by corporations or other profit making entities.

As a consequence of these different methods of rationing (and the inadequacy of the U.S. procedure), meetings of the British Health Service usually discuss the small percentage of the GNP spent on health and such meetings in the U.S. have the opposite concern. U.S. medical economists decry the serious effects of the continuing rise in the costs of medical care and its deleterious effects on the general economy. They rail against the extravagant behavior of their doctors, but never identify the fundamental failing of the U.S. system: its inability to effectively ration medical care[82].

Several years ago (1982-84), when the costs of medical care were being most widely discussed, it was mentioned that cost containment through the rationing of medical care could be an issue in the Presidential campaign of 1988. Nonetheless, while intention to give greater access of the poor to medical care was expressed, rationing was never mentioned - despite concern with severe budget deficits. This was because it has become obvious, even if unspoken, that there was no feasible means in the U.S. of rationing medical care and at the same time achieve greater equality of access. To repeat, in the U.S. where the medical care delivery system is geared to respond to consumer demand, cost containment can be accomplished only by depriving the poor of access to it, and/or by reducing the quality of their care[7]. Until the medical planners in the U.S., when attempting to provide universal access and at the same time control costs, come to grips with the absolute necessity to ration medical care, all of their proposals (usually described as "incremental") will come to naught.

Containing costs by educational programs for physicians to limit the use of diagnostic tests and treatments according to cost-effectiveness soon had proven futile. Controlling treatment by second-opinion programs, too, not only proved unfruitful but, in some instances, may have added to costs. The recommendation to expand the influence of the market-place and introduce more competition into the delivery of medical care in the hope of lowering costs, so far, has only been successful in giving credence to the profit motive in an area where charitable contribution had previously been the dominate theme.

Another means of cost containment being tried in the U.S. was changing the mode of payment for health care by governmental agencies, principally Medicare. The change consisted of prospective payment according to diagnosis rather than retroactive payment for costs. This is a more subtle use of the market-place technique for rationing medical care. Medicare usually sets the pace for private and state (Medicaid) insurance plans in the introduction of changes. It was too early in 1988 to predict the final effects of this change, but costs were still escalating and many claimed there was already a diminution in the quality of care. It certainly had led to premature discharges from hospitals.

These efforts to contain costs by use of the market-place to ration medical care in the U.S. leave no role for doctors to play. It generally has been recognized, for a rationing system to be just at the level of the individual, it has to be done ultimately by physicians[83] who alone are competent to decide who gets care according to their need and its probability of being worthwhile. It is expected that doctors will be governed, and aided, in this task by the ethics of their profession.

Two ethicists, when discussing rationing medical care, raised the issue without offering a solution but seemed sure that rationing was not to be entrusted to physicians: "There is no assurance that the physician is any more fair or just than others in deciding who shall receive so crucially important a resource as health care. Do we as a society really want to give this kind of power to physicians?"[84] Presumably, expertise in a field has no bearing in the rationing of its products; and apparently physicians' ethics cannot be relied upon for rationing, despite the theme of the book, from which this quotation was taken, being an advocacy by these authors in favor of physicians' beneficence.

The medical planners and economists in the U.S., also, do not recommend using the discretion of the doctor as to who receives or does not receive care, nor do they recommend any fundamental change in the medical care delivery system that in most ways maximizes consumer demand. The English National Health System, to the contrary, is organized on the philosophy of responding to professionally defined needs (rather than to consumer demand). The British government sets the limit of expenditure on a system that is accessible to all, and relies on the doctors to allocate the funds at the level of the individual. This is possible because the British public believes in the NHS and trusts their doctors. There is no way that individuals can be told *directly* that they are not eligible for medical treatment, not by governments, not by economists[85,86], nor even by ethicists.

SUMMARY AND CONCLUSIONS TO PART TWO

The data on current bioethical problems, presented in Part Two of this book, lend support to the conclusions drawn from the theoretical considerations offered in Part One. In the first place, solutions to ethical dilemmas are seldom predictable since the variable factors comprehended are generally too numerous to be able to forecast the results of their interplay very far into the future. Secondly, ethical principles are established by what is in the best interests for the welfare of society.

The outcomes of the conflicts between individual rights and the needs of the community - i.e., as in testing for AIDS and testing for the usage of drugs, or with respect to the disabled, or in clinical investigation, or in reproduction, dying, transplantations, and the use of animals for research, while not always immediately apparent - ultimately will be determined by the needs of the community. Premature activities of extremists, in their efforts to force solutions of dilemmas, disturb the equanimity of the community, prevent orderly and proper discussion of the issues, and only delay the arrival at proper conclusions - solutions that are the most beneficial for the welfare of society. To repeat, the solutions to bioethical dilemmas will be determined by experience and experimentation, not merely by *prima facie* pronouncements nor via a *priori* reasoning in favor of individual rights. Admittedly, in 1989, it did appear, in the U.S., that many bioethical dilemmas would be resolved by judicial interpretations of constitutional rights by the courts, rather than by formulation of public policy through public discussion. However, the influence of the latter on judicial opinions could be considerable.

New innovations in medical practice contribute to the constant need for modern societies to ration medical care. That rationing be accomplished in an acceptable, as well as in a just manner, demands that it be done by physicians, and within the framework of a strong doctor-patient relationship. Examination of the doctor-patient relationship suggests that its restoration and strengthening in the U.S. requires that doctor-beneficence once more be recognized as a cardinal principle of medical ethics, and so rewarded. All this only can be achieved if there be a radical change in the U.S. medical-care delivery system.

PART ONE

INTRODUCTION

[1]   R.J. Richards, *Darwin and the Emergence of Evolutionary Theories of Mind and Behavior*, 1987, University of Chicago Press, Chicago.

[2]   R. Boyd and P.J. Richerson, *Culture and the Evolutionary Process*, 1985, University of Chicago Press, Chicago.

[3]   A noted anthropologist recently expressed a similar formulation for the origin of culture: "This is the ultimate product of that evolutionary development that led to the emergence of man - that genetic programing for behavior-that-is-not-genetically-programmed." W. Goldschmidt, *The Human Career. The Self in the Symbolic World*, 1990, Basil Blackwell, Cambridge, Mass, p. 80.

[4]   L.A. White, *The Evolution of Culture*, 1959, McGraw-Hill Book Co., New York.

[5]   "The optimality assumption states that the phenotype(s) characterizing the best adapted individuals possible in a population comes to dominate that population." This is quoted from J.M. Emlen, "Evolutionary ecology and the optimality assumption." In: *The Latest of the Best: Essays on Evolution and Optimality*, Ed. by J. Dupre, 1987, The MIT Press, Cambridge, Massachusetts, p. 164.

[6]   The principal contenders have been E. O. Wilson and his sociobiologic supporters on one side and R. C. Lewontin, S. Rose and L. J. Kamin (*Not in Our Genes*, 1984, Pantheon Books) and others on the opposite side. If the dual inheritance theory for biology and culture as presented by Boyd and Richerson proves to be acceptable, it could be the basis for resolution of this conflict. This is well explained by J. Dupre in: *The Latest of the Best: Essays on Evolution and Optimality*, 1987, MIT Press, Cambridge, Massachusetts, p. 346.

[7]   A good example are the Cook Islanders: they are a population of less than 18,000 and their islands lie in a void of water, with the nearest large society being New Zealand, 2000 miles away. Their islands are ladened with fruit trees and surrounded by waters teeming with fish, yet the islanders walk past fruit rotting on the ground on their way to the supermarket. There they buy cans of fish, pineapple and imported fruit juice. According to *The Economist* for January 16, 1988, page 35, they did well as a subsistence economy because they had good soil and much sun and rain and they were far from invaders. They are not now self-sufficient because of their exposure to the material temptations of the modern world. Indeed, presently they have to be heavily subsidized to exist ($10 million per year and mostly by New Zealand).

[8]   J. Griffin, *Well-being. Its Meaning, Measurement and Moral Importance*, 1986, Oxford University Press, Oxford.

[9]   G. Feaver and F. Rosen (eds.), *Lives, Liberties and the Public Good*, 1987, St. Martin's Press, New York.

[10]   C. Grebogi, E. Ott, and J.A. Yorke, "Chaos, strange attractors, and fractal basin boundaries in non-linear dynamics", *Science* 1987, 238: 632-8.

[11]   R.R. Nelson and S.G. Winter, *An Evolutionary Theory of Economic Change*, 1982, Belknap/Harvard University Press, Cambridge, Mass.

[12]   R.D. Masters, *The Nature of Politics*, 1989, Yale University Press, New Haven.

[13]   E.A. Smith, "Optimization theory in anthropology: applications and critiques." In: *The Latest of the Best: Essays on Evolution and Optimality.* Ed. by J. Dupre, 1987, MIT Press, Cambridge, Mass.

[14]   D.L. Hull, *An Evolutionary Account of the Social and Conceptual Development of Science*, 1988, University of Chicago Press, Chicago.

[15]   C. Levi-Strauss, *Anthropology and Myth: Lectures 1951-82*, Translated by R. Willis, 1987, Oxford-Blackwell, Oxford.

[16]   E. Laszlo, *Evolution, The Grand Synthesis*, 1987, New Science Library\Shambhala, Boston.

[17]   L. Thomas, "A long line of cells," *The Wilson Quarterly*, 1988, XII: 86-97, p. 97.

CHAPTER 1

1   N.C. Fost, "What can a hospital ethics committee do for you?", *Contemporary Pediatrics*, 1986 (Feb.), pp. 119-128.

2   Comment, *Lancet*, 1986, I: 1016.

3   H.K. Beecher, *Experimentation in Man*, 1959, Thomas, Springfield, Illinois.

4   *The Economist* for April 26, 1986, p. 95.

5   J. Bordley and A.M. Harvey, *Two Centuries of American Medicine*, 1976, W. B. Saunders Co., Philadelphia, Pennsylvania.

6   *Institute of Medical Ethics Bull*, Supplement #5, April 1987, p. 15.

7   P.G. Quie, "Health care economics and biomedical ethics," *J Inf Dis*, 1986, 153: 385-389.

8   C.M. Culver, K.D. Clouser, B. Gerr, et al. "Basic curricular goals in medical ethics," *N Engl J Med* 1985, 312: 253-56.

9   D.F. Phillips, "Physicians, journalists, ethicists explore their adversarial, interdependent relationship," *JAMA*, 1988, 260: 751-3.

10   J. La Puma, C.B. Stocking, M.D. Silverstein, A. DiMartini, M. Seigler, "An Ethics consultation service in a teaching hospital," *JAMA*, 1988, 260: 808-11.

11   R.M. Veatch, *A Theory of Medical Ethics*, 1981, Basic Books, Inc., New York, p. 21.

12   B. Lo, "Behind closed doors. Problems and pitfalls of ethics committees," *N Eng J Med*, 1987, 317: 46-50.

13   H.T. Engelhardt, Jr., *The Foundations of Bioethics*, 1986, Oxford University Press, Inc., New York.

14   B. Williams, *Ethics and the Limits of Philosophy*, 1985, Fontana Press/Collins, London.

15   H. Himsworth, *Scientific Knowledge and Philosophic Thought*, 1986, The Johns Hopkins University Press, Baltimore.

16   G.E. Moore, *Principia Ethica*, 1903, Cambridge University Press, Cambridge.

17   A.J. Ayer, *Language, Truth and Logic*, 1936, Victor Gollantz, Ltd., London.

18   D. Hume, *Enquiries Concerning the Human Understanding and Concerning the Principles of Morals* (reprinted from the 1977 edition

and edited by L.A. Selby-Bigge), 1972, Oxford University Press, Oxford.

[19]   W.D. Ross, *The Right and the Good*, 1930, Oxford University Press, Oxford.

[20]   J. Rawls, *A Theory of Justice*, 1971, Harvard University Press, Cambridge, Mass.

[21]   J.J.C. Smart, *Utilitarianism. The Encyclopedia of Philosophy*, Paul Edwards, Editor-in-Chief, 1967, Macmillan Co. & the Free Press, New York, Vol. 8, pp. 206-12.

[22]   J.S. Mill, *Utilitarianism, Liberty, Representative Government*, Ed. by H.B. Acton. 1972, J.M. Dent & Sons, London.

[23]   A.C. Ewing, "Ethics," *Encyclopedia Britannica*, 1961 Ed.

[24]   M. Midgley, *Beast and Man*, 1980, Methuen Co., Ltd., London.

[25]   R.J. Richards, *Darwin and the Emergence of Evolutionary Theories of Mind and Behavior*, 1987, University of Chicago Press, Chicago.

[26]   C. Darwin, *The Descent of Man, and Selection in Relation to Sex*, 2 vols., 1871, Murray, London.

[27]   A.R. Wallace, "The origin of human races and the antiquity of man deduced from the theory of natural selection," *Anthropological Review*, 1864, 2: clviii - clxxxvii.

[28]   P. Kropotkin, Quoted by Richards, 25, pp. 327-30.

[29]   J. Huxley, "Evolutionary Ethics," in *Touchstones for Ethics*, 1893-1943, 1947, Harper, New York.

[30]   T. Nagel, *The View from Nowhere*, 1986, Oxford University Press, Oxford.

[31]   C. Taylor, "Philosophy and the Human Sciences," *Philosophical Papers 2*, 1985, Cambridge University Press, Cambridge, p. 21.

[32]   R. Swinburne, *The Evolution of the Soul*, 1987, Clarendon Press, Oxford.

[32A]   J.C. Eccles, *Evolution of the Brain: Creation of the Self*, 1989, Routledge, London

[33]   J.I.C. Dumond and R.M. Robertson, "Neuronal circuits: an evolutionary perspective," *Science*, 1986, 233: 849-853.

[34]   N. Eldredge and S.J. Gould, "Punctuated equilibria: an alternative to phylogenetic gradualism," In Schopf, ed., *Models in Paleobiology*, 1972, Freeman, Cooper, San Francisco.

[35]   E.O. Wilson, *On Human Nature*, 1978, Harvard University Press, Cambridge.

[36]   E.O. Wilson, *Sociobiology*, 1975, Harvard University Press, Cambridge.

[37]   P. Churchland, *Neurophilosophy: Toward a Unified Science of the Mind/Brain*, 1986, The MIT Press, Cambridge, Mass.

[38]   J. Z. Young, *Philosophy and the Brain*, 1987, Oxford University Press, Oxford and New York.

[39]   F. Hoyle and S. Wickramasinghe, *Evolution from Space: A Theory of Cosmic Creationism*, 1984, Simon and Schuster, Inc., New York.

[40]   R. Penrose, *The Emperor's New Mind: Concerning Computers, Minds and Laws of Physics*, 1989, Oxford University Press, Oxford.

[41]   M. Ruse and E.O. Wilson, "Moral philosophy as applied science," *Philosophy*, 1986, 61: 173-192.

[42]   R.C. Lewontin, S. Rose, and L.J. Kamin, *Not in Our Genes*, 1984, Pantheon Books, New York.

[43]   C. Holden, "The genetics of personality," *Science*, 1987, 237: 598-601.

[43A]   R. Plomin, "The role of inheritance in behavior," *Science*, 1990, 248: 183-8.

[44]   W. Lumsden and E.O. Wilson, *Genes, Minds and Culture*, 1981, Harvard University Press, Cambridge.

[45]   E. Soper, "Forces and dispositions in evolutionary theory," In: *Minds, Machines and Evolution*, Ed. by C. Hookway, 1984, Cambridge University Press, Cambridge.

[46]   N. Chomsky, Quoted by H. Gardner, *The Mind's New Science*, 1985, Basic Books, New York, p. 193.

[47]   R. Boyd and P.J. Richerson, *Culture and the Evolutionary Process*, 1985, University of Chicago Press, Chicago.

[48]   L.A. White, *The Evolution of Culture*, 1959, McGraw-Hill Book Co., New York.

[48A]   S.J. Gould, *Wonderful Life*, 1989, W.W. Norton & Co. Inc., New York.

[49]   R. Boyd and P.J. Richerson, "Simple models of complex phenomena: the case of cultural evolution," In *The Latest of the Best*, Ed. by J. Dupre, 1987, MIT Press, Cambridge, Massachusetts.

[50]   C. Grebogi, E. Ott, J.A. Yorke, "Chaos, strange attractors, and fractal basin boundaries in non-linear dynamics," *Science*, 1987, 238: 632-8.

[51]   F. Crick, *Of Molecules and Men*, 1966, University of Washington Press, Seattle.

[52]   J. Monad, *Chance and Necessity: An Essay on the Natural Philosophy of Modern Biology*, Translated by Austryn Wainhouse, 1971, A.A. Knopf, New York.

[53]   H. Gardner, *The Mind's New Science*, 1985, Basic Books, New York.

[54]   C. Wissler, *Man and Culture*, 1923, Thomas Y. Crowell, New York.

[55]   C. Kluckhohn, "Universal categories of culture," In *Anthropology Today*, Al Kroeber (ed.), 1953, University of Chicago Press, Chicago.

[56]   R. Gillon, "It's All Subjective": Skepticism about the possibility or use of philosophical medical ethics, *Brit Med J*, 1985, 290: 1574-75.

[57]   A.I. Hallowell, "Self, Society and Culture in Phylogenetic Perspective," In *Culture, Man's Adaptive Dimension*, MFA Montague (ed.), 1968, Oxford University Press, Oxford.

[58]   L. Kohlberg, *The Psychology of Moral Development. The Nature and Validity of Moral Stages*, 1984, Harper & Row, San Francisco, p. 282-7.

[59]   *Ibid*, pp. 224-36.

[60]   A.H. Post, Cited by P. Vinogradoff and H. Goitein, In *Comparative Jurisprudence, Encyclopedia Britannica*, 1961.

[61]   J.D. Watson, forward, In H. Himsworth *Scientific Knowledge and Philosophic Thought*, 1986, The Johns Hopkins University Press, Baltimore.

[62]   S.W. Hawking, *A Brief History of Time. From the Big Bang to Black Holes*, 1988, Bantam Books, New York, p. 174-5.

[63]   W.V.D. Quine, *From a Logical Point of View*, 1953, Harvard University Press, Cambridge, Mass.

[64]   R. Rorty, *Philosophy and the Mirror of Nature*, 1979, Princeton University Press, Princeton.

[65]   R. Scruton, "Modern philosophy and the neglect of aesthetics," *Times Literary Supplement* for June 5, 1987, pp. 504, 616-17.

[66]   S. Weinberg, *The First Three Minutes*, 1977, Andre Deutsch, London.

[67]   H.J. Morowitz, *Cosmic Joy and Local Pain: Musings of a Mystic Scientist*, 1987, Charles Scribner's Sons, New York.

[68]   New York Times, June 20, 1986, Op. Ed. page.

[69]   R.B. Redmon, *J Med Ethics*, 1985, 12(2): 77-82.

[70]   H. Shenkin, *Clinical Practice and Cost Containment*, 1986, Praeger Scientific, New York.

[71]   R.M. Veatch, *A Theory of Medical Ethics*, 1981, Basic Books, Inc., New York, p. 125.

[72]   I. Berlin, "On the Pursuit of the Ideal," Speech on the acceptance of Senator Giovanni Agnelli Prize, February 15, 1988, In *The New York Review* for March 17, 1988.

[73]   L. Thomas, "A long line of cells," *The Wilson Quarterly*, 1988, XII: 86-97, p. 97.

[74]   L.L. Emanuel and E.J. Emanuel, In reply to "Letters to the Editor," *JAMA*, 1990, 263: 1070.

CHAPTER 2

[1]   E.W. Patterson, *Jurisprudence: Men and Ideas of the Law*, 1953, The Foundation Press Inc., Brooklyn, New York.

[2]   *Ibid*, pp. 224-5.

[3]   *Ibid*, p. 33.

[4]   R. Dworkin, *Law's Empire*, 1986, Belknap Press/Harvard University Press, Cambridge, Mass.

[5]   J.S. Mill, *Utilitarianism, On Liberty, and Considerations on Representative Government*, Ed. by H.B. Acton, 1972, J.M. Dent and Sons Ltd., London, p, 56.

[6]   R.J. Vincent, *Human Rights and International Relations*, 1986, Cambridge University Press, Cambridge.

[7]   I. Shapiro, *The Evolution of Rights in Liberal Theory*, 1986, Cambridge University Press, Cambridge, p. 18.

[8]   *Ibid*, p. 5.

[9]   F. Rosen, "Bentham and Mill on Liberty and Justice," p. 130, In: *Lives, Liberties and the Public Good*, Ed. by G. Feaver and F. Rosen, 1987, St. Martin's Press, New York.

[10]   H.C. Mansfield, Jr., "Hobbes on Liberty and Executive Power," p. 27, In: *Lives, Liberties and the Public Good*, Ed. by G. Feaver and F. Rosen, 1987, St. Martin's Press, New York.

438   **REFERENCES**

[11]   A. Kuflik, "The utilitarian logic of inalienable rights," *Ethics*, 1986, 97: 75-87.

[12]   R.G. Frey (ed.), *Utility and Rights*, 1985, Oxford Press, Oxford.

[13]   L.J. MacFarlane, *The Theory and Practice of Human Rights*, 1985, Temple Smith, London.

[14]   J. Rawls, *A Theory of Justice*, 1971, Harvard University Press, Cambridge, Mass.

[15]   R. Boyd and P.J. Richerson, *Culture and the Evolutionary Process*, 1985, University of Chicago Press, Chicago.

[16]   *The Economist* for January 23, 1988, p. 9.

[17]   F. Kort, "Considerations for a biological basis of civil rights and liberties," *J Social & Biol Struct*, 1986, 9: 37-51.

[18]   J.S. Mill, *The Subjection of Women*, 1970, The M.I.T. Press, Cambridge, Mass., pp. 51-2.

[19]   *Ibid*, p. 84.

[20]   G. Piel, "Natural philosophy in the Constitution," *Science*, 1986, 233: 1056-60.

[21]   A.N. Whitehead, *Adventures of Ideas*, 1933, MacMillan, New York.

[22]   N.F. Cantor, *Medieval History. The Life and Death of a Civilization*, 1969, MacMillan, New York.

[23]   R. Scruton, *The Meaning of Conservatism*, 1980, MacMillan, London.

[24]   K. Dixon, *Freedom and Equality*, 1986, Routledge and Kegan-Paul, London.

[25]   J. Hobbes, Quoted by R.J. Vincent, *Human Rights and International Relations*, 1986, Cambridge University Press, p. 25.

[26]   J.S. Mill, *Utilitarianism, On Liberty, and Considerations on Representative Government*, Ed. by H.B. Acton, 1972, JM Dent and Sons Ltd., London, p. 115.

[27]   *Ibid*, p. 129.

[28]   *Ibid*, p. 130.

[29]   E.A. Wrigley, *Peoples, Cities and Wealth*, 1987, Blackwell, Oxford.

CHAPTER 3

[1]   "Am Col Phys Ethics Manual," *Ann Int Med*, 1984, 101: 129-137.

[2]   M. Mead, *Cultural Patterns and Technical Change*, 1955, Mentor Books, New York, p. 214.

[3]   *Harvard Magazine* for May-June 1982.

[4]   S. Muller, "The Medical School in the University," *JAMA*, 1984, 252: 1455-57.

[5]   R.L. Landau and J.M. Gustafson, "Death is Not the Enemy," *JAMA*, 1984, 252: 2458.

[6]   R.M. Veatch, "Models for Ethical Medicine in a Revolutionary Age," In *Moral Problems in Medicine*, 2nd Ed., Edited by S. Gorovitz, et al., 1983, Prentice Hall, Engelwood Cliffs, New Jersey.

[7]   *The New York Times* for September 12, 1988. Op-Ed page.

[8]   W.J. Reader, *Professional Men: The Rise of the Professional Classes in Victorian England*, 1966, Weidenfeld and Nicholson, London.

[9]   H.A. Shenkin, *Clinical Practice and Cost Containment*, 1986, Praeger Scientific, N.Y.

[10]   A.J. Barsky, "The paradox of health," *N Eng J Med*, 1988, 318: 414-8.

[11]   A. Relman, Op-Ed Page, *Wall Street Journal* for July 2, 1986.

[12]   J.C. Garnham, "Some observations on informed consent in therapeutic research," *J Med Ethics* 1975, 1: 138-45.

[13]   B.R. Cassileth, R.V. Zupkis, K. Sutton-Smith, and V. March, "Informed Consent: Why Are Its Goals Imperfectly Realized?", *N Engl J Med*, 1980, 302: 896-900.

[14]   D.J. Byrne, A. Napier, and A. Cuschieri, "How informed is signed consent?", *Brit Med J*, 1988, 296: 839-40.

[15]   P. Starr, *The Social Transformation of American Medicine*, 1982, Basic Books, New York.

[16]   E. Friedson, "Concept of a Profession," In *Medical Ethics*, Ed. by N. Abrams, and M.D. Buckner, 1983, The MIT Press, Cambridge, Mass.

[16A]   D.A. Redelmeier and A. Tversky, "Discrepancy between medical decisions for individual patients and for groups," *New Eng J Med*, 1990, 322: 1162-4.

[17]   *Medical Staff News* for September 8, 1986, p. 8.

[18]   R.C. Burchell, R.E. White, H.L. Smith, and N.F. Piland, "Physicians and the organizational evolution of medicine," *JAMA*, 1988, 260: 826-31.

[19]   H. Scovern, "Hired help. A physician's experience in a for-profit staff-model HMO," *New Eng J Med*, 1988, 319: 787-90.

[20]   R.S. Bock, "The pressure to keep prices high at a walk-in clinic," *New Eng J Med*, 1988, 319: 785-7.

[21]   R.W. Evans, "Health care technology and the inevitability of resource allocation and rationing decisions, Part I," *JAMA*, 1983, 249: 2047-53.

[22]   *Ibid*, Part II., pp. 2208-22.

[23]   U.E. Reinhardt, "The future of medical enterprise: perspectives on resource allocation in socialized markets," *J Med Educ*, 1980, 55: 311-24.

[24]   W.G. Schwartz and H.J. Aaron, "Rationing hospital care. Lessons from Britain," *N Engl J Med*, 1984, 310: 52-56.

[25]   W. Winkenwerder and J.R. Ball, "Transformation of American health care. The role of the medical profession," *N Engl J Med*, 1988, 318: 317-19.

[26]   R.H. Nicholson, *Institute of Medical Ethics Bull*, #15, June 1986, p. 6.

[27]   E.D. Pellegrino, "Toward a reconstruction of medical morality," *J Med Humanities and Bioethics* 1987, 8: 7-18.

[28]   H. Brody, "The physician-patient relationship: models and criticisms," *Theoretical Medicine*, 1987, 8: 205-20.

[29]   B.M. Manuel, "The effects of the professional liability crisis on the quality of health care," *Bull Am Col Surg*, 1988, 73: 13-5.

[30]   *The Economist* for February 4, 1989, p. 49-50. [31]A. Enthoven, *Reflections on the Management of the National Health Service*, 1985, Nuffield Provincial Hospitals Trust, London.

[32]   R. Leavey, D. Wilkin, and D.H.H. Metcalfe, "Consumerism and general practice," *Brit Med J*, 1989, 298: 737-9.

[33]   R. Gillon, "Autonomy and the principle of respect for autonomy," *Brit Med J*, 1985, 290: 1806-8.

[34]   J. Rawls, *A Theory of Justice*, 1971, Harvard University Press, Cambridge, Mass.

35   R. Dworkin, *Taking Rights Seriously*, 1977, Harvard University Press, Cambridge, Mass.

36   B.L. Miller, "Autonomy and the Refusal of Lifesaving Treatment," In, *Moral Problems in Medicine*, 2nd Ed., Ed. by S. Gorovitz, et al., 1983, Prentice-Hall, Inc., Englewood Cliffs, N.J.

37   J.S. Mill, *Utilitarianism, On Liberty, and Considerations on Representative Government*, Ed. by H.G. Acton, J.M. Dent & Sons, Ltd., London 1972.

38   *Ibid*, p. 73.

39   R. Lindley, *Autonomy*, 1986, MacMillan Education Ltd., London, p. 51.

40   A.J. Ayer, *Language, Truth and Logic*, 1936, Victor Gollantz, Ltd., London.

41   B. Lo, "Behind closed doors. Problems and pitfalls of ethics committees," *N Eng J Med*, 1987, 317: 46-50.

42   J.E. Connelly and S. Dalle Mura, "Ethical problems in the medical office," *JAMA*, 1988, 260: 812-5.

43   P.S. Applebaum, S.A. Mirkin, and A.L. Bateman, "Empirical assessment of competancy to consent to psychiatric hospitalization," *Am J Psychiatry*, 1981, 138: 1170.

44   T. Hobbes, *Leviathan (1651)*, 1914, Everyman Library, London, p. 2l.

45   R. Lindley, *Autonomy*, 1986, MacMillan Education, Ltd., London, p. 165.

46   *Ibid*, p. 6.

47   H.L. Smith and L.R. Churchill, *Professional Ethics and Primary Care Medicine*, 1986, Duke University Press, Durham, N.C.

48   C. Whitbeck, "Why the Attention to Paternalism in Medical Ethics?", *J of Health Politics, Policy and Law*, 1985, 4: 181-187.

49   D.J. Murphy, "Do-not-resuscitate orders: time for reappraisal in long-term-care institutions," *JAMA*, 1988, 260: 2098-2101.

50   B. Freedman, "Equipoise and the Ethics of Clinical Research," *New Engl J Med*, 1987, 317: 141-45.

51   S.H. Miles, "Paternalism, family duties,and my aunt Maude," *JAMA*, 1988, 259: 2582-3.

52   *Inst of Med Ethics*, Bull. #53 for Sept.-Oct. 1989, p. 7.

53   E.D. Hirsch, Jr., *Cultural Literacy. What Every American Needs to Know*, 1987, Houghton Mifflin, Boston.

[54]   L. Forrow, S.A. Wartman and D.W. Brock, "Science, ethics and the making of clinical decisions. Implications for risk factor intervention," *JAMA*, 1988, 259: 3161-7.

[55]   V. Grant, "Good communications vital for medical practice," *Inst of Med Ethics*, Bull. #44 for November 1988, p. 13-7.

[56]   M.S. Moore, "Some myths about mental illness," *Arch Gen Psychiatry*, 1975, 32: 1483-97.

[57]   T. Szasz, *Psychiatric Slavery*, 1977, Free Press, New York.

[58]   P. Chodoff, "Paternalism versus autonomy in medicine and psychiatry," *Psychiatric Annals*, 1983, 13: 318-20.

[59]   R. Gillon, "Doctors and patients," *Brit Med J*, 1986, 292: 466-9.

[60]   P.S. Grim, P.A. Singer, G.P. Gramelspacher, et al. "Informed consent in emergency research," *JAMA*, 1989, 262: 252-5.

[61]   *The New York Times* for September 27, 1988. p. C9.

[62]   J.J. Paris, R.K. Crone, and F. Reardon, "Physicians' refusal of requested treatment. The case of Baby L," *N Eng J Med*, 1990, 322: 1012-5.

[63]   E.D. Pellegrino and D.C. Thomasma, *For the Patient's Good: The Restoration of Beneficence in Health Care*, 1988, Oxford University Press,

[64]   A.L. Caplan, *Book Review, JAMA*, 1989, 261: 3314-5.

[65]   J.F. Childress, "The place of autonomy in bioethics," *Hastings Center Report*, Jan/Feb 1990, pp. 12-7.

[66]   B. Williams, *Ethics and the Limits of Philosophy*, 1985, Fontana Press, London, p. 180.

[67]   Editorial, *Brit Med J*, 1987, 295: 1583.

[68]   R. Gillon, Consent. *Brit M J*, 1985, 291: 1700-01.

[69]   R. Gillon, "Primum non Nocere" and the Principle of non-maleficence, *Brit Med J*, 1985, 291: 130-31.

[70]   M. Baum, K. Zilkha, and J. Houghton, "Ethics of clinical research: lessons for the future," *Brit Med J*, 1989, 299: 251-3.

[71]   R.M. Veatch, *A Theory of Medical Ethics*, 1981, Basic Books, New York.

[72]   T. Nolan, I. Zvagulis, B. Pless, "Controlled trial of social work in childhood chronic illness," *Lancet*, 1987, ii: 411-415.

[73]   D. Faust, J. Ziskin, "The expert witness in psychology and psychiatry," *Science*, 1988, 241: 31-5.

[74] R. Gillon, "Justice and Medical Ethics," *Brit Med J*, 1985, 291: 201-02.

[75] R. Nozick, *Anarchy, State and Utopia*, 1981, Blackwell, Oxford.

[76] H.T. Engelhardt, Jr., *The Foundation of Ethics*. 1986, Oxford University Press, Oxford.

[77] T.L. Beauchamp and J.F. Childress, "Confidentiality," In *Medical Ethics*, Ed. by N. Abrams and M.D. Buckner, 1984, The MIT Press, Cambridge, Mass.

[78] W. Reich, "Diagnostic Ethics: The Uses and Limits of Psychiatric Explanation," In *Ethical Issues in Epidemiological Research*, Ed. by L. Tancredi, 1986, Rutgers University Press, New Brunswick, New Jersey.

[79] B.L. Rosner, "Psychiatrists, Confidentiality and Insurance Claims," In *Moral Problems in Medicine*, 2nd Edition, Ed. by S. Gorovitz, et al. 1983, Prentice-Hall, Englewood Cliffs, NJ.

[80] *New York Times* for July 17, 1988. p. 15.

[81] W.J. Curran, "The Constitutional right to health care. Denial in the court," *New Eng J Med*, 1989, 320: 788-9.

[82] *N Eng J Med*, 1989, 321: 693.

[83] A.P. Ross, "The case against showing patients their records," *Brit Med J*, 1986, 292: 578.

[84] B.N. Shenkin and D.C. Warner, "Giving the patient his medical record: a proposal to improve the system," *N Eng J Med*, 1973, 289: 688-91.

[85] *New York Times* for September 4, 1986, p. 51.

[86] *Inst of Med Ethics*, Bull. #56, March 1990, p. 4-5.

PART TWO

CHAPTER 4

[1] J. Lederberg, "Medical science, infectious disease, and the unity of humankind," *JAMA*. 1988, 260: 684-5.

[2] R. Rothenberg, M. Woelfel, R. Stoneburner, et al, "Survival with the acute immunodeficiency syndrome," *N Engl J Med*, 1987, 317: 1297-1302.

[3] "Letters to the Editor," *N Eng J Med*, 1988, 318: 1464-5.

[4]   D.B. Barnes, "AIDS: statistics but few answers," *Science*, 1987, 236: 1423-25.

[5]   "Human immunodeficiency virus infection in the United States," *JAMA*, 1988, 259: 478 and 483.

[6]   *The New York Times* for August 17, 1988, p. A14.

[7]   B.A. Evans, K.A. McLean, S.G. Dawson, et al., "Trends in sexual behavior and risk factors for HIV infection among homosexual men, 1984-7," *Brit Med J*, 1989, 298: 215-8.

[8]   R.E. Fay, C.F. Turner, A.D. Klassen, and J.H. Gagnon, "Prevalence and patterns of same-gender sexual contacts among men," *Science*, 1989, 243: 338-48.

[9]   J. Bancroft, "Homosexuality," *Brit Med J*, 1988, 297: 308-9.

[10]   W. Booth, "Another muzzle for AIDS education?", *Science*, 1987, 238: 1036.

[11]   *JAMA*, 1988, 260: 1845-51.

[12]   *JAMA*, 1990, 263: 1538-9.

[13]   J.W. Curran, H.W. Jaffe, Hardy AM, et al., "Epidemiology of HIV infection and AIDS in the United States," *Science*, 1988, 239: 610-616.

[14]   *The New York Times* for August 14, 1988, p. 29.

[15]   *Science*, 1989, 246: 1560.

[16]   *JAMA*, 1989, 261: 201-8.

[17]   R.E. Chaisson, P. Bacchetti, D. Osmond, et al., "Cocaine use and HIV infection in intravenous drug users in San Francisco," *JAMA*, 1989, 261: 561-5.

[18]   *JAMA*, 1988, 260: 893.

[19]   M.F. Goldsmith, "AIDS around the world: analyzing complex patterns," *JAMA* ,1988, 259: 1917-9.

[20]   *New York Times* for January 22, 1988, p. A1.

[21]   *The Economist* for September 30, 1989, p. 64.

[22]   D.C.W. Mabey, R.S. Tedder, A.S.B. Hughes, et al., "Human retroviral infections in the Gambia: prevalence and clinical features," *Brit J Med*, 1988, 296: 83-86.

[23]   T.C. Quinn, F.R.K. Zacarias, R.K. St. John, "AIDS in the Americas: an emerging public health crisis," *N Eng J Med*, 1989, 320: 1005-7.

[24]   *The New York Times* for June 13, 1990, p. A8.

[25]. W. Booth, "AIDS and drug abuse: no quick fix," *Science*, 1988, 239: 717-9.

[26] M.F. Goldsmith, "Sex tied to drugs = STD spread," *JAMA*, 1988, 260: 2009.

[27] *JAMA*, 1989, 261: 353.

[28] D.C. Des Jarlais, S.R. Friedman, "AIDS and IV drug use," *Science*, 1989, 245: 578.

[29] C.A. Raymond. "Combating a deadly combination: intravenous drug abuse, acquired immunodeficiency syndrome," *JAMA*, 1988, 259: 329-32.

[30] L. Bonneux, P. Van der Stuyft, H. Taelman, et al., "Risk factors for infection with human immunodeficiency virus among European expatriates in Africa," *Brit Med J*, 1988, 297: 581.

[31] *New Eng J Med*, 1989, 321: 830-2.

[32] *The New York Times* for April 29, 1990, p. 20E.

[33] J.W. Ward, D.H. Scott, J.R. Allen, et al., "Transmission of human immunodeficiency virus (HIV) by blood transfusions screened as negative for HIV antibody," *N Eng J Med* 1988, 318: 473-8.

[34] A.J. France, C.A. Skidmore, J.R. Robertson, "Heterosexual spread of human immunodeficiency virus in Edinburgh," *Brit Med J*, 1988, 296: 526-9.

[35] M.A. Gainan, A. Hardy, "Epidemiology of AIDS in women in the U.S.," *JAMA*, 1987, 256: 2039-42.

[36] A.M. Johnson, "Heterosexual transmission of human immunodeficiency virus," *Brit Med J* 1988, 296: 1017-20.

[37] *The New York Times* for February 28, 1989, p. C1.

[38] D.C.G. Skegg, "Heterosexually acquired HIV infection," *Brit Med J*, 1989, 298: 401-2.

[39] *Brit Med J*, Editorial, 1987, 295: 1503-4.

[40] *The New York Times* for July 22, 1988, p. B4.

[41] P.D. Cleary, M.J. Barry, K.H. Mayer KH, et al., "Compulsory premarital screening for the human immunodeficiency virus," *JAMA*, 1987, 258: 1757-62.

[42] *JAMA*, 1988, 259: 1011-5. and *Brit Med J*, 1988, 296: 1615-6.

[43] *JAMA*, 1989, 261: 993.

[44] *Lancet*, 1988, i: 1293.

[45] *Ibid*, 1988, ii: 582.

[46]   H.F. Hull, C.J. Bettinger, M.M. Gallaher, et al., "Comparison of HIV prevalence in patients consenting to and declining HIV-antibody testing in an STD clinic," *JAMA*, 1988, 260, 935-8.

[47]   *The New York Times* for February 26, 1988, p. A10.

[48]   *The New York Times* for December 14, 1987, "Letter to the Editor".

[49]   D.S. Burke, J.F. Brundage, R.R. Refield, et al., "Measurement of the false positive rate in a screening program for human immunodeficiency virus infections," *N Eng J Med*, 1988, 319: 961-4.

[50]   A. Ranke, S.L. Valle, M. Krohn, et al., "Long latency precedes overt sero-conversion in sexually transmitted human-immunodeficiency-virus infection," *Lancet* 1987, ii: 589-93.

[51]   D.T. Imagawa, M.H. Lee, S.M. Wolinsky, et al., "Human immunodeficiency virus type 1 infection in homosexual men who remain seronegative for prolonged periods," *N Eng J Med*, 1989, 320: 1458-62.

[52]   D. Brahams, "AIDS in the United States: education and litigation," *Lancet*, 1988, i: 779.

[53]   *The New York Times* for October 14, 1988, p. A12.

[54]   I. Glasser, "Where the A.C.L.U. stands on AIDS," *The New York Times* for May 23, 1987, Op-Ed page.

[55]   R. Gillon, "AIDS and medical confidentiality," *Brit Med J*, 1987, 294: 1675-7.

[56]   *The Wall Street Journal* for April 26, 1988, p. 41.

[57]   W. Booth, A frustrating glimpse of the true AIDS epidemic," *Science*, 1987, 238: 747.

[58]   *The New York Times* for May 12, 1990, p. 38A.

[59]   M. Millo, C.B. Wofsky, and J. Mills, "The acquired immune deficiency syndrome: infection control and public health law," *N Eng J Med*, 1986, 314: 931-36.

[60]   *The New York Times* for March 7, 1987, p. A1.

[61]   *Ibid* for September 28, 1988, p. B2.

[62]   *JAMA*, 1988, 260: 1197.

[63]   *The New York Times* for July 30, 1987, p. 1.

[64]   F.S. Rhame, D.G. Maki, "The case for wider use of testing for HIV infection," *New Eng J Med*, 1989, 320: 1248-54.

[65]   L.F. Novick, D. Berns, R. Stricof, et al., "HIV seroprevalence in newborns in New York State," *JAMA*, 1989, 261: 1745-50.

[66]   R. Hoff, V.P. Berardi, B.J. Weiblen, et al., "Seroprevalence of human immunodeficiency virus among childbearing women," *N Eng J Med*, 1988, 318: 525-30.

[67]   *The Philadelphia Inquirer* for April 4, 1986.

[68]   *The New York Times* for March 4, 1987.

[69]   *Science*, 1990, 247: 1406.

[70]   W. Booth, "An underground drug for AIDS," *Science*, 1988, 241: 1279-81.

[71]   *The New York Times* for January 29, 1989, p. 8.

[72]   *Inst of Med Ethics*, Bull. #32 for November 1987, p. 14.

[73]   *The New York Times* for January 12, 1989, p. A13.

[74]   *The New York Times* for February 12, 1989, p. 22.

[75]   *Brit Med J*, 1990, 300: 934.

[76]   *The Guardian* for May 11, 1988, p. 23.

[77]   G.W. Rutherford GW, "Contact tracing and the control of human immunodeficiency virus infection," *JAMA*, 1988, 259: 3609-10.

[78]   "Partner notification for preventing human immunodeficiency virus (HIV) infection - Colorado, Idaho, South Carolina, Virginia," *JAMA*, 1988, 260: 613-5.

[79]   L. Walters, "Ethical issues in the prevention and treatment of HIV infection and AIDS," *Science*, 1988, 239: 597-603.

[80]   *The New York Times* for September 20, 1988, p. B5.

[81]   *The Wall Street Journal* for December 1, 1988, Editorial, p. A22.

[82]   R. Marcus, et al., "Surveillance of health care workers exposed to blood from patients infected with the human immunodeficiency virus," *New Eng J Med*, 1988, 319: 1118-27.

[83]   *Brit Med J*, 1989, 299: 703.

[84]   *JAMA*, 1990, 263: 1765.

[85]   "Letters to the editor," *JAMA*, 1988, 260: 179-181.

[86]   P. Hodgkin, "HIV infection: the challenge to general practitioners," *Brit Med J*, 1988, 296: 516-7 (also pp. 533, 535, 538).

[87]   T. Richards, "Drug addicts and the GP," *Brit Med J*, 1988, 296: 1082.

[88]   M.B. King, "Psychological and social problems in HIV infection: interviews wit general practitioners in London," *Brit Med J*, 1989, 299: 713-7.

[89]   *USA TODAY* for November 24, 1987, p. 1.

[90] J.G. Bartlett, "Testing for HIV infection: recommendations for surgeons," *Bull Amer Col Surg*, 1988, 73: 4-10.

[91] *The Wall Street Journal* for January 4, 1989, p. B1.

[92] *The Scientist* for March 9, 1987.

[93] D.E. Bloom and G. Carliner, "The economic impact of AIDS in the United States," *Science*, 1988, 239: 604-10.

[94] M.F. Goldsmith, "'Silent epidemics' of 'social disease' makes STD experts raise their voices," *JAMA*, 1989, 261: 3509-10.

[95] *The New York Times* for February 15, 1988, p. A14.

[96] *The New York Times* for February 25, 1988, p. A1.

[97] *JAMA*, 1988, 260: 2620-1.

[98] *The New York Times* for August 12, 1988, p. A1.

[99] N. Hearst and S.B. Hulley, "Preventing the heterosexual spread of AIDS," *JAMA*, 1988, 259: 2428-32.

[100] *Inst Med Ethics*, Bull. #36 for March 1988, p. 3-5.

[101] *Lancet*, 1988, ii: 54-5.

[102] M.M. Waldrop, "AIDS panels converge on a consensus," *Science*, 1988, 240: 1395-6.

[103] *Lancet*, 1988, i: 291.

[104] *The Economist* for March 12, 1988, p. 14.

[105] A. McMillan, "HIV in prisons," *Brit Med J*, 1988, 297: 873-4.

[106] "Number of sex partners and potential risk of sexual exposure to human immunodeficiency virus," *JAMA*, 1988, 260: 2020-1.

[107] *The New York Times* for February 9, 1989, p. A25.

[108] *Inst Med Ethics*, Bull. #41 for August 1988, pp. 5, 6 and 15.

CHAPTER 5

[1] I.J. Chanoff, H.J. Landress, and M.E. Barrett, "The prevalence of illicit-drug or alcohol use during pregnancy and discrepancies in mandatory reporting in Pinella County, Florida," *New Eng J Med*, 1990, 322: 1202-6.

[2] C. Holden, "Is alcohol treatment effective?", *Science*, 1987, 236: 20-2.

[3] M. Gossop, L. Green, G. Phillips, and B. Bradley, "What happened to opiate addicts immediately after treatment: a perspective follow-up study," *Brit Med J*, 1987, 294: 1377-80.

⁴   D.B. Barnes, "Breaking the cycle of drug addiction," *Science*, 1988, 241: 1029-30.

⁵   J. Grabowski, L. Lasagna, "Screening for drug use: technical and social aspects," Issues in *Science and Technology*, Winter 1987 (National Academy of Sciences).

⁶   *The New York Times* for December 5, 1989, p. D1.

⁷   *Lancet*, 1990, i: 963.

⁸   *The Economist* for March 5, 1988, p. 23-4.

⁹   *JAMA*, 1988, 259: 1615.

¹⁰   *The New York Times* for July 13, 1989, p. A1.

¹¹   C. Holden, "Alcoholism and the medical cost crunch," *Science*, 1987, 235: 1132-3.

¹²   *JAMA*, 1990, 263: 358.

¹³   *Science*, 1990, 247: 810.

¹⁴   Editorial in *Lancet* for November 28, 1987, pp. 1249-50.

¹⁵   *The New York Times* for December 13, 1987, p. E26.

¹⁶   M. Hayashida, A.I. Alterman, A.T. McLellan, et al., "Comparative effectiveness and costs of inpatient and outpatient detoxification of patients with mild-to-moderate alcohol withdrawal syndrome," *New Eng J Med*, 1989, 320: 358-65.

¹⁷   M.P.I. Weller, P.C. Ang, D.T. Latimer-Sayer, and A. Zachary, "Drug abuse and mental illness," *Lancet*, 1988, i: 997.

¹⁸   *The New York Times* for October 16, 1989, op-ed, p. A21.

¹⁹   *Brit Med J*, 1990, 300: 57.

²⁰   E.A. Nadelmann, *Science*, 1989, 246: 1104-5.

²¹   T.F. Kirn, "Stronger laws and stiffer penalties aimed at keeping drivers safely sober," *JAMA*, 1988, 259: 2059-60.

²²   *Lancet*, 1988, ii: 1292-3.

²³   T.F. Kirn, "In time of change, USSR seeks to end tradition of extensive alcohol use by majority of citizens," *JAMA*, 1987, 258: 883-5.

²⁴   *The Economist* for September 26, 1987, p. 71.

²⁵   *JAMA*, 1990, 263: 352.

²⁶   E. Gordis, B. Tabakoff, D. Goldman, and K. Berg, "Finding the gene(s) for alcoholism," *JAMA*, 1990, 263: 2094-5.

²⁷   *The New York Times* for August 12, 1988, p. A8.

²⁸   D.J. Boone, "Reliability of urine drug testing," *JAMA*, 1987, 258: 2587-8.

[29]   E. Marshall, "Testing urine for drugs," *Science*, 1988, 241: 150-2.

[30]   N.B. Person, J.R.L. Ehrenkranz, "Fake urine samples for drug analysis: hot but not hot enough," *JAMA*, 1988, 259: 841.

[31]   *The New York Times* for March 5, 1986, p. A24.

[32]   *Ibid* for April 23, 1987, p. A16.

[33]   C. Holden, "Doctors square off on employee drug testing," *Science*, 1987, 238: 744-5.

[34]   C. Holden, "NIH scientists balk at random drug tests," *Science*, 1988, 239: 724.

[35]   K.H. Davis, R.L. Hawks, R.V. Blanke, "Assessment of laboratory quality in urine drug testing," *JAMA*, 1988, 260: 1749-54.

[36]   *The New York Times* for March 12, 1987, p. A24.

[37]   *Ibid* for January 12, 1989, p. A25.

[38]   *The Philadelphia Inquirer* for December 11, 1986, Ed. page.

[39]   I. Glasser, "Letter to the editor," *The New York Times* for April 1, 1986.

[40]   G.T. Marx, "Drug foes aren't high on civil liberties," *The New York Times* for February 24, 1986, Op-Ed page.

[41]   *The New York Times* for May 18, 1987.

[42]   *Ibid* for March 3, 1988, p. A16.

[43]   *Ibid* for June 10, 1987, p. A13.

[44]   J.A. Dunbar, A. Porttila, and J. Pikkareinen, "Drinking and driving: success of random breath testing in Finland," *Brit Med J*, 1987, 295: 101-3.

[45]   *The New York Times* for January 19, 1988, p. 1A.

[46]   *Ibid* for January 22, 1988, p. 1A.

[47]   *The Economist* for July 22, 1989, p. 43.

[48]   *The New York Times* for September 7, 1988, p. A18.

[49]   T.F. Kirn, "Methadone maintenance treatment remains controversial even after 23 years of experience," *JAMA*, 1988, 260: 2970-5.

[50]   G.F. Koob and F.E. Bloom, "Cellular and molecular mechanisms of drug dependence," *Science*, 1988, 242: 715-23.

[51]   *The New York Times* for June 6, 1987, Editorial.

[52]   *The Economist* for October 8, 1988, p. 21-4.

[53]   *The New York Times* for February 21, 1990, p. A3.

[54]   E.A. Nadelmann, "Drug prohibition in the United States: costs, consequences, and alternatives," *Science*, 1989, 245: 939-47.

[55]   B. Fozouni and I. Siassi, *Science*, 1989, 246: 1102-3.

[56]   *The New York Times* for November 6, 1989, Editorial, p. A22.

[57]   E. Marshall, "Drug wars: legalization gets a hearing," *Science*, 1988, 241: 1157-9.

[58]   D.E. Koshland, Jr, "Thinking tough," *Science*, 1988, 241: 1273.

[59]   *The New York Times* for July 28, 1988, p. A26.

[60]   E. Marshall, "The drug of champions," *Science*, 1988, 242: 183-4.

[61]   V.S. Cowart, "Support lags for research on steroid effects," *JAMA*, 1989, 262: 2500-2.

[62]   W.E. Buckley, C.E. Yesalis, III, K.E. Friedl, et al., "Estimated prevalence of anabolic steroid use among male high school seniors," *JAMA*, 1988, 260: 3441-5.

[63]   *The New York Times* for November 17, 1988, p. A1.

[64]   *Lancet*, 1987, i: 667-8.

[65]   *Lancet*, 1988, i: 612.

[66]   *Inst of Med Ethics Bull*, Supplement No. 7, "Drugs in sport," August 1987.

[67]   V.S. Cowart, "Athlete drug testing receiving more attention than ever before in history of competition," *JAMA*, 1989, 261: 3510-6.

CHAPTER 6

[1]   W. Reich, "Diagnostic ethics: the use and limits of psychiatric explanation," In *Ethical Issues in Epidemiological Research*, Ed. by L. Tancredi, 1986, Rutgers University Press., New Brunswick, New Jersey.

[2]   D. Faust, J. Ziskin, "The expert witness in psychology and psychiatry," *Science*, 1988, 241: 31-5.

[3]   M.B. Parloff, "Psychotherapy and research: an anaclitic depression," *Psychiatry*, 1980, 43: 279-93.

[4]   T. Szasz, *Law, Liberty and Psychiatry*, 1963, MacMillan Co., New York.

[5]   R.D. Laing, *The Divided Self*, 1969, Pantheon, New York.

[6]   R. Porter, *A Social History of Madness. Stories of the Insane*, 1987, Weidenfeld and Nicholson, London.

[7]   P. Chodoff, "The case for involuntary hospitalization of the mentally ill," *Am J Psychiatry*, 1976, 133: 496-501.

⁸ P. Chodoff, "The case for involuntary hospitalization of the mentally ill," In *Medical Ethics*, Ed. by N. Abrams and M.D. Buckner, 1983, The M.I.T. Press, Cambridge, Mass.

⁹ R. Michels and S. Eth, "Ethical issues in psychiatric research on communities: a case study of the Community Mental Health Center Program," In *Ethical Issues in Epidemiologic Research*, Ed. by L. Tancredi, 1986, Rutgers University Press, New Brunswick, New Jersey.

¹⁰ *Ibid*, pp. 81-83.

¹¹ *Brit Med J*, 1988, 296: 1466.

¹² P.H. Rossi, J.D. Wright, G.A. Fisher, and G. Willis, "The urban homeless: estimating composition and size," *Science*, 1987, 235: 1336-41.

¹³ L. Merccs and N.L. Cohen, "Taking the suspected mentally ill off the streets to public general hospitals," *N Eng J Med*, 1986, 315: 1158-61.

¹⁴ *The Economist* for April 11, 1987.

¹⁵ *The New York Times* for September 11, 1988, p. 52.

¹⁶ C. Holden, "Health problems of the homeless," *Science*, 1988, 242: 188-9.

¹⁷ W.R. Breakey, P.J. Fischer, M. Kramer, et al., "Health and mental health problems of homeless men and women in Baltimore," *JAMA*, 1989, 262: 1352-7.

¹⁸ M. Marshall, "Collected and neglected: are Oxford hostels for the homeless filling up with disabled psychiatric patients?", *Brit Med J*, 1989, 299: 706-9.

¹⁹ I. Marks and G. Thornicroft, "Private inpatient psychiatric care: A two tier system is developing in Britain," *Brit Med J*, 1990, 300: 892.

²⁰ T. Groves, "Who needs long term psychiatric care?", *Brit Med J*, 1990, 300: 999-1001.

²¹ *The New York Times* for January 29, 1989, p. E5.

²² *JAMA*, 1989, 262: 1376.

²³ *The Wall Street Journal* for July 16, 1987, "Letter to the Editor".

²⁴ *The Philadelphia Inquirer* for February 28, 1990, p. 1-A.

²⁵ D. Cohen, *Forgotten Millions. The Treatment of the Mentally Ill - A Global Perspective*, 1988, Palladin, London.

²⁶ "Letters to the editor," *N Eng J Med*, 1988, 318: 1544-5.

[27] R.J. Wyatt and E.G. DeRenzo, "Scienceless to homeless," *Science*, 1986, 234: 1309.

[28] *The Los Angeles Times* for November 12, 1987, p. 14.

[29] *The New York Times* for June 17, 1983, Editorial.

[30] *Ibid* for May 27, 1990.

[31] *Ibid* for August 14, 1989, p. B6.

[32] *Ibid* for January 21, 1988, p. A24.

[33] C. Dyar, "Decisions from the House of Lords," *Brit Med J*, 1987, 294: 1219.

[34] *The New York Times* for November 21, 1989, p. A1.

[35] *The New York Times* for May 31, 1988, p. B3.

[36] D. Faust and J. Ziskin, "The expert witness in psychology and psychiatry," *Science*, 1988, 241: 31-5.

[37] W.L. Holleman and M.C. Holleman, "School and work release evaluations," *JAMA*, 1988, 260: 3629-34.

[38] A.P. Read and D. Donnai, "Preimplantation diagnosis with polymerase chain reaction," *Brit Med J*, 1989, 299: 3.

[39] "Medical news," *JAMA*, 1985, 254: 3160.

[40] "Medical news," *JAMA*, 1987: 258: 1132-3.

[41] C.G. Cole, A. Coyne, K.A. Hart, et al., "Prenatal testing for Duchenne and Becker muscular dystrophy," *Lancet*, 1988, i: 262- 4.

[42] Editorial. *Lancet*, 1987, ii: 663-4.

[43] J.S. Thompson and M.W. Thompson, "Genetics in Medicine", (4th Ed.), 1986, W. B. Saunders Co., Philadelphia.

[44] *Science*, 1990, 240: 18.

[45] *The Wall Street Journal* for September 14, 1987, p. 27.

[46] *The New York Times* for August 27, 1988, p. 7.

[47] *JAMA*,1989, 261: 3108-14.

[48] P.S. Harper and A. Clarke, "Should we test children for "adult" genetic diseases?", *Lancet*, 1990, 335: 1205-6.

[49] M. Goldsmith, "Trial appears to confirm safety of chorionic villus sampling procedure," *JAMA*, 1988, 259: 3521-2.

[50] M. d'A Crawford, "Prenatal diagnosis of common genetic disorders," *Brit Med J*, 1988, 297: 502-6.

[51] L. Pijpers, M.G.H. Jahoda, A. Reuss A, et al., "Transabdominal chorionic villus biopsy in second and third trimesters of pregnancy to determine fetal karytype," *Brit Med J*, 1988, 297: 822.

[52] "Letters to the editor," *N Eng J Med*, 1988, 318: 926-9.

[53] S.M. Pueschel, "Maternal alpha-fetoprotein screening for Down's syndrome," *N Eng J Med*m 1987, 317: 376-8.

[54] N.J. Wald, H.S.Cuckle, J.W. Densem, et al., "Maternal serum screening for Down's syndrome in early pregnancy," *Brit Med J*, 1988, 297: 883-7.

[55]. "King's Fund forum consensus statement: screening for fetal and genetic abnormalities," *Brit Med J*, 1987, 295: 1551-3.

[56] J.R. Botkin, "The legal concept of wrongful life," *JAMA*, 1988, 259: 1541-5.

[57] M. Midgley, *Beast and Man*, 1980, Methuen Co., Ltd., London.

CHAPTER 7

[1] H.E. Beecher, "Ethics and clinical research," *N Engl J Med*, 1966, 274: 1354-60.

[2] P.S. Appelbaum, L.H. Roth, C.W. Lidz, et al., "False hopes and best data: research and the therapeutic misconception," *Hastings Cent Rep*, 1987, 17: 20-4.

[3] W.J. MacKillop, G.K. Ward, and B. O'Sullivan, "The use of expert surrogates to evaluate clinical trials in non-small-cell lung cancer," *Br J Cancer*, 1986, 54: 661-3.

[4] F.J. Ingelfinger, "Informed (but uneducated) consent," *N Eng J Med*, 1972, 287: 465-6.

[5] B. Freedman, "Equipoise and the ethics of clinical research," *N Eng J Med*, 1987, 317: 141-5.

[6] J. Goldman and M.D. Katz, "Inconsistency and institutional review boards," *JAMA*, 1982, 248: 197-202.

[7] *The New York Times* for March 18, 1987, p. 1.

[8] *Science*, 1987, 235: 1319.

[9] "The shocking American report with lessons for all, editorial, *Brit Med J*, 1987, 295: 73.

[10] "Research ethics," *Inst of Med Ethics*, Bull. #19, Oct 1986, pp. 3-6.

[11] *Inst of Med Ethics*, Bull. #56, March 1990, pp. 8-10.

[12] *Inst of Med Ethics*, Bull. #33, Dec 1987, pp. 2-3.

[13] C. Marwick, "Philosophy on trial: examining ethics of clinical investigations," *JAMA*, 1988, 260: 749-51.

[14]   M. Baum, "Do we need informed consent?", *Lancet*, 1986, 2: 911-2.

[15]   M. Baum, K. Zilkha, and J. Houghton, "Ethics of clinical research: lessons for the future," *Br Med J*, 1989, 299: 251-3.

[16].   D. Brahams, "Randomized trials and informed consent," *Lancet*, 1988, ii: 1033-4.

[17]   "Letters to the editor," *Lancet*, 1988, ii: 1194-5.

[18]   J.W. Warren, J. Sobal, J.H. Tenney, et al., "Informed consent by proxy. An issue in research with elderly patients," *N Eng J Med*, 1986, 315: 1124-8.

[19]   G.L. Annas, L.H. Glantz, "Rules for research in nursing homes," *N Eng J Med*, 1986, 315: 1157-8.

[20]   *The New York Times* for October 30, 1986, p. A20.

[21]   *The Wall Street Journal* for August 6, 1987, Editorial.

[22]   "Research ethics committees," *Inst of Med Ethics Bull*, Supplement #2, September 1986.

[23]   *JAMA*, 1989, 262: 348.

[24]   *Inst of Med Ethics*, Bull. #37, April 1988, p. 4.

[25]   D.J. Rothman, "Ethics and human experimentation," *N Engl J Med*, 1987, 317: 1195-99.

[26]   C. Holden, "A pivotal year for lab animal welfare," *Science*, 1986, 232: 147-50.

[27]   *The New York Times* for August 30, 1987, p. E7.

[28]   G. Chui, "Activists beset UC, Stanford labs," *Science*, 1988, 239: 1229-1232.

[29]   M. Daly, "All heaven in a rage," *History Today*, May, 1987, pp. 7-9.

[30]   D. Kennedy, "The anti-scientific method," *The Wall Street Journal* for October 29, 1987, p. 32.

[31]   M. Prowse, "The last moral frontier," *Financial Times (England)* for December 22, 1989, p. 17B.

[32]   *The New York Times* for January 14, 1989, p. 1.

[33]   *Ibid* for May 3, 1990, p. B1.

[34]   *Inst of Med Ethics*, Bull. #1, April 1985, p. 5.

[35]   D.M. Jackson, "Letter to the editor," *JAMA*, 1988, 260: 2062.

[36]   B.E. Rollin, *Animal Rights and Human Morality*, 1981, Prometheus Books, Buffalo, N.Y.

[37]   T.E. Regan, *The Case for Animal Rights*, 1983, University of California Press, Berkeley, Cal.

[38]   *Inst of Med Ethics*, Bull. #22, January 1987, p. 13.

[39]   *The Wall Street Journal* for June 6, 1987, Ed. page.

[40]   C. Norman, "Cat study halted amid protests," *Science*, 1988, 242: 1001-2.

[41]   C. Holden, "Animal regulations: so far so good," *Science*, 1987, 238: 880-2.

[42]   C. Holden, "Billion dollar price tag for new animal rules," *Science*, 1988, 242: 662-3

[43]   C. Holden, "Experts ponder simian well-being," *Science*, 1988, 1753-5.

[44]   C. Holden, "Compromise in sight on animal regulations," *Science*, 1989, 245: 124-5.

[45]   *The New York Times* for May 23, 1987.

[46]   *The New York Times* for March 21, 1987, "Letters to editor."

[47]   W.E. Seidelman, "Animal experiments in Nazi Germany," *Lancet*, 1986, ii: 1214.

[48]   *The Wall Street Journal* for June 3, 1988, p. 18.

[49]   *The New York Times* for November 19, 1985, p. C1.

[50]   *Science*, 1988, 241: 777.

[51]   *The New York Times* for January 17, 1989, p. C13.

[52]   *JAMA*, 1989, 262: 2649.

[53]   J.B. Callicott, In: *The Preservation of the Species*, Ed. by B.G. Norton, 1986, Princeton University Press, Princeton, NJ. pp. 138-172.

[54]   E. Sober, *Ibid*, pp. 173-194.

[55]   D.H. Regan, *Ibid*, pp. 195-220.

[56]   D.E. Koshland, Jr, "For whom the bell tolls," *Science*, 1988, 241: 1405.

[57]   *The New York Times* for May 1, 1990, p. A22.

[58]   *Science*, 1989, 243: 11-2.

[59]   H. Jonas, "Freedom of scientific inquiry and the public interest," *Hastings Center Report 6*, August 1976, p. 15-17.

[60]   D.H.L. Bishop, "Release of genetically altered viruses into the environment," *Brit Med J*, 1988, 296: 1685-6.

[61]   A. Skolnick, "Gene replacement therapy for hereditary emphysema?", *JAMA*, 1989, 262: 2499.

62 M. Crawford, "Religious groups join animal patent battle," *Science*, 1987, 237: 480-1.

63 *The New York Times* for June 9, 1987, p. C1.

64 Y. Blumenfeld, "Frankenstein by accident?", *The New York Times* for February 25, 1987, Op-Ed page.

65 "Gene Therapy," Editorial, *Lancet*, 1989, i: 193-4.

66 *The Economist* for June 27, 1987, p. 88.

67 *Science*, 1987, 236: 1179.

68 P.H. Abelson, "World competition in biotechnology," *Science*, 1988, 240: 701.

69 R. Lewin, "Ecological invasions offer opportunities," *Science*, 1987, 238: 752-3.

70 S.J.M. Davis, *The Archeology of Animals*, 1987, Yale University Press, New Haven, CT.

71 *The New York Times* for June 19, 1986, p. A25.

72 *The New York Times* for July 24, 1988, p. 19.

73 M. Crawford, "Court rules the cells are the patient's property," *Science*, 1988, 241: 653-4.

74 *Science*, 1987, 237: 840

75 R.C. Cowen, *The Philadelphia Inquirer* for September 9, 1987, Op-Ed page.

76 *Science*, 1990, 248: 546-7.

77 *Science*, 1987, 235: 741.

78 *Science*, 1989, 244: 1251-2.

79 D. Dickson, "Europe splits over gene regulation," *Science*, 1987, 238: 18-9.

80 D.E. Koshland, Jr., "Frontiers in recombinant DNA," *Science*, 1987, 236: 1157, Editorial.

81 "Gene therapy in man. Recommendations of European medical research councils," *Lancet*, 1988, i: 1271-2.

82 *The New York Times* for October 22, 1988, p. B9.

83 L. Roberts, "Rifkin battles gene transfer experiment," *Science*, 1989, 243: 734.

84 G. Kolata, "Genetic screening raises questions for employers and insurers," *Science*, 1986, 232: 317-9.

85 D.E. Koshland, Jr., "Sequences and consequences of the human genome," *Science*, 1989, 246: 189.

[86]   *Times Literary Supplement* (London) for December 15-21, 1989, p. 1384.

[87]   B. Dixon, "Charting the genome," *Brit Med J*, 1989, 299: 574.

[88]   R. Kanigel, "The genome project," *The New York Times* for December 13, 1987.

[89]   R.A. Weinberg, "The case against gene sequencing," *The Scientist* for November 16, 1987, p. 11.

[90]   L. Roberts, "Academy backs genome project," *Science*, 1988, 239: 725-6.

[91]   L. Roberts, "Carving up the human genome," *Science*, 1988, 242: 1244-6.

[92]   D. Dickson, "Genome research gets rough ride in Europe," *Science*, 1989, 243: 599.

[93]   *Lancet*, 1989, i: 856.

[94]   P.H. Abelson, "Soviet science," *Science*, 1988, 239: 961.

CHAPTER 8

[1]   *The New York Times* for October 6, 1988, p. A22.

[2]   T. Smith, "Late abortions and the law," *Brit Med J*, 1988, 296: 446-7.

[3]   C. Woodroffe and V. Beral, "Cost of limiting abortion," *Brit Med J*, 1988, 296: 62.

[4]   *The New York Times* for November 10, 1986, "Letter to the editor."

[5]   D. Brahams, "A baby's life or a mother's liberty: A United States case," *Lancet*, 1988, i: 1006.

[6]   *The New York Times* for November 23, 1987, p. 1.

[7]   L.J. Nelson and N. Milliken, "Compelled treatment of pregnant women. Life, liberty and law in conflict," *JAMA*, 1988, 259: 1060-6.

[8]   M.A. Warren, "On the moral and legal status of abortion," In: *Contemporary Issues In Bioethics*, Ed. by T.L. Beauchamp and L. Walters, 2nd Edition, 1982, Wadsworth Publishing Co., Belmont, California.

[9]   D. Holbrook, "Medical ethics and the potentialities of the living being," *Brit Med J*, 1985, 291: 459-62.

[10]   C. Holden, "Koop finds abortion evidence 'inconclusive'", *Science*, 1989, 243: 730-1.

[11]   N.E. Adler, H.P. David, B.N. Major, et al., "Psychological responses after abortion," *Science*, 1990, 248: 41-4.

[12]   *Inst of Med Ethics*, Bull. #19, p. 12.

[13]   *Ibid*, Bull. #23, p. 3.

[14].   C. Tietze, S.K. Henshaw, "Induced abortion: a world review," 6th ed., 1986, Alan Guttmacher Institute, New York.

[15]   *Inst of Med Ethics*, Bull. #34, p. 10.

[16]   *The New York Times* for December 25, 1988, p. 1.

[17]   *The New York Times* for November 26, 1988, p. 1.

[18]   *Ibid* for December 15, 1988, Editorial, p. A38.

[19]   *The New York Times* for February 23, 1986, Op-Ed page.

[20]   *Ibid* for March 15, 1986, "Letter to the editor."

[21]   *Ibid* for April 26, 1989, p. A1.

[22]   *The Wall Street Journal* for July 30, 1986, Op-Ed page.

[23]   *The New York Times* for January 21, 1988, p. A18.

[24]   *Ibid* for November 13, 1986, Op-Ed Page.

[25]   *Ibid* for December 13, 1988, p. A20.

[26]   "The abortion act twenty years on," Editorial, *Lancet*, 1988, i: 91-2.

[27]   *The Economist* for October 31, 1987, p. 51.

[28]   *Inst of Med Ethics*, Bull. #31 for October 1987, p. 13.

[29]   *The New York Times* for May 27, 1988, Op-Ed page, p. A31.

[30]   I. Gentles, "Good news for the fetus," *Policy Review for Spring*, 1987.

[31]   B.L. Maciak, A.M. Spitz, L.T. Strauss, et al., "Pregnancy and birth rates among sexually experienced U.S. teenagers - 1974, 1980 and 1983," *JAMA*, 1987, 258: 2069-71.

[32]   C. Holden, "Networks nix contraceptive ads," *Science*, 1987, 238: 887.

[33]   "WHO/UNICEF/UNFPA. The reproductive health of adolescents: a strategy for action," 1989, WHO, Geneva.

[34]   *The New York Times* for March 7, 1990, p. 19.

[35]   *The Los Angeles Times* for November 20, 1987, Ed. page. [36]*Inst of Med Ethics*, Bull #15, June 1986, p. 13.

[37]   *The New York Times* for June 9, 1988, p. B17.

[38]   *The New York Times* for October 6, 1988, p. A24.

[39]   *The New York Times* for July 5, 1985, p. 1.

[40]   *Lancet*, 1990, ii: 1189-90.

[41]   *Inst of Med Ethics*, Bull. #32, November 1987, p. 15.

[42]   C. Djerassi, "The bitter pill," *Science*, 1989, 245: 356-61.

[43]   L. Roberts, "U.S. lags on birth control development," *Science*, 1990, 247: 909.

[44]   J. Cook and D. Maine, "Spousal veto over family planning services," *Amer J Pub Health*, 1987, 77: 339-44.

[45]   *The New York Times* for June 12, 1986, p. A1.

[46]   *Ibid* for September 9, 1987, p. A18.

[47]   *The New York Times* for August 9, 1988, p. A1.

[48]   *Ibid* for January 25, 1988, p. A1.

[49]   J.C. Hobbins, "Selective reduction - a perinatal necessity?", *New Eng J Med*, 1988, 318: 1062-3.

[50]   *The Times* (London) for May 14, 1988, p. 3.

[51]   *Inst of Med Ethics*, Bull. #29, August 1987, p. 4.

[52]   *The New York Times* for October 28, 1988, p. A1.

[53]   *The New York Times* for October 30, 1988, p. 1.

[54]   *The Wall Street Journal* for December 1, 1988, Editorial, p. A22.

[55]   M.N. Cohen, *Health and the Rise of Civilization*, 1989, Yale University Press, New Haven, p. 131.

CHAPTER 9

[1]   *The New York Times* for July 15, 1988, p. A12.

[2]   *Science*, 1988, 241: 895.

[3]   T. Ziporyn, "'Artificial' human reproduction poses medical, social concerns," *JAMA*, 1986, 255: 13-5

[4]   *The New York Times* for October 30, 1988, p. 1.

[5]   S. Elias and G.J. Annas, "Social policy considerations in noncoital reproduction," *JAMA*, 1986, 255: 62-8.

[5A]   P. Braude, M.H. Johnson, and R.J. Aitken, "Human Fertilization and Embryology Bill goes to report stage," *Brit Med J*, 1990, 300: 1410-12.

[6]   *The Wall Street Journal* for April 4, 1987, p. 31.

[7]   M.G. Wagner, St. Clair, PA, "Are in-vitro fertilization and embryo transfer of benefit to all?", *Lancet*, 1989, ii: 1027-30.

[8]   M. Gold, "Franchising test-tube babies," *Science*, 1986, for April, p. 16-7.

[9]   *New Eng J Med*, 1989, 321: 1052.

[10]   *The New York Times* for April 11, 1989, p. C5.

[11]   *JAMA*, 1988, 260: 1181.

[12]   *Lancet*, 1989, ii: 342.

[13]   *JAMA*, 1989, 262: 1158.

[14]   *The New York Times* for April 19, 1990, p. A19.

[15]   B. Dixon, "*In vitro* fight looms Down Under," *The Scientist*, 1987, 1: 1-2.

[16]   K. Dawson, "*In vitro* fertilization: legislation and problems of research," *Brit Med J*, 1987, 295: 1184-6.

[17]   D. Bartels, "The moral costs of IVF research," *The Scientist* for April 6, 1987.

[18]   D. Kirk, "West Germany moving to make IVF research a crime," *Science*, 1988, 241: 406.

[19]   *Inst of Med Ethics*, Bull. #51, June 1989, p. 13.

[20]   *The New York Times* for March 12, 1987, Editorial.

[21]   *Inst of Med Ethics*, Bull. #20 for November 14, 1986, p. 14.

[22]   *The New York Times* for June 26, 1988, p. 1.

[23]   *Inst of Med Ethics*, Bull. #4, May 1986, p. 14.

[24]   *The New York Times* for February 4, 1987, p. B1.

[25]   D. Brahams, "Surrogacy, adoption and custody," *Lancet*, 1987, ii: 817.

[26]   R. Deitch, "Commentary from Westminster," *Lancet*, 1985, ii: 994-5.

[27]   *Inst of Med Ethics Bull*, Supplement #1, May 1986, p. 19-20.

[28]   *The New York Times* for December 13, 1987, p. A42.

[29]   *Ibid* for September 20, 1988, p. A15.

[30]   *Ibid* for March 12, 1989, p. 40.

[31]   *Science*, 1990, 247: 1183.

[32]   *The New York Times* for June 14, 1990, p. A9.

[33]   C. Holden, "A revisionist look at population and growth," *Science*, 1986, 231: 1493-4.

[34]   N. Eberstadt, "Population and economic growth," *The Wilson Quarterly* for Winter 1986, p. 95-127.

[35]   *Science*, 1990: 248, 680.

[36]   *The New York Times* for September 5, 1988, p. 1.

[37]   S. Uniacke, "*In vitro* fertilization and the right to reproduce," *Bioethics*, 1987, 1: 241-54.

CHAPTER 10

[1]   J. Rachels, "Active and passive euthanasia," *N Engl J Med*, 1975, 292: 78-80.

[2]   T. Engelhardt, "Ethical issues in aiding the death of young children," In *Contemporary Issues in Bioethics*, 2nd Ed, Edited by T.L. Beauchamp and L. Walters, 1982, Wadsworth Publishing Co., Belmont, California.

[3]   "The prognosis for babies with meningomyelocele and high lumbar paraplegia at birth. Comment by an Ethical Working Group," *Lancet*, 1985, ii: 996-7.

[4]   H. Kuhse and P. Singer, "Should the baby live?: The problem of handicapped infants," 1985, Oxford University Press, Oxford.

[5]   D. Brahams, "Severely handicapped babies and the law," *Lancet* 1986, i: 984-5.

[6]   C. Bull, M.L. Rigby, and E. Shinebourne, "Should management of complete atrioventricular canal defect be influenced by coexistent Down syndrome?", *Lancet*, 1985, i: 1147-9.

[7]   D.K. Stevenson, R.L. Ariagno, J.S. Kutner, T.A. Raffin, and E.W.D. Young, "The 'Baby Doe' rule," *JAMA*, 1986, 255: 1909-12.

[8]   "Limitations of care for very-low-birthweight infants," *Lancet*, 1988, i: 1257-8.

[9]   *The New York Times* for July 26, 1985.

[10]   *The New York Times* for June 12, 1986, Editorial.

[11]   "High Court says no to Administration's Baby Doe rules," *Science*, 1986, 232: 1595.

[12]   M. Angell, "The Baby Doe rules," *N Eng J Med*, 1986, 314: 642-4.

[13]   L.M. Koppelman, T.G. Irons, and A.E. Koppelman, "Neonatologists judge the "Baby Doe" regulations," *N Eng J Med*, 1988, 318: 677-83.

[14]   A.F. Fischer and D.K. Stevenson, "The consequences of uncertainty: An empirical approach to medical decision making in neonatal intensive care," *JAMA*, 1987, 258: 1929-31.

[15]   *The New York Times* for June 18, 1985, p. 19.

[16]   *Ibid*, December 12, 1987, p. 38.

[17]   D. Brahams, "Court of Appeal endorses medical decision to allow baby to die," *Lancet*, 1989, i: 969-70.

[18]   G.C. Lang, "'Baby Doe' - a medical ethical issue," *West J Med*, 1985, 142: 837-41.

[19].   M.N. Cohen, *Health and the Rise of Civilization*, 1989, Yale University Press, New Haven.

[20]   D. Callahan, *Setting Limits*, 1987, Simon and Schuster, New York, pp. 130-1.

[21]   J. Lubitz and R. Prihoda, "The use and costs of Medicare services in the last 2 years of life," *Health Care Financ Rev*, 1984, 5: 117-131.

[22]   *Inst of Med Ethics*, Bull. #38, May 1988, p. 15.

[23]   M.E. Charlson, F.L. Sax, C.R. MacKenzie, et al., "Resuscitation: How do we decide? A prospective study of physicians' preferences and the clinical course of hospitalized patients," *JAMA*, 1986, 255: 1316-22.

[24]   *The New York Times* for August 13, 1987.

[25]   K. Prager, "High hopes and many morals," *JAMA*, 1990, 263: 2297.

[26]   J.E. Ruark, T.A. Raffin, and the Stanford University Medical Center Committee on "Ethics. Initiating and withdrawing life support," *New Eng J Med*, 1988, 318: 25-30.

[27]   D. Frankl, R.K. Oye, and P.E. Bellamy, "Attitudes of hospitalized patients toward life support: a survey of 200 medical inpatients," *Am J Med*, 1989, 86: 645-8.

[28]   G.E. Taffet, T.A. Teasdale, and R.J. Luchi, "In-hospital cardiopulmonary resuscitation," *JAMA*, 1988, 260: 2069-2072.

[29]   D.J. Murphy, "Do-not-resuscitate orders: time for reappraisal in long-term-care facilities," *JAMA*, 1988, 260: 2098-2101.

[30]   S.J. Youngner, "Who defines futility?", *JAMA*, 1988, 260: 2094-5.

[31]   D.L. Schiedermayer, "The decision to forgo CPR in the elderly patient," *JAMA*, 1988, 260: 2096-7.

[32]   T. Tomlinson and H. Brody, "Ethics and communications in do-not-resuscitate orders," *N Engl J Med*, 1988, 318: 43-6.

[33]   *President's Commission for the Study of Ethical Problems in Medicine and Biomedical and Behavioral Research. Deciding to forego life-sustaining treatment*, 1983, U.S. Government Printing Office, Washington, p. 3-9.

[34]   D.E. Levy, J.J. Caronna, B.H. Singer, et al., "Predicting outcome from hypoxic-ischemic coma," *JAMA*, 1985, 253: 1420-6.

[35] P.M. Black, "Predicting the outcome from hypoxic-ischemic coma: medical and ethical implications," Editorial, *JAMA*, 1985, 254: 1215-6.

[36] E.O. Jorgensen and R. Rosenberg, "Predicting the outcome from hypoxic-ischemic coma," *JAMA*, 1986, 255: 1569-70.

[37] S.H. Wanzer, S.J. Adelstein, R.E. Cranford, et al., "The physician's responsibility to hopelessly ill patients," *N Eng J Med*, 1984, 310: 955-9.

[38] N.G. Smedira, B.H. Evans, L.S. Grais, et al., "Withholding and withdrawal of life support from the critically ill," *N Engl J Med*, 1990, 322: 309-15.

[39] R. Higgs, "Living wills and treatment refusal," *Brit Med J*, 1987, 295: 1221-2.

[40] F. Rouse, *Inst. of Med. Ethics*, Bull. Supplement #5, April 1987. p. 1-6.

[41] R.M. Veatch, "Doctor's orders," *JAMA*, 1985, 254: 3468.

[42] J.N. Zinberg, "Advance directives: do they provide direction?", *JAMA*, 1990, 263: 1764.

[43] D. Callahan, *What Kind of Life*, 1989, Simon & Schuster, New York.

[44] *The New York Times* for November 17, 1987, p. 22.

[45] *The New York Times* for January 12, 1988, p. A12.

[46] *The New York Times* for May 27, 1988, p. A12.

[47] D. Callahan, "On feeding and dying," 1983, *13 Hastings Center Rep*, 22.

[48] J. Lynn and J.F. Childress, "Must patients always be given food and water?", 1983, *13 Hastings Center Rep*, 17.

[49] E.J. Emanuel, "Should physicians withhold life-sustaining care from patients who are not terminally ill?", *Lancet*, 1988, i: 106-8.

[50] W.J. Curran, "Defining appropriate medical care: providing nutrients and hydration for the dying," *N Eng J Med*, 1985, 313: 940-2.

[51] A.R. Somers, "Nursing homes and ethics committees," *N.J. Med*, 1989, 86: 45-9.

[52] *The Philadelphia Inquirer* for August 11, 1987, Editorial.

[53] E.J. Emanuel, "What criteria should guide decision makers for incompetent patients?", *Lancet*, 1988, i: 170-1.

[54] *The New York Times* for October 15, 1988, p. 1.

[55] *Ibid* for July 25, 1989, p. A1.

[56]   T.B. Brewin, "Voluntary euthanasia," *Lancet*, 1986, i: 1085-6.

[57]   *The Philadelphia Inquirer* for April 27, 1987, p. 1A.

[58]   *The New York Times* for December 13, 1987, p. 38.

[59]   *Ibid* for February 2, 1988, p. C9.

[60]   J. Dawson, "Easeful death," *Brit Med J*, 1986, 293: 1187-8.

[61]   *Inst of Med Ethics*, Bull. #38, May 1988, p. 17-19.

[62]   *The Wall Street Journal* for August 21, 1987, p. 1.

[63]   *Ibid* for September 29, 1987, "Letter to the editor."

[64]   J.H. Segers, "Elderly persons on the subject of euthanasia," *Issues Law Med*, 1988, 3: 407-24.

[65]   *Brit Med J*, 1990, 300: 69.

[66]   C.B. Golin, "Euthanasia feared as 'solution' to rising health costs," *American Medical News* for May 17, 1985, p. 3.

[67]   T. Wetle, Age as a risk factor for inadequate treatment. *JAMA* 1987, 258: 516.

[68]   *The Wall Street Journal* for January 22, 1988, p. 29.

[69]   C.T. Currie, "Doctors and ageism," *Brit Med J*, 1987, 295: 1586.

[70]   H.A. Shenkin, *Clinical Practice and Cost Containment*, 1986, Praeger, New York.

[71]   G. Silver, "The old, the very old, and the too old," *Lancet*, 1987, ii: 1453.

[72]   C.T. Currie, *Brit Med J*, 1988, 296: 711.

[73]   L. Volicer, Y. Rheaume, J. Brown, et al., "Hospice approach to the treatment of patients with advanced dementia of the Alzheimer type," *JAMA*, 1986, 256: 2210-3.

[74]   J. Lynn, "Dying and dementia," *JAMA*, 1986, 256: 2244-5.

[75]   *The Philadelphia Inquirer* for February 7, 1988, p. 3A.

[76]   *The New York Times* for April 9, 1987, "Letter to the editor."

[77]   *Inst of Med Ethics*, Bull. #25 for April, 1987, p. 8.

[78]   *Ibid*, Bull. #27 for June 1987, p. 13.

[79]   G.D. Lundberg, "'It's Over, Debbie' and the euthanasia debate," *JAMA*, 259: 2142-3.

[80]   W. Reichel and A.J. Dyck, "Euthanasia: a contemporary moral quandry," *Lancet*, 1989, ii: 1321-3.

[81]   W.B. Schwartz and H.J. Aaron, "Rationing hospital care. Lessons from Great Britain," *N Eng J Med*, 1984, 310: 52-6.

[82]   V.R. Fuchs, "The 'rationing' of medical care," *N Eng J Med*, 1984, 311: 1572-3.

[83]   W.A. Knaus, "Rationing, justice and the American physician," *JAMA*, 1986, 255: 1176-7.

[84]   D.S. Grimes, "Rationing health care," *Lancet*, 1987, i: 615-6.

CHAPTER 11

[1]   H.T. Engelhardt, Jr., "Allocating scarce medical resources and the availability of organ transplantation," *N Eng J Med*, 1984, 311: 66-71.

[2]   J.B. Reinhart and J.P. Kemph, "Renal transplantation for children: another view," *JAMA*, 1988, 260: 3327-8.

[3]   R.M. House and T.L. Thompson, II, "Psychiatric aspects of organ transplantation," *JAMA*, 1988, 260: 535-9.

[4]   *American Medical News* for September 9, 1988, p. 2.

[5]   "Report of Organ Transplant Panel: corneal transplantation," *JAMA*, 1988, 259: 719-21.

[6]   P.W. Eggers, "Effect of transplantation on Medicare end-stage renal disease program," *N Eng J Med*, 1988, 318: 223-9.

[7]   H.A. Shenkin, *Clinical Practice and Cost Containment: A Physician's Perspective*, 1986, Praeger, New York.

[8]   "Renal transplantation in children," Editorial, *Lancet*, 1987, ii: 434.

[9]   *Forbes Magazine* for May 28, 1990, pp. 365-72.

[10]   *The Economist* for June 21, 1986, p. 31.

[11]   *The New York Times* for February 24, 1988, Editorial page.

[12]   A. Bodenham, J.C. Berridge, and G.R. Park, "Brain stem death and organ donation," *Brit Med J*, 1989, 299: 1009-10.

[13]   *Lancet*, 1990, i: 80-2.

[14]   *The New York Times* for September 6, 1987, p. 1.

[15]   *Brit Med J*, 1989, 298: 276.

[16]   J.C. McDonald, "The National Organ Procurement and Transplantation Network," *JAMA*, 1988, 259: 725-6.

[17]   J. Firshein, "Transplant panel wants criteria on performance set," *Hospitals* for June 5, 1986.

[18]   J.F. Childress, "Wilson Center Colloquium on Organ Transplantation: Easing the Bottlenecks," Held on July 9, 1985, In: *The Wilson Center Reports* for September 1985.

[19]   *The New York Times* for August 10, 1985, p. 1.

[20] S. Woolhander, D.U. Himmelstein, B. Labar, and S. Lang, "Transplanted technology: third world options and first world science," *N Eng J Med* 1987, 317: 505-6.

[21] D.H. Cowan, J.A. Kantorowitz, J. Moskowitz, and P.H. Rheinstein, Eds., *Human Organ Transplantation: Societal, Medical-Legal, Regulatory, and Reimbursement Issues*, 1986, Health Administration Press, Ann Arbor, Michigan.

[22] P.J. Held, M.V. Pauly, R.R. Bovbjerg, et al., "Access to kidney transplantation," *Arch Int Med*, 1988, 148: 2594-2600.

[23] *The New York Times* for January 24, 1989, p. C1.

[24] *Ibid* for August 1, 1989, p. C1.

[25] *Ibid* for April 3, 1990, p. C3.

[26] L.H. Edmunds, Jr., "Cardiac surgery," *Bull Amer Col Surg*, 1988, 73: 5-10.

[27] J.S. Schroeder and S. Hunt, "Cardiac transplantation, update 1987," *JAMA*, 1987, 258: 3142-5.

[28] *The New York Times* for December 1, 1987, p. C3.

[29] W.C. DeVries, "The permanent artificial heart," *JAMA*, 1988, 259: 849-59.

[30] "Special report," *Science 86*, June, p. 10.

[31] D. Callahan, "The artificial heart: bleeding us dry," *The New York Times* for September 17, 1988, Op-Ed page, p. 27.

[32] *The New York Times* for September 9, 1986, p. C1.

[33] A. Capron, "Anencephalic donors: separate the dead from the dying," *Hasting Center Report*, 1987, 17: 5-9.

[34] *American Medical News* for November 6, 1987, p. 3.

[35] *The Los Angeles Times* for November 11, 1987, p. 3.

[36] *The New York Times* for December 14, 1987, p. A18.

[37] *Ibid* for August 20, 1988, p. 7.

[38] *American Medical News* for September 23/30, 1988, p. 1.

[39] J.R. Salaman, "Anencephalic organ donors," *Brit Med J*, 1989, 298: 622-3.

[40] *The New York Times* for September 18, 1988, p. 8E.

[41] W. Holzgreve, F. Beller, B. Buchholz, et al., "Kidney transplantation from anencephalic donors," *N Eng J Med*, 1987, 316: 1069-70.

[42] *The New York Times* for October 28, 1984, p. 1.

[43]	O. Jonasson and M.A. Hardy, "The case of Baby Fae," *JAMA*, 1985, 254: 3358-9.

[44]	E. Knoll and G.D. Lundberg, "Informed consent and Baby Fae," *JAMA*, 1985, 254: 3359-60.

[45]	A.L. Caplan, "Ethical issues raised by research involving xenografts," *JAMA*, 1985, 254: 3339-43.

[46]	*The New York Times* for December 15, 1987, p. C3.

[47]	*Ibid* for January 30, 1990, p. C1.

[48]	L.H. Edmunds, Jr., "What's new in cardiac surgery," *Bull Amer Col Surg*, 1988, 73: 5-10.

[49]	*The Wall Street Journal* for October 14, 1986, p. 1.

[50]	H. Bismuth, B.G. Ericzon, K. Rolles, et al., "Hepatic transplantation in Europe," *Lancet*, 1988, ii: 674-6.

[51]	D.K. Flavin, R.G. Niven, and J.E. Kelsey, "Alcoholism and orthotopic liver transplantation," *JAMA*, 1988, 259: 1546-7

[52]	T.E. Starzl, D. Van Thiel, A.G. Tzakis, et al., "Orthoptic liver transplantation for alcoholic cirrhosis," *JAMA*, 1988, 260: 2542-4.

[53]	*Lancet*, 1987, ii: 1015.

[54]	D. Pyke, "Pancreas transplantation for diabetes?", *Lancet*, 1988, i: 816-7.

[55]	W.R. Kennedy, X. Navarro, F.C. Goetz, et al., "Effects of pancreatic transplantation on diabetic neuropathy," *N Eng J Med*, 1990, 322: 1031-7.

[56]	D.E.R. Sutherland, K.C. Moudry, and D.S. Fryd, "Results of pancreas transplant registry," *Diabetes*, 1989, 38: Suppl 1: 46-54.

[57]	R. Tattersall, "Is pancreas transplantation for insulin-dependent diabetes worthwhile?", *N Engl J Med*, 1989, 321: 112-4.

[58]	*The New York Times* for January 12, 1988, p. C1.

[59]	T.E. Starzl, M.I. Rowe, S. Todo, et al., "Transplantation of multiple abdominal viscera," *JAMA*, 1989, 261: 1449-57.

[60]	J.W. Williams, H.N. Sankary, P.F. Foster, et al., "Splanchnic transplantation," *JAMA*, 1989, 261: 1458-62.

[61]	*JAMA*, 1989, 261: 1397.

[62]	F.D. Moore, "The desperate case: CARE (costs, applicability, research, ethics)," *JAMA*, 1989, 261: 1483-4.

[63]	*Science*, 1988, 242: 1379.

[64]	O. Lindvall, et al., "Fetal dopamine-rich mesencephalic grafts in Parkinson's disease," *Lancet*, 1988, ii: 1483.

65   O. Lindvall, P. Brundin, H. Widner, et al., "Grafts of fetal dopamine neurons survive and improve motor function in Parkinson's disease," *Science*, 1990, 247: 574-7.

66   E. Carpenter, "NIH probing use of fetal tissue," *The Scientist* for October 5, 1987.

67   *The New York Times* for August 16, 1987, p. 1.

68   *The New York Times* for March 15, 1988, p. C6.

69   R. Lewin, "Ethical issues raised," *Science*, 1988, 240: 391.

70   *Inst of Med Ethics*, Bull. #51, June 1989, p. iv.

71   *JAMA*, 1988, 260: 2012-5.

72   B.J. Culliton, "Panel backs fetal tissue research," *Science*,1988, 242: 1625-6.

73   *The New York Times* for November 2, 1989, p. A1.

74   *The New York Times* for November 19, 1989, p. 1.

75   D. Dickson, "Fetal tissue transplants win U.K. approval," *Science*, 1989, 245: 464-5.

76   *The New York Times* for January 14, 1988, p. B7.

77   *The New York Times* for April 24, 1988, p. 22.

78   J.D. Arras and S. Shinnar, "Anencephalic newborns as organ donors: a critique," *JAMA*, 1988, 259: 2284-5.

79   H.G. Welch and E.B. Larson, "Dealing with limited resources. The Oregon decision to curtail funding for organ transplants," *N Eng J Med*, 1988, 319: 171-3.

80   *JAMA*, 1989, 262: 176-7.

81   H.A. Shenkin, *Clinical Practice and Cost Containment: A Physician's Perspective*, 1986, Praeger, New York, pp. 60-1.

82   *Brit Med J*, 1990, 300: 765-6.

83   R.H. Blank, *Rationing Medicine*, 1988, Columbia University Press, New York.

84   E.D. Pellegrino and D.C. Thomasma, *For the Patient's Good: The Restoration of Beneficence in Health Care*, 1988, Oxford University Press, New York, pp. 180-7.

85   L.B. Russell, "Some of the tough decisions required by a national health plan," *Science*, 1989, 246: 892-6.

86   J.M. Eisenberg, "Clinical economics: a guideline to the economic analysis of clinical practices," *JAMA*, 1989, 262: 2879-86.

NAME INDEX

Episteme

A SERIES IN THE FOUNDATIONAL,
METHODOLOGICAL, PHILOSOPHICAL, PSYCHOLOGICAL, SOCIOLOGICAL, AND
POLITICAL ASPECTS OF THE SCIENCES, PURE AND APPLIED

KLUWER ACADEMIC PUBLISHERS – DORDRECHT / BOSTON / LONDON